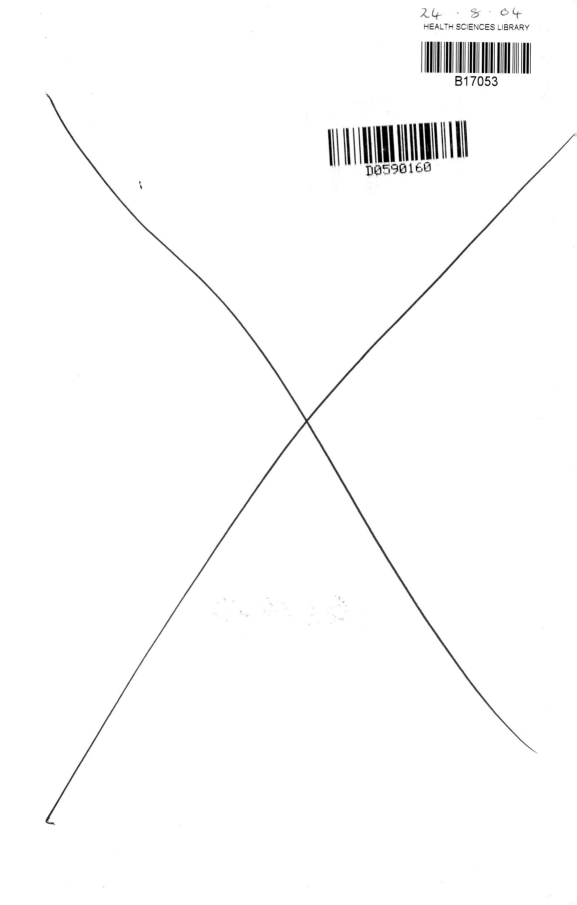

Oxford Medical Publications

Stroke Genetics

Stroke Genetics

Edited by

Hugh S. Markus

Clinical Neuroscience, St George's Hospital Medical School,
London, UK

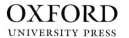

OXFORD
UNIVERSITY PRESS

OXFORD

UNIVERSITY PRESS

Great Clarendon Street, Oxford OX2 6DP

Oxford University Press is a department of the University of Oxford.
It furthers the University's objective of excellence in research, scholarship,
and education by publishing worldwide in

Oxford New York

Auckland Bangkok Buenos Aires Cape Town Chennai
Dar es Salaam Delhi Hong Kong Istanbul Karachi Kolkata
Kuala Lumpur Madrid Melbourne Mexico City Mumbai Nairobi
São Paulo Shanghai Taipei Tokyo Toronto

Oxford is a registered trade mark of Oxford University Press
in the UK and in certain other countries

Published in the United States
by Oxford University Press Inc., New York

© Oxford University Press, 2003

© Hugh Markus Figures 1.3, 1.4b, 1.6, 1.7, 2.1, 2.2a, 2.2b, 6.2, 8.1, 8.2, 8.4,
10.3A–C, 13.1–8

The moral rights of the authors have been asserted
Database right Oxford University Press (maker)

First published 2003

A catalogue record for this title is available from the British Library

Library of Congress Cataloging in Publication Data
(Data available)

ISBN 0 19 8515863 (Hbk)
10 9 8 7 6 5 4 3 2 1

Typeset by Newgen Imaging Systems (P) Ltd., Chennai, India
Printed in Great Britain
on acid-free paper by
T. J. International Ltd., Padstow, Cornwall

Dedication

For Philippa and Helen

Preface

Stroke causes an enormous health burden in both developed and developing societies. It is the major cause of adult neurological disability in the developed world, and in most countries the third most common cause of adult mortality. In addition to stroke, cerebrovascular disease causes vascular dementia, which is the second commonest cause of dementia after Alzheimer's disease. Despite its importance on a population basis, research into the genetics of stroke, particularly for multifactorial stroke, has lagged behind that for other polygenic disorders such as diabetes, asthma, and ischaemic heart disease. However, the situation is beginning to change. Increasing evidence suggests that genetic factors are important in the stroke risk, often via interactions with conventional risk factors. A small proportion of stroke cases are caused by single gene disorders and the genetic basis of a number of these has been described in recent years including CADASIL, perhaps the most common monogenic cause of ischaemic stroke. An increasing number of studies, primarily candidate gene association studies, have suggested possible genetic risk factors for multifactorial stroke. Recently the location of the first stroke specific gene (STRK1), acting independently of conventional risk factors, has been described. The availability of current neuroimaging and other investigation techniques for accurately classifying stroke phenotype, in combination with the revolution in genotyping technology and statistical analysis, makes this a highly fruitful area for future research.

This book is intended as an introduction to stroke genetics for both the interested clinician seeing stroke patients, and the basic scientist entering this field of research. Chapter 1 provides an introduction to stroke with a particular focus on pathophysiological mechanisms and pathways which may provide clues as to which candidate gene systems are implicated in stroke. The importance of treating stroke as a syndrome, which includes a number of phenotypes, which may have very different genetic risk factor profiles, is discussed. Chapter 2 describes the genetic approaches and techniques involved in investigating stroke genetics, with a particular focus on those applicable to the more common forms of multifactorial or polygenic stroke. Chapter 3 discusses the genetic epidemiology of stroke, reviewing the evidence that genetic factors are indeed important in stroke risk. Many conventional risk factors for stroke, such as hypertension, appear to have a genetic basis, and many studies have investigated this; these are reviewed in Chapter 4. Animal models of stroke have provided important clues to the genetic basis of polygenic ischaemic stroke and have provided possible candidate loci. This is discussed in Chapter 5.

The genetics of ischaemic stroke are covered in Chapters 6–8. In Chapter 6, single gene disorders associated with ischaemic stroke are reviewed, with a particular focus both on their clinical features and how to diagnose them, and on the underlying genetic defects. The genetics of polygenic ischaemic stroke, including new approaches to investigate this area are reviewed in Chapter 7. A potentially powerful technique for investigating the complex pathophysiological processes which may lead to ischaemic stroke is the use of intermediate phenotypes. Two of the most widely used have been carotid artery intima-media thickness as an intermediate phenotype for large vessel stroke, and magnetic resonance imaging of high signal intensities as an intermediate phenotype for small vessel disease stroke. These approaches are reviewed in Chapter 8.

The genetics of cerebral haemorrhage are reviewed in Chapters 9–11. Chapter 9 deals with intracerebral haemorrhage including both single gene disorders such as amyloid angiopathy, and multifactorial intracerebral haemorrhage. A significant proportion of cerebral haemorrhage is caused by subarachnoid haemorrhage, most commonly secondary to aneurysms, and this appears to have a significant genetic component. The underlying genetics, and approaches to screening for familial aneurysms, are discussed in Chapter 10. Arteriovenous malformations including angiomas can cause cerebral haemorrhage. Recently significant advances have been made in the genetic basis of familial angiomas. This is discussed in Chapter 11. The spectrum of genetic disorders present in childhood differs somewhat from that in adults and this is discussed in Chapter 12. The last Chapter 13, presents a practical approach to investigating a patient presenting with stroke for underlying genetic disorders, including an introduction to genetic counselling which is particularly important when performing diagnostic tests for monogenic stroke disorders.

February 2003   *Hugh S. Markus*

Contents

Contributors

Robert D. Brown, Jr.
Department of Neurology
Mayo Clinic,
Jacksonville, FL,
Mayo Medical School,
Rochester, MN,
USA.

Angela M. Carter
Academic Unit of Molecular Vascular
Medicine,
Research School of Medicine,
G Floor, Martin Wing,
Leeds General Infirmary,
University of Leeds,
UK.

Andrew J. Catto
Academic Unit of Molecular Vascular
Medicine,
G Floor, Martin Wing,
Leeds General Infirmary,
University of Leeds,
Leeds LS1 3EX,
UK.

Martin Dichgans
Department of Neurology,
Klinikum Großhadern,
Marchioninistraße 15,
81377 München,
Germany.

Bruna Gigante
Department of Experimental Medicine
and Pathology,
University La Sapienza,
Rome,

IRCCS Neuromed (Is),
Polo Molisano University La Sapienza,
Rome,
Italy.

Joost Haan
Department of Neurology K5Q,
Leiden University Medical Center,
PO Box 9600,
2300 RC Leiden,
Department of Neurology,
Rijnland Hospital,
Simon Smitweg 1,
2353 GA Leiderdorp,
The Netherlands.

Ahamad Hassan
Clinical Neuroscience,
St George's Hospital Medical School,
Cranmer Terrace,
London SW17 0RE,
UK.

Paula Jerrard-Dunne
Clinical Neuroscience,
St George's Hospital Medical School,
Cranmer Terrace,
London SW17 0RE,
UK.

Fenella Kirkham
Neurosciences Unit,
Institute of Child Health
(University College, London),
The Wolfson Centre,
Mecklenburgh Square,
London WC1N 2AP,
UK.

Pierre Labauge
Department of Neurology,
CHU de Montpellier-Nîmes,
CHU Caremeau,
30029 Nîmes Cedex 4,
INSERM EPI 99-21,
Laboratoire de Génétique des Maladies
Vasculaires,
Faculté de Médecine Lariboisière,
10 Avenue de Verdun,
75010 Paris,
France.

Hugh S. Markus
Clinical Neuroscience,
St George's Hospital Medical School,
Cranmer Terrace,
London SW17 0RE,
UK.

James F. Meschia
Department of Neurology
Mayo Clinic,
Jacksonville, FL,
Mayo Medical School,
Rochester, MN,
USA.

Mara Prengler
Neurosciences Unit,
Institute of Child Health (University
College, London),
The Wolfson Centre,
Mecklenburgh Square,
London WC1N 2AP,
UK.

Speranza Rubattu
Department of Experimental Medicine
and Pathology,
University La Sapienza,
Rome,
IRCCS Neuromed (Is),
Polo Molisano University La Sapienza,
Rome,
Italy.

Giuseppe A. Sagnella
Blood Pressure Unit,
St George's Hospital Medical School,
Cranmer Terrace,
London SW17 0RE,
UK.

Wouter I. Schievink
Vascular Neurosurgery Program,
The Maxine Dunitz Neurosurgical
Institute,
Cedars-Sinai Medical Center,
8631 West Third Street, Suite 800E,
Los Angeles, CA 90048,
USA.

Rosita Stanzione
Department of Experimental Medicine
and Pathology,
University La Sapienza,
IRCCS Neuromed (Is),
Polo Molisano University La Sapienza,
Rome,
Italy.

Massimo Volpe
Department of Experimental Medicine
and Pathology,
University La Sapienza,
Rome,
IRCCS Neuromed (Is),
Polo Molisano University La Sapienza,
Rome,
Italy.

Chapter 1

An introduction to stroke

Hugh S. Markus

1.1 Introduction

The genetics of stroke is still in its infancy. However a considerable amount is known about the epidemiology of stroke and the role of conventional risk factors. A knowledge of this area is essential in planning genetic studies, particularly when the study of gene–environment interactions are planned. A brief review of this area follows. Stroke is a heterogenous disease and accurate and reproducible definitions and classifications are essential for risk factors studies. Different stroke subtypes and phenotypes have different pathogenic mechanisms and an understanding of these is essential in planning and interpreting candidate gene studies. This area is also reviewed in this chapter.

1.2 Definitions

Stroke is a clinical syndrome describing a range of disorders which result in focal cerebral ischaemia. A uniform definition of stroke is vital for epidemiological studies. The World Health Organisation (WHO) definition of stroke has been widely used. Stroke is defined as 'rapidly developing clinical signs of focal (or global) disturbance of cerebral function, with symptoms lasting 24 h or longer, or leading to death, with no apparent cause other than of vascular origin'. This definition includes stroke due to both cerebral infarction or intracerebral and subarachnoid haemorrhage. An arbitrary time window of 24 h distinguishes stroke from transient ischaemic attack (TIA), which has the same definition but is defined as a neurological deficit lasting less than 24 h. The two are best thought of as a continuum, and in fact neuroimaging studies show that many cases of TIA are accompanied by cerebral infarction. The term cerebrovascular disease covers all vascular disease affecting the brain including stroke, vascular dementia, and asymptomatic cerebrovascular disease.

1.3 The heterogeneity of stroke and its classification

Stroke is best thought of as a syndrome, representing a collection of disease processes which all result in cerebral ischaemia. The different processes have different clinical phenotypes, different aetiological mechanisms, and different risk factor profiles. Increasing evidence suggests that different subtypes of stroke may have both different degrees of heritability, and different underlying genetic risk factor profiles. For example, the autosomal dominant condition CADASIL (Section 6.2.1) causes exclusively, or almost exclusively, stroke due to small vessel disease (lacunar) stroke. Therefore when looking for underlying aetiological causes, including genetic causes, the most appropriate classification of stroke is into pathophysiological subtypes.

New techniques for imaging the brain and vascular system have transformed the ability to accurately phenotype or subtype stroke. However even in series in which extensive investigations are performed, the underlying cause of stroke cannot be identified in 20–30 per cent of individuals. A pathophysiological classification of stroke is shown in Table 1.1. This divides stroke into its two main subtypes of cerebral haemorrhage and cerebral ischaemia, and subdivides each of these. The division of ischaemic stroke is based on those of the Stroke Data Bank classification (Kunitz *et al*. 1984) and the more recent trial of ORG 10172 in acute stroke treatment (TOAST) classification (Adams *et al*. 1993). Although the TOAST classification has been shown to have good inter-observer reproducibility, particularly when a computerized algorithm and standardized data collection procedures are used (Goldstein *et al*. 2001), it is important to remember that this is not 100 per cent. An important consideration, particularly when deciding whether to focus on particular stroke subtypes in aetiological studies, is whether the different types really do represent different disease processes. Strong

Table 1.1 Pathophysiological classification of stroke[a]

Ischaemic stroke
Large artery
Cardioembolic
Lacunar (small vessel disease)
Other determined aetiology
Undetermined aetiology
Multiple possible aetiologies
Cerebral haemorrhage
Primary subarachnoid haemorrhage
Primary intracerebral haemorrhage

Definitions

Large artery stroke: Occlusion or stenosis (>50%) in large extracranial or intracranial cerebral artery (carotid, vertebral, basilar, anterior cerebral, middle cerebral, posterior cerebral), with ischaemia in that arterial territory.

Cardioembolic stroke: One or more of the following conditions: Mechanical prosthetic heart valve, atrial fibrillation, myocardial infarction within last 2 months, dilated cardiomyopathy/congestive heart failure at stroke onset, endocarditis, sick sinus syndrome, atrial myxoma, left ventricular thrombus.

Lacunar stroke: Lacunar syndrome (pure motor stroke, pure sensory stroke, ataxic hemiparesis, clumsy hand dysarthria) with either no lesion on brain imaging or a deep infarct (≤1.5 cm diameter) in a location consistent with the clinical syndrome.

[a] This classification is based on, but modified from, the TOAST and Stroke Data Bank classifications.

support for this is provided by studies looking at recurrent strokes. The pathological subtype of recurrence is usually the same as the index case; for example, this was the case for 88 and 68 per cent of recurrences in two population based studies (Hankey *et al.* 1998, Petty *et al.* 2000). This figure is high, particularly when one considers inter-observer errors in assigning subtypes, and that shared risk factors such as hypertension may predispose to more than one subtype.

Another classification which has been widely used is the Oxfordshire Community Stroke Project (OCSP) classification (Bamford *et al.* 1991). This divides cerebral infarction into four categories: total anterior circulation infarction (TACI), partial anterior circulation infarction (PACI), lacunar infarction (LACI) and posterior circulation infarction (POCI). This classification is based on a combination of the apparent location of clinical symptoms and signs, and pathophysiology. For example, LACI represents a particular pathophysiological subtype, while both TACI and PACI can include patients with large artery stroke from carotid stenosis, as well as patients with cardioembolic stroke. For this reason it is less well suited to aetiological studies.

1.4 Stroke epidemiology

World Health Organisation data indicates that deaths from circulatory disease kill more of the worlds population than any other disease group, accounting for 15 million deaths annually, or 30 per cent of the annual total. Stroke accounts for 4.5 million of these (Murray and Lopez 1996). Of all deaths in industrialized countries 10–12 per cent are due to stroke, and about 88 per cent of the deaths attributed to stroke are amongst people over 65 years of age. There is a marked variation in stroke mortality rates in both men and women in different countries, with the highest incidence countries having about a five times greater rate than the lower incidence countries. In most industrialized countries death rates from stroke, and ischaemic heart disease, have fallen markedly over the last few decades, although there is some evidence that this may be levelling off. In contrast, stroke rates in some Eastern European countries have increased over the same period. It is uncertain whether this fall is due to a decline in incidence or a lower case fatality. However when community stroke registers have been specifically set up, as in the WHO MONICA project, the evidence suggests that for the purposes of international comparisons, there is good agreement between mortality rates from official statistics and stroke incidence registers (Thorvalsden *et al.* 1995). In the past, stroke was thought of as mainly affecting industrialized countries. However recent studies suggest that stroke in the developing countries is also becoming a major health problem, and two thirds of stroke deaths now occur in non-industrialized countries (Wolfe 2000).

The incidence of stroke is defined as the number of first in a lifetime strokes occurring per unit time. Evaluation of the incidence of stroke in a given population requires both the use of a standard definition, and prospective ascertainment of cases using

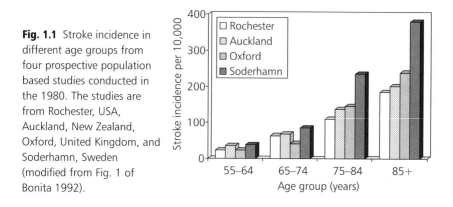

Fig. 1.1 Stroke incidence in different age groups from four prospective population based studies conducted in the 1980. The studies are from Rochester, USA, Auckland, New Zealand, Oxford, United Kingdom, and Soderhamn, Sweden (modified from Fig. 1 of Bonita 1992).

comprehensive case finding methods to identify non-fatal cases treated both in hospital and out of hospital, as well as patients who have died very shortly after the acute stroke event. Few studies meet these criteria, but data from four studies which do is summarized in Fig. 1.1 (Bonita 1992). Such studies show that stroke incidence rises exponentially with age. Almost one in four men and one in five women aged 45 years can expect to have a stroke if they live to their 85th year (Wolfe 2000). Although the stroke risk is higher in men than in women, more women die secondary to stroke due to their greater life expectancy. Typically first ever strokes account for about 75 per cent of all strokes.

Stroke is responsible for a great burden of disability in the community. It is the major cause of adult neurological disability and this results in enormous cost. In the United Kingdom stroke accounts for about 5 per cent of all in hospital costs, and as much as 12 per cent of health costs when community care costs are included (Wolfe 2000). Therefore small reductions in stroke incidence will have great population benefits.

Epidemiological studies have allowed identification of a large number of risk factors of varying proportions, many of which could be modified by life-style alterations or specific pharmacological treatment. However interpretation of stroke epidemiological studies is hampered by a number of difficulties. First, in many studies diagnosis has been largely clinical without investigations to both confirm the diagnosis and identify the aetiological subtype. Second, in most studies there has been a low rate of post-mortems in stroke fatalities. The diagnosis of stroke on death certification has been shown to be inaccurate, even in the best controlled studies (Corwin *et al.* 1982). Additional difficulties are created by the heterogenous nature of stroke and the fact that it can be caused by quite different pathogenic mechanisms, which may have different risk factor profiles. Without brain imaging, reliable separation of cerebral haemorrhage from cerebral infarction is not possible, except in the case of subarachnoid haemorrhage. In many large epidemiological studies cerebral haemorrhage and cerebral infarction have not been separated. This means that the results are weighted very much in favour of the more common cerebral infarction. Furthermore, cerebral infarction itself is caused by very different pathogenic processes, predominantly cardiac embolism, large vessel atherosclerotic disease and lacunar stroke. Without more detailed investigation including brain imaging, and imaging of the cerebral vessels and heart, reliable separation of these different phenotypes is impossible. Therefore much of the information on the relative role of risk factors in different groups has been gained from hospital-based case control studies rather than more representative population-based studies.

1.5 **Stroke risk factors**

The most reliable identification of stroke risk factors comes from prospective cohort studies such as the Framingham study. However, in most of these studies there has been little or no division of stroke into cerebral haemorrhage and cerebral ischaemia, let alone any division of cerebral ischaemia into its different pathogenic subtypes. Therefore because most strokes are due to infarction, these studies primarily tell us the risk factors for infarction rather than haemorrhage. Similarly, because a large number of ischaemic strokes are related to the complications of atherosclerosis (e.g. carotid artery stenosis, embolism secondary to myocardial infarction, atrial fibrillation secondary to coronary heart disease) these studies have similar risk factor profiles to those of coronary heart disease. However there do seem to be some differences, particularly in the relative importance of different risk factors, for coronary heart disease and stroke. More recent studies have included imaging, allowing differentiation of different stroke subtypes, and this suggests that the risk factor profile of the different subtypes may vary. Case control studies allow much more detailed evaluation of each individual stroke in a standardized fashion, and therefore differentiation between different stroke subtypes. However they are subject to potential bias, both in selection of cases and controls. Nevertheless they provide useful information, particularly on relationships with particular stroke subtypes. More recently imaging techniques such as carotid duplex ultrasound and MRI have allowed associations to be determined between individual components of the pathological process, referred to as intermediate phenotypes (such as carotid atherosclerosis), and risk factors, on a population basis.

1.5.1 **Strength of association and attributable risk**

A risk factor for stroke is a characteristic of that individual, indicating that he or she has an increased risk of stroke compared with an individual without that characteristic. Such an association does not necessarily imply causality. Determining causality depends upon a number of factors including the strength of the association, its consistency over different studies and populations, its independence from confounding factors, temporal sequence between risk factor and stroke, presence of biological and epidemiological plausibility, and demonstration that removal or reduction of that risk factor in randomised trials reduces stroke risk.

The strength of an association between a risk factor and stroke can be expressed as the relative risk or relative odds ratio. This figure describes the number of times greater that the frequency of stroke is in an individual or population with that risk factor, compared with its frequency in an individual or population without that same risk factor. The importance of any risk factor on a population basis will depend both upon its relative risk and also the prevalence of that risk factor in the population. Population risk can be indicated using the concept of 'attributable risk' or 'absolute risk'. Absolute risk difference between a population with, and a population without, the risk factor can be calculated as shown in Table 1.2. The dependence of absolute or attributable risk upon the population prevalence of the risk factor can be illustrated with hypertension. For example, elevation of systolic blood pressure to greater than 180 mmHg confirms a greatly increased relative risk of stroke, which is much greater that the relative risk of stroke due to a blood pressure in the range 160–180 mmHg. However such marked elevations of blood pressure are rare while more modest elevations are much more common. Therefore the population attributable risk associated with a blood pressure elevation in the range 160–180 mmHg is greater than that due to blood pressure elevation of greater than 180 mmHg.

Table 1.2 Methods for calculation of relative risk, relative odds and absolute risk difference for a stroke risk factor[a]

		Stroke	
		Yes	No
	Yes	A	B
Risk factor			
	No	C	D

Risk of stroke in those with the risk factor $(R^+)=A/A+B$

Risk of stroke in those without the risk factor $(R^0)=C/C+D$

Relative risk $=R/R^0$

Absolute risk difference $= (R^+) - (R^0)$

Odds of stroke in those with the risk factor $(O^+)=A/B$

Odds of stroke in those without the risk factor $(O^-)=C/D$

Relative odds (or odds ratio)$=O^+/O^-$

[a] In this hypothetical longitudinal study some subjects have the risk factor for stroke $(A + B)$, and some develop stroke $(A + C)$ (modified from Table 6.6 in Walton 1993).

1.6 **Risk factors for stroke**

A number of conventional risk factors for stroke are well recognized. Many of these, themselves have a genetic predisposition, and the genetics of hypertension, diabetes and hyperlipidaemia are reviewed in detail in Chapter 4. The relative importance of the more important risk factors is shown in Table 1.3.

1.6.1 **Age**

Age is the strongest risk factor for both cerebral infarction and primary intracerebral haemorrhage. The incidence of stroke approximately doubles with each successive decade over the age of 55 years (Wolfe 2000). For example, the risk of stroke in people aged 75–84 is approximately 25 times the risk in people aged 45–54. This increase in age is seen across different populations.

1.6.2 **Gender**

Male gender is a risk factor for stroke but overall, due to their greater life expectancy and the greater importance of age as a risk factor, more women will suffer stroke during their lifetime. The excess risk seen in men is less than that seen in ischaemic heart disease.

Table 1.3 Approximate relative risks associated with well recognized risk factors for stroke[a]

Risk factor	Relative risk for stroke
Age (55–64 versus >75 years)	5
Blood pressure: 160/95 versus 120/80 mmHg	7
Smoking (current status)	2
Diabetes mellitus	2
United Kingdom social class (I versus V)	1.6
Ischaemic heart disease	3
Heart failure	5
Atrial fibrillation	5
Past TIA	5
Physical activity (little or none versus some)	2.5
Oral contraceptives	3

[a] The estimates of relative risk given are representative figures derived from a number different studies of each risk factor.

1.6.3 **Hypertension**

Increasing blood pressure is a major risk factor for stroke. It is strongly and independently associated with both ischaemic and haemorrhagic stroke (Collins and MacMahon 1994). The relationship between diastolic blood pressure and subsequent stroke is log-linear throughout the normal range and there appears to be no threshold below which the stroke risk becomes stable, at least not over the normal range of blood pressures studied from 70–100 mmHg diastolic. This is supported by clinical trial data suggesting that antihypertensive agents reduce recurrent stroke risk, even in individuals with normal blood pressure (PROGRESS Investigators 2001). The proportional increase in stroke risk associated with a given increase in blood pressure is similar in both sexes and almost doubles with each 7.5 mmHg increase in diastolic blood pressure. There is less data on the relationship between stroke and systolic blood pressure but this may be even stronger than that with diastolic blood pressure and even 'isolated' systolic hypertension, with a normal diastolic blood pressure, is associated with increased stroke risk. Approximately 40 per cent of strokes can be attributed to systolic blood pressure of more than 140 mmHg. The causal nature of the relationship is strongly supported by the results of randomized controlled studies demonstrating that stroke can be prevented by treating blood pressure (Collins and MacMahon 1994).

1.6.4 **Smoking**

Studies have demonstrated that cigarette smoking is a risk factor of stroke with a relative risk of approximately 2. It is important in both males and females, and studies have shown that it is a risk factor specifically for ischaemic stroke as well as all strokes.

1.6.5 **Diabetes mellitus**

Diabetes is associated with a relative risk of stroke of approximately 2–2.5. It has also been demonstrated to be a risk factor for carotid atherosclerosis. Some studies, based on stroke mortality, have led to an over-estimation of the strength of any association between diabetes and stroke because there appears to be an increased stroke mortality in diabetic patients.

1.6.6 **Cholesterol**

Increased total cholesterol and low-density lipoprotein cholesterol are strong risk factors for ischaemic heart disease while high levels of high-density lipoprotein cholesterol appear to be protective. The relationship to stroke appears to be weaker. A meta-analysis involving 13,000 strokes in 450,000 people in 45 prospective cohorts found that, after standardization for age, there was no association between blood cholesterol and stroke except, perhaps, in those under 45 years of age when screened.

(Prospective Studies Collaboration 1995). However, because the subtypes of strokes were not available in most studies, the lack of any overall relationship might conceal a positive association with ischaemic stroke together with a negative association with haemorrhagic stroke. This is supported by recent trials which have demonstrated that cholesterol reduction, with statin therapy, reduces stroke risk (Byington *et al.* 2001, Heart Protection Study Collaborative Group 2002). Although this effect is likely to be due to cholesterol lowering, statins do have additional therapeutic effects which could reduce stroke incidence, including atherosclerotic plaque stabilization and upregulation of endothelial nitric oxide synthase.

1.6.7 Body mass index

Body mass index has been shown to be an independent risk factors for stroke in both smokers and non-smokers. Much of the association between body mass index and stroke in studies is reduced when confounding variables such as hypertension, diabetes, cigarette smoking, and lack of exercise are introduced into the analysis. However, it may be that some of these, such as hypertension and diabetes, are the mechanisms through which obesity exerts its influence on increasing stroke risk. In addition adipose tissue has been associated with increased cytokine levels and it has been suggested that a secondary increase in inflammation could be a mechanism via which obesity increases stroke risk.

1.6.8 Physical exercise

A number of studies, both cohort and case-controlled, have demonstrated that lack of exercise is associated with an increased risk of stroke. Such an effect could act, at least partly, through reducing blood pressure.

1.6.9 Plasma fibrinogen

There is a strong and consistent association between increased plasma fibrinogen and stroke. This relationship is partly confounded by smoking although it is possible that smoking exerts part of its increased stroke risk via increased fibrinogen. Fibrinogen is also affected by obesity, exercise, alcohol (negatively), diabetes, psychosocial factors, and inflammation and infection. Due to this confounding, it is not certain to what extent plasma fibrinogen is the causal factor or an indicator of other risk factors.

1.6.10 Alcohol

There is increasing evidence that moderate alcohol consumption may protect against both ischaemic heart disease and ischaemic stroke, with a J-shaped curve best describing the relationship. However, heavy alcohol consumption is a risk factor for stroke. This may act by increasing blood pressure and also leading to atrial fibrillation or myocardial damage secondary to cardiomyopathy. Alcohol consumption is a particularly strong risk factor for cerebral haemorrhage.

1.6.11 Ethnicity

There are marked differences in both the incidence of stroke, and the relative distribution of stroke subtypes, among different ethnic groups. The incidence of stroke is increased in Black Americans and United Kingdom African Caribbeans compared with Caucasians (Gillum *et al.* 1999). The incidence in a population-based study in South London was doubled (Wolfe *et al.* 2002). The distribution of stroke subtypes appears to differ from Caucasians with both increased cerebral haemorrhage and ischaemic small vessel disease, but less large vessel stroke. This is likely to be explained, at least partly, by the increased prevalence of hypertension, although this could not fully account for the increased incidence in the South London study (Stewart *et al.* 1999). United Kingdom Asian populations have a higher stroke mortality than Caucasians, and this may partly be due to an increased incidence of central obesity, insulin resistant and diabetes mellitus. Stroke incidence also appears to be higher in Chinese (Thorvaldsen *et al.* 1995), and intracranial atherosclerosis appears to be more common.

1.6.12 Homocysteine

Very high levels of serum homocysteine, associated with the autosomal recessive condition homocysteinuria, are associated with an increased risk of stroke and other arterial thrombosis at an early age (see Section 6.4.2). More recently considerable evidence suggests that moderately elevated levels of homocysteine are associated with stroke on a population basis (Hankey and Eikelboom 2001) Such an association could be mediated via a number of mechanisms including endothelial dysfunction and accelerated atherogenesis, or increased thrombosis. Some recent evidence suggests homocysteine may be a particular risk factor for small vessel cerebral damage and large vessel stroke, but not for cardioembolic stroke (Fassbender *et al.* 1999, Eikelboom *et al.* 2000).

1.6.13 Socio-economic conditions

There is a strong association between social class or other markers of socio-economic status and stroke risk. However this is likely to act through a number of factors; smoking, poor diet and lack of exercise are all associated with low socio-economic status.

1.6.14 Recent infection and inflammation

A number of case control studies of ischaemic stroke have shown an association between recent infection, as determined both by history of recent respiratory tract or other symptoms, and by serological testing (Grau *et al.* 1995). The association appears, at least to a degree, to be non-specific for type of infection and may result from inflammatory changes leading to a prothrombotic state and acute endothelial dysfunction. It may partially account for the increased incidence of stroke seen in the winter months. Chronic inflammation may also contribute to stroke risk. A large number of cross-sectional and prospective studies have shown that chronic inflammation, often estimated by measurement of C-reactive protein, is an independent risk factor for ischaemic heart disease (Danesh *et al.* 2000, Ridker *et al.* 2000). Fewer, and mostly less rigorous studies, have suggested a similar association with stroke (Feigin *et al.* 2002, van Exel *et al.* 2002). Considerable evidence suggest these association are mediated, at least in part, by increased atherosclerosis (de Boer *et al.* 2000).

1.6.15 Diet

A large number of studies demonstrate that increased salt intake is associated with increased blood pressure although the strength of this association has been debated. It has been estimated that a 100 mmol increase in sodium intake will increase blood pressure by 10 mmHg leading to about a 34 per cent increased risk of stroke (Law 1996). It has been suggested that a number of other dietary factors may increase or reduce stroke risk but the evidence for this is less robust. A number of studies have suggested that higher vitamin C levels are associated with a lower risk of stroke. This may act through an anti-oxidant effect. The relationship with vitamin C may also explain the reports of a lower incidence of stroke associated with high fruit and vegetable intake. Folate may reduce stroke risk by reducing homocysteine concentration (Homocysteine Lowering Trialists' Collaboration 1998).

1.6.16 Oral contraceptives

Studies have shown a definite increased stroke risk associated with the oral contraceptive pill. The risk associated with early combined oral contraceptive preparations has been known for some time, but evidence linking the second and third generation combined oestrogen/progesterone oral contraceptives has more recently been published. A recent meta-analysis of 73 studies found current oral contraceptive use was associated with increased risk of ischemic stroke with a relative risk of 2.75 (95% CI, 2.24–3.38). Smaller oestrogen dosages were associated with lower risk but risk was significantly elevated for all dosages (Gillum *et al.* 2000). Their use has also been associated with an increase in risk of cerebral haemorrhage, although of lower magnitude (WHO Collaborative Study of Cardiovascular Disease and Steroid Hormone Contraception 1996).

1.6.17 Migraine

Occasionally stroke may complicate a migrainous attack. In addition migraine itself appears to be a risk factor for stroke, particularly in young women. A number of studies have investigated the relationship between migraine and stroke risk, that is, have determined whether migraine is a risk for strokes which do not necessarily occur during the migraine attack. These studies have tended to show a positive association (Tietjen 2000, Tzourio *et al.* 2000).

1.6.18 Vascular disease elsewhere

Much of stroke relates either directly or indirectly from atheromatous disease which also causes ischaemic heart disease and peripheral vascular disease. Therefore, it is not surprising that other evidence of cardiovascular disease is a risk factor for stroke. Furthermore some risk factors such as hypertension are risk factors both for cerebral haemorrhage and atheromatous disease increasing the strength of such associations. An increased risk of stroke has been associated with the presence of ischaemic heart disease as determined by history of myocardial infarction, angina, or electrocardiographic abnormalities, with peripheral vascular disease, with cardiac failure, and with atrial fibrillation.

Both non-rheumatic and rheumatic atrial fibrillation are important risk factors for stroke. Part of this association may be coincidental because atrial fibrillation is also caused by ischaemic heart disease and hypertension, which themselves are both risk factors for stroke. However at least part of the association appears to be causal, and there is an approximately 40–60 per cent reduction in stroke risk following anticoagulation in patients with non-valvular atrial fibrillation (Segal *et al.* 2001). Not surprisingly, carotid bruits, or asymptomatic carotid atherosclerosis demonstrated ultrasonically, are risk factors for stroke.

1.7 Risk factors and genetics: implications for planning candidate gene studies

The conventional risk factors described above account for about 40–50 per cent of the risk of stroke (Sacco *et al.* 1989). However a significant proportion of stroke risk remains unexplained. Considerable evidence, reviewed in Chapter 3, suggests that at least part of this is explained by genetic factors, particularly in younger individuals. Such genetic influences may act independent of conventional risk factors, or by interacting with conventional risk factors. For example, one individual with hypertension may develop small vessel cerebrovascular disease in the absence of significant large vessel atherosclerosis, while another individual with hypertension of the same severity may develop carotid stenosis with no evidence of small vessel disease on MRI scanning. A third individual with similar hypertension may develop neither. Therefore there must be modulating factors which may well be genetic.

1.8 Specific stroke subtypes

Risk factors for stroke, including genetic factors, could predispose to stroke either by increasing the risk of the onset of cerebral ischaemia, or modulating the extent of ischaemic damage. Such modulating risk factors might affect the collateral blood supply particularly the integrity of the Circle of Willis, the ischaemic cascade, and repair processes. Many of these modulating processes will influence the severity of all types of cerebral ischaemia, although others such as the integrity of the Circle of Willis will predispose only to ischaemic events occurring proximal to this site. To date there has been relatively little work on the role of genetic factors influencing the cerebral response to injury. It has been suggested that the e4 allele of the Apo E4 gene may worsen outcome following subarachnoid haemorrhage (Dunn *et al.* 2001, Leung *et al.* 2002), but there have been few other studies in this area.

In contrast most stroke genetic studies have focused on genetic factors which predispose to the onset of cerebral ischaemia itself. Here different pathophysiological mechanisms are involved in the different stroke subtypes. In view of this, and increasing evidence that genetic factors may predispose to particular stroke subtypes, an understanding of the pathophysiological processes involved is essential in planning appropriate candidate gene studies. This is covered in the next section.

1.8.1 Ischaemic stroke subtypes

Small artery stroke (lacunar infarction)

Occlusion of a single deep perforating artery results in a restricted area of deep infarction known as a 'lacune'. The perforating arteries supply both the white matter and the deep grey matter nuclei and are end-arteries. This lack of collateral supply means that ischaemia results in a predictable small discreet region of infarction. Lacunar infarction can frequently be asymptomatic, but if it occurs in a strategically important region it will results in symptoms; for example, a lacunar infarct in the posterior limb of the internal capsule may cause contralateral hemiparesis. Because of their location, single lacunar infarcts do not usually result in loss of higher 'cortical' cognitive functions including speech or visual function. The most common lacunar syndromes are pure motor stroke, pure sensory stroke, sensorimotor stroke, and ataxic hemiparesis or clumsy hand syndrome.

The pathogenesis of lacunar infarction is incompletely understood. This is partly due to a paucity of pathological studies. An important factor influencing this is the low early mortality rate. Pathological studies have shown both a diffuse arteriopathy affecting the small perforating arteries, and microatheroma (Lammie 2002). The diffuse arteriopathy has been referred to as lipohyalinosis (Fig. 1.2). This is a destructive small vessel (40–200 µmol diameter) lesion characterized in the acute phase by fibrinoid necrosis, and in the more commonly observed healed phase by loss of normal wall architecture, collagenous sclerosis, and mural foam cells (Lammie 2002). This lesion is thought to cause primarily smaller (3–7 mm diameter), and less often symptomatic, infarcts than those caused by atherosclerosis. In contrast intracranial atherosclerosis, affecting arteries 200–800 µm in diameter, is thought to more often cause larger (5 mm or more in

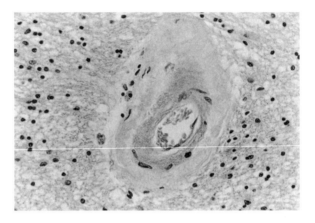

Fig. 1.2 A penetrating arteriole showing marked hyalinization and thickening of the vessel wall (Fig. 5.2(d) in Donnan *et al.* 2002).

diameter), and more often symptomatic, lacunar infarcts. In Fisher's (1969) landmark clinicopathological studies of lacunes, he identified stenotic or occlusive plaques either in the proximal portion of the relevant perforating artery (microatheroma), at its junction (junctional atheroma), or in the parent artery itself (mural atheroma). The mechanism of infarction in such cases appeared to be either due to occlusive thrombus complicating a plaque, or to severely stenotic, non-occlusive plaque (Lammie 2002). In the latter case it has been assumed that infarction occurs secondary to post-stenosis hypoperfusion.

In contrast to stroke in patients with large vessel disease, there is little evidence to suggest that embolism plays an important role in lacunar stroke. Epidemiological evidence suggests that there is a low frequency of significant carotid stenosis or cardiac sources of embolism, and more recently transcranial Doppler studies have shown that asymptomatic circulating emboli in the middle cerebral artery are rare in this stroke subtype (Kapostza *et al.* 1999). It is of course possible that local embolism from the atherosclerotic lesion either at the perforating vessel origin or within the vessel itself, could play a role in pathogenesis.

Many patients with lacunar stroke also have evidence of more chronic ischaemia on neuroimaging. This is seen as areas of low density in the periventricular and deep white matter lesions on CT imaging or high signal on MRI imaging (best seen on T2-weighted or FLAIR sequences). This appearance, referred to as leukoaraiosis, is thought to represent chronic ischaemia in the perforating arteries territory (Fig. 1.3). This hypothesis is supported by a number of lines of evidence (Ward and Brown 2002). First, leukoaraiosis first occurs in the regions furthest from the origin of the perforating arteries (i.e. the internal watershed regions). These are the regions in which perfusion pressure is lowest and therefore any diffuse arteriopathy resulting in reduced perfusion would first lead to ischaemia in these territories (Fig. 1.4). Second, cerebral blood flow studies, using a number of modalities, have shown reduced perfusion in

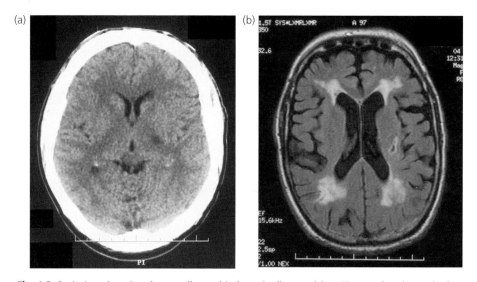

Fig. 1.3 Brain imaging showing small vessel ischaemic disease: (a) A CT scan showing a single lacunar infarct in the posterior limb of the left internal capsule. (b) A FLAIR MRI scan showing a combination of lacunar infarction and leukoaraiosis. The FLAIR sequence is essentially a T2-weighted sequence in which free water appears as low, not high, signal. An old lacunar infarct is seen in the left subcortex (right side of image on paper). This appears as low density due to a central region of cavitation containing free water. Leukoaraiosis is seen as high signal around the horns of both lateral ventricles. This combination of a clinical lacunar syndrome and radiological leukoaraiosis has been referred to as 'ischaemic leukoaraiosis' (see text), and has been used as a phenotype for genetic studies of extensive cerebral small vessel disease. (Copyright with author).

the white matter territories (Ward and Brown 2002). Most studies have not had the resolution to differentiate regions of normal appearing white matter from regions of ischaemic white matter. In the latter hypoperfusion may be occurring secondary to tissue damage, via vasoneuronal coupling, rather than being a causal link in the disease process. However more recent MRI studies, with higher spatial resolution, have shown reduced perfusion not only within the leukoaraiotic lesions, but also in normal appearing white matter (O'Sullivan *et al.* 2002). Third, studies have shown impaired cerebral autoregulation in the white matter territories (Kuwabara *et al.* 1996).

The most attractive disease hypothesis is that the diffuse arteriopathy results in hypoperfusion and impaired autoregulation. Acute ischaemia in a single perforating artery territory then results in lacunar infarction, while more diffuse ischaemia occurring over a prolonged period (perhaps due to transient reductions in blood pressure) results in leukoaraiosis. It has been suggested that in patients with widespread leukoaraiosis and lacunar infarction, the pathology may be primarily in the smaller arterioles and lipohyalinosis may be more important, while in patients with one or a few larger lacunar infarcts without leukoaraiosis, intracranial atherosclerosis may be more important.

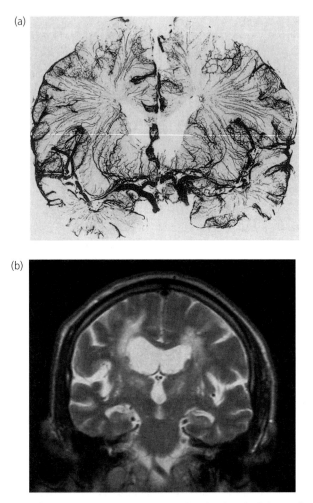

Fig. 1.4 Leukoaraiosis first occurs in brain regions at the distal end of the perforating arteries supply. This is illustrated by the microinjection radiological plate showing the arteriolar blood supply of the periventricular region (Salamon 1973). An MRI scan of a similar coronal view is also shown. The high signal on the MRI scan (leukoaraiosis) first develops in those regions furthest from the origin of the perforating arteries, i.e. those which have lowest perfusion pressure. These regions can be thought of as internal watershed regions. (a) Fig 5.4(a) in Donnan *et al.* (2002); (b) MRI scan. ((b) Copyright with author).

There is some preliminary evidence to suggest different risk factor profiles in the two groups, although much further work needs to be carried out in this area.

The disease processes causing lacunar stroke remain uncertain. Hypertension is the predominant risk factor but not all hypertensive patients develop either symptomatic lacunar infarction or asymptomatic small vessel disease on MRI imaging. Recently homocysteine has been implicated as a risk factor in patients with small vessel disease, and it may be particularly important for the leukoaraiosis phenotype (Fassbender *et al.* 1999). Increasing evidence suggests that endothelial dysfunction may be an important step in disease pathogenesis (Hassan *et al.* in press). Neuropathological studies have demonstrated endothelial disruption. Plasma markers of endothelial dysfunction including thrombomodulin, intercellular adhesion molecule 1 (ICAM1) and Von Willibrand factor are elevated (Hassan *et al.* in press). Mice lacking the endothelial nitric oxide synthase gene develop cerebral vascular lesions resembling that seen in human small vessel disease (Rudic and Sessa 1999). Nitric oxide derived from the endothelium is responsible for maintenance of white matter cerebral blood flow in man (White *et al.* 1998), and probably also dynamic autoregulation (White *et al.* 2000). One possible disease mechanism is that endothelial dysfunction results in impaired nitric oxide release exacerbating both the hypoperfusion and dysautoregulation. It has also been suggested that elevated homocysteine acts as a risk factor for disease via endothelial dysfunction.

There are a number of important considerations when phenotyping cases of small vessel disease. First lacunar infarction, is usually defined as an infarct in the subcortical structures with a diameter of less than 1.5 cm. Larger subcortical infarction can frequently occur from embolic mechanisms secondary to both large artery disease and cardioembolic stroke. Occasionally smaller subcortical infarcts can also occur in patients with such embolic sources, and the stroke subtype in such cases is usually described as tandem or combined rather than small vessel disease itself. Second, it is important to remember that leukoaraiosis itself is a radiological term (Hachinski *et al.* 1987). It can be caused by a number of diverse pathologies, although on a population basis an ischaemic pathology appears to be far the most common. One approach to identifying a group of patients in whom the leukoaraiosis is likely to have an ischaemic basis is the use of the definition 'ischaemic leukoaraiosis' (Jones *et al.* 1999). This refers to patients who have radiological leukoaraiosis in combination with a clinical lacunar stroke.

Cardioembolic stroke

About 20 per cent of ischaemic strokes are caused by cardioembolism. A number of different cardiac pathologies may result in intracardiac thrombus and subsequent embolism. On a population basis, particularly in the elderly, the most common underlying lesion is atrial fibrillation, which results in stasis and thrombosis within the left atrium and atrial appendage. Left ventricular dysfunction secondary to cardiac failure, and/or areas of left ventricular hypokinesia secondary to myocardial infarction, may predispose to left ventricular thrombus. Thrombus may also arise on cardiac valves particularly the mitral valve, which may also become infected resulting in infective emboli. A large number of other cardiac lesions can result in cerebral embolism. Some of these, such as patent foramen ovale, are common in the normal population. While they have an increased prevalence in patients with stroke, in an individual patient it can be difficult to know whether the particular lesion has been responsible for stroke in that patient.

Thrombus, rather than platelet aggregation, is thought to play a major role in many cases of cardioembolism. This is supported by the findings that anticoagulation with warfarin is much more effective than the antiplatelet agent aspirin in patients with atrial fibrillation, and some other forms of cardioembolism. This is in contrast to recent studies which have shown that antiplatelet agents are as effective, and possibly more effective, for other types of stroke (The Stroke Prevention in Reversible Ischemia Trial (SPIRIT) Study Group 1997, Mohr *et al.* 2001).

Due to the large number of different lesions that can cause cardioembolism, finding underlying genes responsible for this type of stroke is likely to be difficult. A more productive approach may be to identify genes which are responsible for the underlying cardiac disorders, such as atrial fibrillation, themselves. However genes which predispose to thrombosis may be risk factors for all types of cardioembolism.

Atheroma in the ascending arch of the aorta is now recognized as an important cause of embolic stroke. Case control studies have shown that it is more common in patients with otherwise unexplained stroke, and larger atheromatous plaques are particularly associated with stroke (The French Study of Aortic Plaques in Stroke Group 1996). Although this is sometimes included under the category cardioembolic stroke, the pathogenesis is likely to be different, and may be more similar to that for large vessel stroke. There is little data comparing the relative efficacy of anticoagulants with antiplatelet agents in this patient group. However if the unstable aortic atherosclerotic plaque behaves in a similar manner to the active carotid plaque, platelet aggregation may play a more important role. Consistent with this, the pattern of asymptomatic embolization in this condition is more similar to that seen in carotid disease, rather than other cardioembolic diseases such as atrial fibrillation (Rundek *et al.* 1999).

Large artery stroke

Large artery stroke (carotid and vertebral artery stenosis) accounts for about a quarter of all ischaemic stroke. Many patients with stroke have some degree of carotid plaque and carotid stroke is usually defined as the presence of a carotid stenosis ≥50 per cent in the symptomatic artery territory. In almost all cases stenosis occurs secondary to atherosclerosis, although in rare cases it may occur secondary to carotid dissection or other processes such as post radiotherapy. The carotid bulb is a site of predilection for atherosclerosis, perhaps due to flow patterns occurring at the site of bifurcation. There may be slightly different processes predisposing to atherosclerosis at the carotid bulb, compared with those causing systemic atherosclerosis. This is supported by a recent study finding that increased intima-media thickness of the carotid bulb is more strongly associated with stroke than myocardial infarction. In contrast intima-media thickness of the common carotid artery is similarly associated with both stroke and myocardial infarction (Jerrard-Dunne *et al.* 2003).

In a patient with an asymptomatic carotid stenosis the stroke risk is only about 2 per cent per year. In contrast, when a carotid stenosis become symptomatic the risk of stroke over the next 2 years is approximately 30 per cent. Prospective studies, largely from the medical arms of the carotid endarterectomy trials, have shown that the risk of recurrent stroke is greatest in the first couple of months and is much reduced by 6 months. The risk has returned to that of asymptomatic stenosis by about 2 years (Fig. 1.5) (European Carotid Surgery Trialists' Collaborative Group 1998). The mechanisms converting a plaque from asymptomatic to symptomatic are incompletly understood, but ulceration or erosion of the plaque surface with subsequent thrombus formation and embolism is thought to play a crucial role (Rothwell 2000).

In patients with carotid stenosis, embolism rather than hypoperfusion, is believed to be the primary mechanism causing stroke. This is supported by a number of lines of evidence. Angiographic studies have demonstrated emboli in patients with acute stroke secondary to carotid stenosis. In patients with symptomatic carotid stenosis, emboli can sometimes be seen in the retinal vessels, which are supplied by the ophthalmic artery, which is the first branch of the internal carotid artery. Transcranial Doppler studies have demonstrated that asymptomatic embolization is common in patients with symptomatic carotid disease (Siebler *et al.* 1994, Markus *et al.* 1995), occurring in as many as 40 per cent of cases during a single hours recording. Its frequency rapidly tails off in the days and weeks following the last clinical event. Asymptomatic embolization in this patient group has been shown to independently predict subsequent stroke and TIA risk (Molloy and Markus 1999). Consistent with

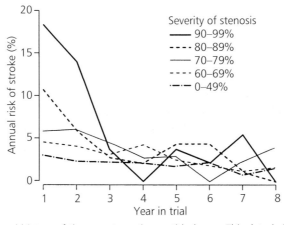

Fig. 1.5 The natural history of the symptomatic carotid plaque. This data is from the medical arm of the European Carotid Endarectomy Study (European Carotid Surgery Trialists' Collaborative Group 1998 Fig. 3). After a stroke or TIA the risk of recurrent ischaemic stroke is high but falls rapidly over the first two years. By the end of the second year the risk is similar to that seen in asymptomatic stenosis. The figure also illustrates that risk is higher as the degree of stenosis increases.

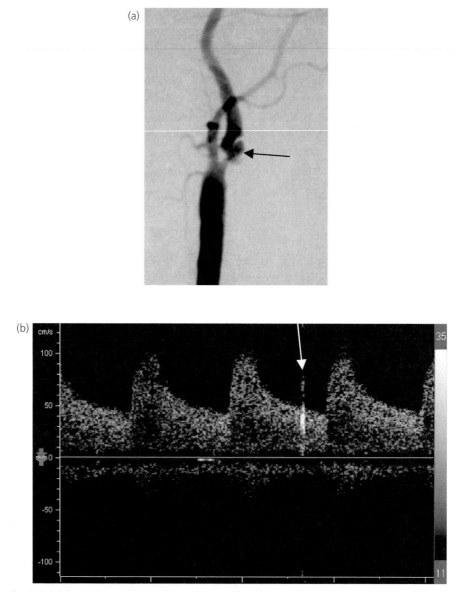

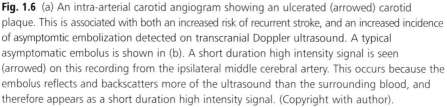

Fig. 1.6 (a) An intra-arterial carotid angiogram showing an ulcerated (arrowed) carotid plaque. This is associated with both an increased risk of recurrent stroke, and an increased incidence of asymptomtic embolization detected on transcranial Doppler ultrasound. A typical asymptomatic embolus is shown in (b). A short duration high intensity signal is seen (arrowed) on this recording from the ipsilateral middle cerebral artery. This occurs because the embolus reflects and backscatters more of the ultrasound than the surrounding blood, and therefore appears as a short duration high intensity signal. (Copyright with author).

the importance of embolization, plaque ulceration has emerged as a strong risk factor for stroke (Fig. 1.6). Detected either histologically on endarterectomy specimens or angiographically, it is more common in patients with symptomatic stenosis, and is an independent predictor of subsequent stroke risk (Rothwell *et al.* 2000). Platelet aggregation appears to play a crucial role in embolization secondary to surface erosions or ulceration in this patient group. Aspirin is as effective, if not more effective, than anticoagulation with warfarin. Antiplatelet agents have been shown to reduce asymptomatic embolization, detected by transcranial Doppler ultrasound. More potent antiplatelet agents, such as the novel nitric oxide donor S-nitrosoglutathione, can almost completely abolish embolization in this group (Kapostza *et al.* 2002).

The finding that asymptomatic embolization is very common, and much more common than clinical events, in patients with symptomatic carotid stenosis, may seem at first surprising. However previous studies have demonstrated frequent asymptomatic retinal embolization or small asymptomatic infarcts on neuroimaging. Why some emboli result in symptoms and others do not remains uncertain. This may depend largely on embolus size, but collateral supply and the reactivity of the intracerebral vessels may play an important role. Haemodynamic factors may interact with embolization by resulting in impaired clearance of emboli (Caplan and Hennerici 1998).

While in most patients with carotid stenosis embolism is the cause of stroke, occasionally haemodynamic stroke can occur. This is particularly the case in patients with tight carotid stenosis who have an episode of severely reduced perfusion pressure, for example hypotension during a cardiac operation. In addition patients with carotid occlusion suffer an increased risk of stroke, although it is less than that in patients with tight carotid stenosis. In this patient group impaired cerebral haemodynamics is a risk factor for stroke (Markus and Cullinaine 2001), and haemodynamic factors, rather than embolism, are thought to be the predominant pathogenic process.

The collateral supply, and in particular the patency of the Circle of Willis, can play a crucial role in determining the outcome of carotid stenosis and occlusion. For example, in a patient with an incomplete Circle of Willis internal carotid artery occlusion can result in massive stroke. In contrast, a patient with both a patent anterior communicating artery and posterior communicating artery can suffer carotid occlusion and remain asymptomatic without cerebral infarction. Factors determining the patency of the Circle of Willis have not been determined but it is possible that genetic factors play an important role.

1.8.2 Cerebral haemorrhage (Table 1.4)

Subarachnoid haemorrhage

Subarachnoid haemorrhage describes primary haemorrhage into the subarachnoid space. If stroke is defined as a focal neurological deficit only a proportion of patients with subarachnoid haemorrhage develop stroke. The key clinical feature is a sudden

Table 1.4 Aetiological classification of cerebral haemorrhage

Subarachnoid haemorrhage
- Saccular aneurysms
- Normal angiogram
- Rare causes

Primary intracerebral haemorrhage
- Malformations or changes in cerebral vessels
  - Lipohyalinosis/microaneurysms in perforating arteries
  - Amyloid angiopathy
  - Cerebral arteriovenous malformations
  - Saccular aneurysms
  - Cerebral venous thrombosis
  - Moya–moya syndrome
  - Cerebral arteriovenous malformations
  - Cavernomas
  - Mycotic aneurysms
  - Vasculitis
- Hypertension
- Haematological factors
  - Treatment related
    – Anticoagulants
    – Thrombolysis
    – Antiplatelet agents
  - Haemophilia
  - Leukaemia
  - Thrombocytopenia
- Drugs
  - Alcohol
  - Amphetamines
  - Cocaine
- Other causes
  - Cerebral tumours

onset headache often described as a 'thunderclap'. Other features include loss of consciousness in about 50 per cent of patients, epileptic seizures in about 10 per cent, and on examination signs of meningism including neck stiffness. Focal neurological deficits may arise acutely from associated focal haematoma such as subarachnoid clot in the sylvian fissure, secondary to a middle cerebral artery aneurysm, which results in hemiparesis. More commonly they may result from secondary vasospasm. This usually occurs between days 4 and 12.

Approximately 85 per cent of all spontaneous subarachnoid haemorrhages are due to rupture of saccular aneurysms at the base of the brain. This is a serious disorder with a high mortality and morbidity, and unselected hospital series have shown case fatality rates after 3 months as high as 50 per cent. Morbidity may occur from the initial bleed itself but there is also a high rebleed rate, which is the rational behind early neuro-surgical and neuroradiological intervention. The underlying saccular aneurysm is identified by intra-arterial angiography. However in 10 per cent of all subarachnoid patients there is no aneurysm detected. These patients present a different clinical picture with a more benign outcome. In two thirds of these cases the centre of the haemorrhage is around the mid brain, commonly ventral to it, and the pathophysiological mechanism is largely unknown. It has been speculated this peri-mesencephalic subarachnoid haemorrhage may arise from a ruptured vein rather than being arterial, and possibly from a varicose vein or venous malformation (Warlow *et al.* 1996*a*). The remaining 5 per cent of spontaneous subarachnoid haemorrhages are due to a variety of other diseases including arterial dissection and various other rare conditions.

Genetic studies have primarily concentrated on the genetics of aneurysmal sub-arachnoid haemorrhage. A major advantage in studying this condition is that new magnetic resonance angiography techniques can detect asymptomatic aneurysms in a large proportion of cases (Fig. 1.7). This technique can be used to determine whether other family members have aneuryms, and reduces problems due to incomplete pene-trance. The genetics of aneurysmal subarachnoid haemorrhage is covered in detail in Chapter 10.

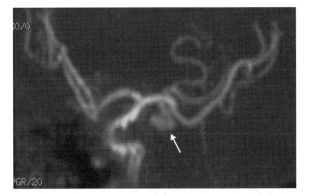

Fig. 1.7 MRA of an asymptomatic left middle cerebral artery aneurysm (arrowed). This technique can be used to identify asymptomatic aneurysms in families with an index case of subarachnoid haemorrhage secondary to a saccular aneurysm. Although not as sensitive for small aneurysms as intra-arterial angiography, it is non-invasive, and therefore does not have the 1 per cent stroke risk associated with conventional angiography. (Copyright with author).

Primary intracerebral haemorrhage

Primary intracerebral haemorrhage accounts for about 10 per cent of strokes. Bleeding into the brain parenchymal tissue usually results in symptoms with the onset of a focal neurological deficit. Therefore most primary intracerebral haemorrhages result in stroke itself. However neuroimaging data suggests that asymptomatic micro haemorrhages may be common, particularly in patients with ischaemic small vessel disease.

Primary intracerebral haemorrhage results for a number of different mechanisms and in many cases no one single cause can be identified. Hypertension is the major risk factor for intracerebral haemorrhage. Both the relative and absolute incidence of intracerebral haemorrhage is increased in Black individuals, particularly Africans, and this may partly reflect the increased prevalence and severity of hypertension in this ethnic group. Hypertensive intracerebral haemorrhage usually occurs in the subcortical structures particularly the basal ganglia. The underlying mechanism is controversial but it is thought to result from degenerative changes in the small perforating arteries (Warlow et al. 1996b). These are found mostly in the deep regions such as the basal ganglia, cerebellum and brainstem, and this explains the distribution of hypertensive intracerebral haemorrhage. Microaneurysms measuring 300–900 μm in diameter, appearing on small perforating arteries of 100–300 μm in diameter, have been described in a number of pathological studies and have been suggested as the underlying lesion resulting with haemorrhage. Their importance and prevalence has been controversial, but they certainly do appear to be a cause of haemorrhage in many patients. However other degenerative disease of the small perforating vessels may also predispose to haemorrhage. This is supported by studies which have found fibrinoid necrosis of the walls of the small vessels as an almost invariable phenomena in patients with hypertensive intracerebral haemorrhage, while electron microscopic study of specimens obtained at autopsy or emergency surgery have shown that the most common site of rupture is at distal bifurcations of the lenticulostriate arteries, and rarely in the wall of a microaneurysm (Warlow et al. 1996b). It is possible therefore that microaneurysms may be primarily a marker of degenerative changes in the small perforating arteries rather than the source of bleeding. The underlying pathology in this group of patients shows many similarities to the small vessel arteriopathy seen in patients with lacunar stroke. It is possible that lacunar stroke and primary hypertensive intracerebral haemorrhage are facets of the same disease. This is supported by more recent studies using gradient echo magnetic resonance imaging. This technique is very sensitive to the presence of small regions of haemosiderin, resulting from past haemorrhage. Such studies, both in patients with hypertensive small vessel cerebral ischaemic disease (Kato et al. 2002), and in patients with the small vessel arteriopathy CADASIL (Dichgans et al. 2002), have shown evidence of multiple microhaemorrhages in the perforating arteries territories (Fig. 1.8).

Another important cause of primary intracerebral haemorrhage, which is being increasingly recognized particularly in the elderly, is amyloid angiopathy. This is

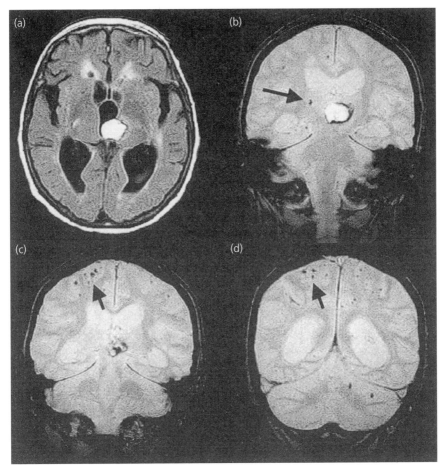

Fig. 1.8 MR imaging in a patient with primary intracerebral haemorrhage. In (a) on a FLAIR sequence an area of high signal, consistent with an subacute haemorrhage in the left thalamus can be clearly seen. On the gradient echo images in b–d multiple areas of low signal, consistent with old microbleeds can be seen (Fig. 25.3 in Donnan *et al.* 2002).

primarily a cause of lobar haemorrhages. The underlying abnormality consists of patchy deposits of amyloid in the muscle layer of small and medium sized arteries in the lepto-meninges of the cerebral cortex, and the subcortical white matter. In unselected autopsy studies in patients who have not suffered cerebral haemorrhage, the presence of cerebral arterial amyloid becomes increasingly frequent with age ranging from 5 to 10 per cent in those aged 60–69 years to 25 per cent in individuals aged 70–79 years, 40 per cent between ages 80–89, and more than 50 per cent in those aged over 90 years (Warlow *et al.* 1996*b*). Despite the frequency of these changes in normal individuals, there is convincing evidence that they are associated with intracerebral haemorrhage. Amyloid angiopathy is frequently associated with multiple or recurrent haemorrhages. This cause of stroke is dealt with in more detail in Chapter 9. In a minority of patients the amyloid results from an autosomal dominant disorder due to mutations in the amyloid precursor protein gene, but in the majority of cases the disease appears to be sporadic.

Cerebral arteriovenous malformations (AVMs) are an important cause of cerebral haemorrhage particularly in the young, in which age group they account for up to a third of intracerebral haemorrhages. AVMs are conglomerates of dilated arteries and veins without a capillary network joining them. This is embedded in a stroma devoid of normal brain tissue. They are usually single, being multiple in only 4 per cent of cases unless there is some underlying systemic disorder such as hereditary haemorrhagic telangiectasia. The familial occurrence of AVMs has been reported but is very rare. Haemorrhages from AVMs are mostly lobar (in the cortex) but they can also occur in the deep nuclei. AVMs can usually be clearly seen on MRI and are further defined by angiography, on which large feeding arteries and rapid shunting of blood to veins that are often tortuous and enlarged can be seen. Aneurysms are often found on the feeding arteries and are believed to be secondary to the flow disturbance. They are associated with an increased risk of rebleeding. The annual risk of rebleeding for AVMs is about 2 per cent per year, but in the presence of associated aneurysms may be 5–7 per cent.

Other rare causes of cerebral haemorrhage include cavernous angiomas (see Chapter 11), Moya-Moya syndrome (Section 6.3.1) where haemorrhage occurs from rupture of new vessel formation which occurs secondary to large intracerebral vessel occlusion in young individuals, underlying intracerebral tumours, vasculitis, and drug and alcohol abuse. The risk of intracerebral haemorrhage is also markedly increased in patients with bleeding disorders, particularly those on anticoagulant therapy or those who have been administered thrombolytic therapy.

References

Adams, H.P., Jr., Bendixen, B.H., Kappelle, L.J., *et al.* (1993). Classification of subtype of acute ischemic stroke. Definitions for use in a multicenter clinical trial. TOAST. Trial of Org 10172 in Acute Stroke Treatment. *Stroke*, **24**, 35–41.

Bamford, J., Sandercock, P., Dennis, M., Burn, J., and Warlow, C. (1991). Classification and natural history of clinically identifiable subtypes of cerebral infarction. *Lancet*, **337**, 1521–6.

Bonita, R. (1992). Epidemiology of stroke. *Lancet*, **339**, 342–4.

Byington, R.P., Davis, B.R., Plehn, J.F., White, H.D., Baker, J., Cobbe, S.M., and Shepherd, J. (2001). Reduction of stroke events with pravastatin: the Prospective Pravastatin Pooling (PPP) Project. *Circulation*, **103**, 387–92.

Caplan, L.R. and Hennerici, M. (1998). Impaired clearance of emboli (washout) is an important link between hypoperfusion, embolism, and ischemic stroke. *Archives of Neurology*, **55**, 1475–82.

Collins, R. and MacMahon, S. (1994). Blood pressure, antihypertensive drug treatment and the risks of stroke and of coronary heart disease. *British Medical Bulletin*, **50**, 272–98.

Corwin, L.T., Wolf, P.A., Kannel, W.B., and McNamara, P.M. (1982). Accuracy of death certification of stroke: the Framlingham Study. *Stroke*, **13**, 816–8.

Danesh, J., Whincup, P., Walker, M., *et al.* (2000). Low grade inflammation and coronary heart disease: prospective study and updated meta-analyses. *British Medical Journal*, **321**, 199–204.

de Boer, O.J., van der Wal, A.C., and Becker, A.E. (2000). Atherosclerosis, inflammation, and infection. *Journal of Pathology*, **190**, 237–43.

Dichgans, M., Holtmannspötter, M., Herzog, J., Peters, N., Bergmann, M., and Yousry, T.A. (2002). Cerebral microbleeds in CADASIL: a gradient-echo magnetic resonance imaging and autopsy study. *Stroke*, **33**, 67–71.

Donnan, G., Norrving, B., Bamford, J., and Bogousslavsky, J. (eds) (2002). *Subcortical stroke*, 2nd edn. Oxford University Press, Oxford.

Dunn, L.T., Stewart, E., Murray, G.D., Nicoll, J.A., and Teasdale, G.M. (2001). The influence of apolipoprotein E genotype on outcome after spontaneous subarachnoid hemorrhage: a preliminary study. *Neurosurgery*, **48**, 1006–10.

Eikelboom, J.W., Hankey, G.J., Anand, S.S., Lofthouse, E., Staples, N., and Baker, R.I. (2000). Association between high homocyst(e)ine and ischemic stroke due to large- and small-artery disease but not other etiologic subtypes of ischemic stroke. *Stroke*, **31**, 1069–75.

European Carotid Surgery Trialists' Collaborative Group. (1998). Randomised trial of endarterectomy for recently symptomatic carotid stenosis: final results of the MRC European Carotid Surgery Trial (ECST). *Lancet*, **351**, 1379–87.

Fassbender, K., Mielke, O., Bertsch, T., *et al.* (1999). Homocysteine in cerebral macroangiography and microangiopathy. *Lancet*, **353**, 1586–7.

Feigin, V.L., Anderson, C.S., and Mhurchu, C.N. (2002). Systemic inflammation, endothelial dysfunction, dietary Fatty acids and micronutrients as risk factors for stroke: a selective review. *Cerebrovascular Disease*, **13**, 219–24.

Fisher, C.M. (1969). The arterial lesion underlying lacunes. *Acta Neuropathologica (Berlin)*, **12**, 1–15.

Gillum, R.F., Gorelick, P.B., and Cooper, E.S. (eds.) (1999). *Stroke in Blacks*. Karger, Basel.

Gillum, L.A., Mamidipudi, S.K., and Johnston, S.C. (2000). Ischemic stroke risk with oral contraceptives. A meta-analysis. *Journal of the American Medical Association*, **284**, 72–8.

Goldstein, L.B., Jones, M.R., Matchar, D.B., Edwards, L.J., Hoff, J., Chilukuri, V., Armstrong, S.B., and Horner, R. (2001). Improving the reliability of stroke subgroup classification using the Trial of ORG 10172 in Acute Stroke Treatment (TOAST) criteria. *Stroke*, **32**, 1091–7.

Grau, A.J., Buggle, F., Steichen-Wiehn, C., Heindl, S., Banerjee, T., Seitz, R., *et al.* (1995). Clinical and biochemical analysis in infection-associated stroke. *Stroke*, **26**, 1520–6.

Hackniski, V.C., Potter, P., and Merskey, H. (1987). Leukoaraiosis. *Archives of Neurology*, **44**, 21–3.

Hankey, G., Jamorozik, K., Braodhurst, R., *et al.* (1998). Long-term risk of first recurrent stroke in the Perth community stroke study. *Stroke*, **29**, 2491–500.

Hankey, G.J. and Eikelboom, J.W. (2001). Homocysteine and stroke. *Current Opinion in Neurology*, **14**, 95–102.

Hassan, A., Hunt, B., O'Sullivan, M., Parmar, K., Bamford, J., Briley, D., Brown, M.M., Thomas, D., and Markus, H.S. (2003). The role of endothelial dysfunction in lacunar infarction and ischaemic leukoaraiosis. *Brain*. **126**, 424–32.

Heart Protection Study Collaborative Group. (2002). MRC/BHF Heart Protection Study of cholesterol lowering with simvastatin in 20,536 high-risk individuals: a randomised placebo-controlled trial. *Lancet*, **360**, 7–22.

Homocysteine Lowering Trialists' Collaboration. (1998). Lowering blood homocysteine with folic acid based supplements: meta-analysis of randomised trials. *British Medical Journal*, **316**, 894–8.

Jerrard-Dunne, P., Markus, H.S., Steckel, D.A., Buehler, A., von Kegler, S., and Sitzer, M. (2003). Early carotid atherosclerosis and family history of myocardial infarction and stroke—specific effects on arterial sites have implications for genetic studies: The Carotid Atherosclerosis Progression Study (CAPS). *Arteriosclerosis, Thrombosis and Vascular Biology*, 13, 302–6.

Jones, D.K., Lythgoe, D., Horsfield, M.A., Simmons, A., Williams, S.C.R., and Markus, H.S. (1999). Characterisation of white matter damage in ischaemic leukoaraiosis with diffusion tensor magnetic resonance imaging. *Stroke*, 30, 393–7.

Kaposzta, Z., Martin, J.F., and Markus, H.S. (2002). Switching off embolisation from the symptomatic carotid plaque using s-nitrosoglutathione. *Circulation*, 105, 1480–4.

Kaposzta, Z., Young, E., Bath, P.M.W., and Markus, H.S. (1999). The clinical application of asymptomatic embolic signal detection in acute stroke: a prospective study. *Stroke*, 30, 1814–8.

Kato, H., Izumiyama, M., Izumiyama, K., Takahashi, A., and Itoyama, Y. (2002). Silent cerebral microbleeds on T2*-weighted MRI: correlation with stroke subtype, stroke recurrence, and leukoaraiosis. *Stroke*, 33, 1536–40.

Kunitz, S.C., Gross, C.R., Heyman, A., Kasse, C.S., Mohr, J.P., Proce, T.R., and Wolf, P.A. (1984). The pilot Stroke Data Bank: definition, design, and data. *Stroke*, 15, 740–6.

Kuwabara, Y., Ichiya, Y., Sasaki, M., Yoshida, T., Fukumura, T., Masuda, K., Ibayashi, S., and Fujishima, M. (1996). Cerebral blood flow and vascular response to hypercapnia in hypertensive patients with leukoaraiosis. *Annals of Nuclear Medicine*, 10, 293–8.

Law, M. (1996). Commentary: evidence on salt is consistent. *British Medical Journal*, 312, 1284–5.

Lammie, G.A. (2002). Pathology of lacunar infarction. In *Subcortical stroke* (eds G. Donnan, B. Norrving, J. Bamford, and J. Bogousslavsky), 2nd edn. pp. 37–46. Oxford University Press, Oxford.

Leung, C.H., Poon, W.S., Yu, L.M., Wong, G.K., and Ng, H.K. (2002). Apolipoprotein e genotype and outcome in aneurysmal subarachnoid hemorrhage. *Stroke*, 33, 548–52.

Markus, H. and Cullinane, M. (2001). Severely impaired cerebrovascular reactivity predicts stroke and TIA risk in patients with carotid artery stenosis and occlusion. *Brain*, 124, 457–67.

Markus, H.S., Thomson, N., and Brown, M.M. (1995). Asymptomatic cerebral embolic signals in symptomatic and asymptomatic carotid artery disease. *Brain*, 118, 1005–11.

Mohr, J.P., Thompson, J.L., Lazar, R.M., Levin, B., Sacco, R.L., Furie, K.L., Kistler, J.P., Albers, G.W., Pettigrew, L.C., Adams, H.P., Jackson, C.M., and Pullicino, P. (2001). Warfarin–Aspirin Recurrent Stroke Study Group. A comparison of warfarin and aspirin for the prevention of recurrent ischemic stroke. *New England Journal of Medicine*, 345, 1444–51.

Molloy, J. and Markus, H.S. (1999). Asymptomatic embolization predicts stroke and TIA risk in patients with carotid artery stenosis. *Stroke*, 30, 1440–3.

Murray, C.J.L. and Lopez, A.D. (eds). (1996). *The global burden of disease: a comprehensive assessment of mortality and disability from disease, injuries, and risk factors in 1990 and projected to 2020.* Harvard University Press, Boston, MA.

O'Sullivan, M., Lythgoe, D.J., Periera, A.C., Summers, P.E., Jarosz, J.M., Williams, S.C.R., and Markus, H.S. (2002). Patterns of cerebral blood flow reduction in patients with ischaemic leukoaraiosis. *Neurology*, 59, 321–6.

Petty, G.W., Brown, R.D., Whisnant, J.P., Sicks, J.D., O'Fallon, M., and Wiebers, D.O. (2000). Ischaemic stroke subtypes. A population-based study of functional outcome, survival, and recurrence. *Stroke*, 31, 1062–8.

PROGRESS Investigators. (2001). Randomised trial of a perindopril-based blood-pressure-lowering regimen among 6,105 individuals with previous stroke or transient ischaemic attack. *Lancet*, 358, 1033–41.

Prospective Studies Collaboration. (1995). Cholesterol, diastolic blood pressure and stroke: 13,000 strokes in 250,000 people in 45 prospective cohorts. *Lancet*, **346**, 1647–53.

Ridker, P.M., Hennekens, C.H., Buring, J.E., and Rifai, N. (2000). C-reactive protein and other markers of inflammation in the prediction of cardiovascular disease in women. *New England Journal Medicine*, **342**, 836–43.

Rothwell, P.M., Gibson, R., and Warlow, C.P. (2000). Interrelation between plaque surface morphology and degree of stenosis on carotid angiograms and the risk of ischemic stroke in patients with symptomatic carotid stenosis. On behalf of the European Carotid Surgery Trialists' Collaborative Group. *Stroke*, **31**, 615–21.

Rudic, D.R. and Sessa, W.C. (1999). Nitric Oxide in endothelial dysfunction and vascular remodelling. *American Journal of Human Genetics*, **64**, 673–7.

Rundek, T., Di Tullio, M.R., Sciacca, R.R., Titova, I.V., Mohr, J.P., Homma, S., and Sacco, R.L. (1999). Association Between Large Aortic Arch Atheromas and High-Intensity Transient Signals in Elderly Stroke Patients. *Stroke*, **30**, 2683–6.

Sacco, R.L., Ellenberg, J.H., Mohr, J.P., Tatemichi, T.K., Hier, D.B., and Price, T.R. (1989). Infarcts of undetermined cause: the NINCDS stroke data bank. *Annals of Neurology*, **25**, 382–90.

Salamon, G. (1973). *iAtlas de la vascularisation arterielle du cerveau chez l'homme*, 2nd edn. Sandoz, Paris.

Segal, J.B., McNamara, R.L., Miller, M.R., Powe, N.R., Goodman, S.N., Robinson, K.A., and Bass, E.B. (2001). Anticoagulants or antiplatelet therapy for non-rheumatic atrial fibrillation and flutter. *Cochrane Database Systematic Reviews*, **1**, CD001938.

Siebler, M., Kleinschmidt, A., Sitzer, M., *et al.* (1994). Cerebral microembolism in symptomatic and asymptomatic high-grade internal carotid artery stenosis. *Neurology*, **44**, 615–8.

Stewart, J., Dundas, R., Howard, R., Rudd, A., and Wolfe, C.D.A. (1999). Ethnic differences in stroke incidence. The south London Stroke register. *British Medical Journal*, **318**, 967–71.

The French Study of Aortic Plaques in Stroke Group. (1996). Atherosclerotic disease of the aortic arch as a risk factor for recurrent ischemic stroke. *New England Journal of Medicine*, **334**, 1216–21.

The Stroke Prevention in Reversible Ischemia Trial (SPIRIT) Study Group. (1997). A randomized trial of anticoagulants versus aspirin after cerebral ischemia of presumed arterial origin. *Annals of Neurology*, **42**, 857–65.

Thorvaldsen, P., Asplund, K., Kuulasmaa, K., Rajakangas, A.M., and Schroll, M. (1995). Stroke incidence, case fatality, and mortality in the WHO MONICA project. World Health Organization Monitoring Trends and Determinants in Cardiovascular Disease. *Stroke*, **26**, 361–7.

Tietjen, G.E. (2000). The relationship of migraine and stroke. *Neuroepidemiology*, **19**, 13–9.

Tzourio, C., Kittner, S.J., Bousser, M.G., and Alperovitch, A. (2000). Migraine and stroke in young women. *Cephalalgia*, **20**, 190–9.

van Exel, E., Gussekloo, J., de Craen, A.J., Bootsma-van der Wiel, A., Frolich, M., and Westendorp, R.G. (2002). Inflammation and stroke: the Leiden 85-Plus Study. *Stroke*, **33**, 1135–8.

Walton, J. (ed.) (1993). *Brain's diseases of the nervous system*, 10th edn. p. 203. Oxford University Press, Oxford, UK.

Ward, N.S. and Brown, M.M. (2002). Leukoaraiosis. In *Subcortical stroke* (eds Donnan, G. Norrving, B. Bamford, J. and Bogousslavsky, J.), 2nd edn. pp. 4746–66. Oxford University Press, Oxford.

Warlow, C.P., Dennis, M.S., van Gijn, J., Hankey, G.J., Sandercock, P.A.G., Bamford, J.M., and Wardlaw, J. (1996a). What caused this subarachnoid haemorrhage? In *Stroke. A practical guide to management*, pp. 322–59. Blackwell Science, Oxford, UK.

Warlow, C.P., Dennis, M.S., van Gijn, J., Hankey, G.J., Sandercock, P.A.G., Bamford, J.M., and Wardlaw, J. (1996*b*). What caused this intracerebral haemorrhage? In *Stroke. A practical guide to management*, pp. 287–321. Blackwell Science, Oxford, UK.

White, R.P., Deane, C., Vallance, P., and Markus, H.S. (1998). Nitric oxide synthase inhibition in humans reduces cerebral blood flow but not the hyperaemic response to hypercapnia. *Stroke*, **29**, 467–72.

White, R., Vallance, P., and Markus, H.S. (2000). The effect of nitric oxide synthase inhibition on dynamic cerebral autoregulation in man. *Clinical Science*, **99**, 555–60.

WHO Collaborative Study of Cardiovascular Disease and Steroid Hormone Contraception. (1996). Haemorrhagic stroke, overall stroke risk and combined oral contraceptives; results of an international, multi centre, case-controlled study. *Lancet*, **348**, 505–10.

Wolfe, C.D.A. (2000). The impact of stroke. *British Medical Bulletin*, **56**, 275–86.

Wolfe, C.D.A., Rudd, A.G., Howard, R., Coshall, C., Stewart, J., Lawrence, E., Hajat, C., and Hillen, T. (2002). The incidence and case fatility of stroke subtypes in a multi ethnic population. The South London Stroke Register. *Journal of Neurology Neurosurgery and Psychiatry*, **72**, 211–6.

Chapter 2

Genetic principles and techniques

Andrew J. Catto and Angela M. Carter

2.1 **Introduction**

Considerable progress has been made in defining the underlying genetic basis of many Mendelian and mitochondrial diseases which can cause stroke and other cerebrovascular diseases. Examples include cerebral autosomal dominant arteriopathy with subcortical infarcts and leucoencephalopathy (CADASIL), familial angiomas, Fabry's disease, and mitochondrial encephalopathy with lactic acidosis and stroke-like syndrome (MELAS). These diseases were discovered either by working back from a known biochemical defect, or thorough linkage (or segregation) analysis, in informative multiplex pedigrees. The routine techniques used in such stroke studies, and as applied to numerous others Mendelian disorders, are covered in standard textbooks (Strachan and Read 1999). However, although the monogenic stroke disorders provide important insights into stroke mechanisms, they account for only a minority of cases of stroke. What remains is the daunting task of defining the genetic variants that contribute to the inherited component of risk for so-called 'common' or 'sporadic' stroke.

Most cases of stroke have a multifactorial aetiology, and any genetic contribution to risk is likely to be polygenic. In such cases the identification of the genetic variants predisposing to stroke is hampered by a number of factors; most important is the high degree of heterogeneity in stroke disease aetiology, the difficulty in establishing clearly defined subtypes, and complex gene–environment interactions. These factors make it difficult to identify the contribution of genetic variants to the pathogenesis of disease, even when there are clear relationships between genetic variants and the intermediate phenotype. Genetic heterogeneity may also confound interpretation, as a number of quite different genes might result in the same outward stroke phenotype. As stroke is a disease of old age (presenting on average 10 years later than acute myocardial infarction), there are likely to be fewer relatives (and very few parents) available for study. As the development of stroke is dependent on multiple risk factors, such as diabetes and ischaemic heart disease, these are likely to confound and possibly mask the expression of any stroke gene. Furthermore, subjects without a 'stroke genotype' will still go on to develop a stroke, probably through as yet unrecognized environmental influences and/or gene–gene interactions. By contrast, even if the individual does inherit one of the 'stroke genes', it does not follow that they will express the stroke phenotype (variable penetrance).

What can genetic analyses add to our understanding of the pathogenesis of common stroke? Genetic information can provide far more information than just susceptibility to disease; genetic factors are likely to also influence the severity of disease or the disease outcome in terms of residual defect or mortality. Genetics in the context of stroke may well help in defining different subtypes of the disease, which itself would assist in the design of new therapeutics targeted to specific subtypes of ischaemic stroke in particular.

This chapter focuses on genetic approaches and techniques used in the investigation of polygenic stroke. We describe the most common forms of polymorphism encountered in the human genome and describe their potential influence on gene function. We have included examples, where appropriate, for those polymorphisms which have been reported to be related to stroke. We go on to outline the different types of clinical/epidemiological study which can be utilized to evaluate the influence of polymorphisms on disease development. We conclude this chapter by indicating some of the methods currently employed to identify common polymorphisms and give a brief outline of the functional studies which can be carried out to determine the functionality of identified polymorphisms.

2.2 **Common types of polymorphic variant**

Short sequence repeats (SSRs) are a common form of polymorphism, these comprise repeats of (most commonly) 2–4 nucleotides which are highly variable in length (from a few to hundreds of repeats). The differences in length in the population reflect slippage of DNA-polymerase during replication and can be useful for differentiating paternal and maternal alleles. SSRs are estimated to occur on average every 2 kb and comprise approximately 3 per cent of the human genome (Lander *et al.* 2001). There are thousands of these repeat elements interspersed throughout the human genome which have been well characterized, and these have been utilized to form a genetic map of the human genome that has facilitated the identification of at least 100 disease genes; common examples include (CA)n and (CGG)n.

The most commonly occurring genetic variants are single nucleotide polymorphisms (SNPs), where one single nucleotide is substituted for another, for example, CTG to TTG, with C to T transitions being the most frequently encountered. SNPs have been estimated to occur with a frequency of at least 1 per 1000 base pairs in the human genome (Sachidanandam *et al.* 2001). A publicly available map of 1.42 million SNPs mapping the human genome, with an average density of 1 SNP every 1.9 kb, has been compiled (a list of internet resources is included later in this chapter). This is an invaluable resource for candidate-gene studies and for genome-wide association scans. Other types of polymorphic variant include variable number tandem repeats (VNTRs), which comprise shorter repeats of approximately 10–60 nucleotides, and insertions or deletions of from a single base pair to the insertion of transposable elements including Alu repeat and LINE elements.

2.3 Influence of polymorphisms on gene function

Clearly not all polymorphisms are functional; however, the potential influence of a polymorphism on gene function can be inferred by its location within the gene locus.

2.3.1 Coding region polymorphisms

Polymorphisms occurring within the coding region of a gene can be silent (where no change in the encoded amino acid is induced), or missense (resulting in a change in the encoded amino acid), or can influence splice sites. Missense polymorphisms can have an influence on the structure and/or function of the encoded protein. For example, those occurring in key areas of protein function may influence the folding of a protein, ligand–receptor binding, or enzyme–substrate interactions. Furthermore, introduction of a premature stop codon can result either in the truncation of the protein, leading to altered protein function, or will cause the induction of nonsense-mediated decay of the mRNA resulting in an absence of the protein (Schell *et al.* 2002). Polymorphisms occurring at or in the vicinity of splice junctions may influence splicing mechanisms therefore leading to the generation or abolition of splice variants. Thus, variants influencing the exons of a gene can influence the amino acid composition of the encoded protein leading to qualitative differences in gene function; the severity of any associated phenotype would be dependent upon the nature of the amino acid change and its location.

Examples of functional coding region polymorphisms associated with thrombosis include the misense mutation in codon 506 (Arg^{506}–Gln) of the factor V Leiden gene (G1691A). This polymorphism is directly associated with resistance to activated protein C (APC) (Zoller and Dahlback 1994), conferring a procoagulant state through prolongation of the action of factor Va. The frequency of the mutation is 2–7 per cent in the general population and it is regarded as the commonest inherited form of venous thrombosis, occurring in 10–40 per cent of cases with venous thromboembolism. Our group (Catto *et al.* 1995) and the prospective US Physicians Study (Ridker *et al.* 1995) found no evidence that G1691A polymorphism is a significant risk factor for arterial thrombosis causing stroke. The α-fibrinogen Thr312Ala polymorphism occurs in close proximity to several sites important for factor XIIIa-dependent cross-linking, which raises the possibility that it affects fibrin clot stability. In a study in stroke subjects (Carter *et al.* 1999), there was a significant interaction between the Thr312Ala polymorphism and atrial fibrillation in relation to post-stroke mortality ($P = 0.002$). The Thr312Ala polymorphism may give rise to an increased susceptibility for embolization of intra-atrial clot.

2.3.2 Non-coding region polymorphisms

Non-coding region polymorphisms can influence gene function if they occur in the promoter and distal 5′ regions of gene regulation, within introns or within the 3′UTR. Regulatory elements, both within the 5′ and 3′ regulatory regions of genes, are involved in the determination of steady-state levels of the corresponding protein. These elements can act to enhance or suppress gene transcription or affect the stability of the transcribed mRNA, and sequence variation within, or in the vicinity of, these regulatory elements may influence steady-state levels of the encoded protein. Polymorphisms occurring within the 5′ gene regulatory region may create or destroy a DNA binding site motif thereby influencing the transcriptional regulation of the gene. Gene regulatory elements have also been shown to exist within intronic and exonic sequences, and polymorphisms within these regions would be expected to have similar consequences. Finally, since the 3′UTR of a gene frequently carries RNA binding protein motifs which influence mRNA processing and stability, polymorphisms occurring within this region of a gene may influence the steady-state levels of mRNA and consequently the amount of protein produced by translation of the mRNA. Therefore polymorphisms in either the 5′ or 3′ gene regulatory regions may give rise to quantitative differences in the encoded protein.

2.4 Phenotype associated with genetic polymorphisms

The phenotypic consequences of polymorphisms will depend upon the severity of the disruption of gene function caused by the polymorphism and represents one of the discriminating factors between mono- and polygenic disorders. Monogenic disorders are, on the whole, more likely to arise as a consequence of a coding mutation, particularly those introducing premature stop codons or those occurring in key functional regions of the translated protein, or a splice site mutation, that is, those resulting in a profound disruption in gene function. Mutations occurring in the vital regulatory regions of the gene, particularly those occurring in the core promoter, may also give rise to drastically reduced protein levels. In contrast, in polygenic disorders the influence of polymorphisms tend to be additive in their effects and as a single entity would be expected to have only a very modest influence on gene function; disease manifests itself as a consequence of the presence of an accumulation of other genetic variants and environmental factors. Therefore in complex polygenic disorders it seems most likely that common variants giving rise to quantitative differences in candidate genes (i.e. those arising in the 5′ and 3′ gene regulatory regions), and coding region polymorphisms giving rise to more conservative amino acid changes, are more likely to influence disease development and progression.

2.5 Information gained from analysis of common polymorphisms

Many of the benefits of SNP maps remain largely speculative at the present time. They may be useful for identifying multiple genes, which make relatively small contributions to the pathogenesis of multifactorial disease. Polymorphisms may also provide a means for better classification of disease subtypes, allow identification of both those most likely to benefit from certain types of therapy and those susceptible to complications of stroke, and give greater understating of the aetiology and pathogenesis of stroke. However, whether they will reliably 'predict' risk of stroke disease is far more speculative. It is plausible that common genetic variants might explain some of the inter-individual variations in the susceptibility to common multifactorial diseases, disease severity and response to therapies and developing novel therapeutic targets. The area of pharmacogenetics is both interesting and exciting and further developments in the field of stroke disease are awaited (McCarthy 2001). In future, monitoring of individual drug response profiles with DNA tests throughout life will be standard practice (Roses 2000).

The clustering of risk factors is to an extent population specific and this explains in part the inconsistent findings of studies looking at single polymorphic variants and their relationship to disease. The methods used to identify the complex genetic contributions are by no means trivial and the presence of gene–environment interactions clearly adds to the complexity in identifying genetic risk factors and the numbers of cases to be included in any study. Study design and strict classification are important features of any clinical study and these are addressed below.

2.6 Study designs used to identify genetic risk factors for stroke

A variety of techniques can be used to investigate the genetic basis of common stroke. These include linkage based techniques, candidate gene association studies, and with the recent mapping of the human genome, genome-wide association studies. These approaches are discussed below.

2.7 Linkage analysis

The application of linkage analysis to complex disorders presents the investigator with the problem that there is seldom any clear pattern of inheritance, enabling the cosegregation of marker and disease loci to be analysed. Stroke disease is characterized by multiple uncertainties. For example, when does high blood pressure become hypertension, the remarkably heterogeneous nature of stroke disease (in marked contradistinction to coronary artery disease), and the variable age of onset. It is taken as a 'given' that stroke is a polygenic disorder and therefore a defined mode of inheritance cannot readily be assigned in tracking marker systems. At present, linkage analysis in multifactorial disorders has to employ simplified procedures. These include sib-pair analysis, random mapping of major genes in subsets with possible Mendelian inheritance or candidate-gene linkage analysis.

2.7.1 Sibling-pair analysis

Sibling (or sib) pair analysis (or affected sib-pair—ASP) is a model-free form of analysis and is being used more frequently to study polygenic disorders, including stroke (Meschia *et al.* 2002). It involves the collection of pairs of siblings who are both affected by the condition of interest (perhaps with an available parent) to confirm 'identical by descent' or IBD. A sib-pair analysis assumes that in the absence of linkage between a marker and disease, there should be equal proportions of siblings in the groups. If the marker is linked to a major locus responsible for at least some part of the disease phenotype, there may be significant deviations from the expected ratios. No assumption is made about the mode of inheritance. In the analysis, proportions of 0, 1, or 2 alleles inherited IBD at each locus are compared to the proportions that would be expected under the null hypothesis of no linkage (0.25, 0.50, and 0.25, respectively). Therefore, if a given locus were to be related to the disorder, we would expect to see ASPs sharing more alleles IBD than would otherwise be expected. This is referred to as a model-free analysis (Farrall 1997). Full genetic models are implicit in all allele sharing models (Whittemore 1996).

There are a number of possible approaches to the analysis of data from ASP studies (Hardwick *et al.* 1997). These can use χ^2 statistics or likelihood methods. The likelihood method can be analysed using computer packages such as MAPMAKER/SIBS (Kruglyak and Lander 1995). Statistical approaches have also been developed to study quantitative traits, for example the method of Haseman and Elston (1972). The ASP approach has been used successfully in the investigation of stroke risk factors. Jeunemaitre *et al.* (1992) conducted an ASP study on two sibships from the USA and France. There was significant linkage between the angiotensinogen gene (Caulfield *et al.* 1994) and hypertension in the French, but not US, sibship.

Whether quantitative or qualitative traits are chosen, the design of the study must take into account the availability and extent of pedigrees. As stroke is a disease of old age there may be insufficient subjects available to study, especially parents, and even fewer subjects in large pedigrees. There is some evidence to suggest that this approach is feasible, and Meschia and colleagues (Meschia *et al.* 2001) have reported that in 310 probands (median age, 75 years; range, 26–97 years; 48% women), 75 per cent had at least 1 living sibling; 10 per cent, at least 1 concordant living sibling; 2 per cent, at least 1 concordant sibling living in the same city; and 7 per cent, at least 1 concordant living and 1 discordant living sibling. Although feasible, such an approach would need to be multicentre. The process could also be simplified by employing a structured telephone interview, and Meschia *et al.* (2000) have validated such a model with a high degree of confidence.

Another important consideration is the power to detect linkage between the susceptibility locus and the marker. A number of factors including marker heterozygosity, sample size, effect size and the distance from marker to susceptibility locus are of importance (Risch 1990).

2.7.2 Linkage-disequilibrium studies

This study design is based on the assumption that a mutation in a founder of the population of interest is still causative for the disease (Kruglyak 1997). In a small region close to the mutation, alleles present in the founder haplotype should be maintained in the same haplotype at meiosis and passed down through succeeding generations and unaffected by recombination. The regions over which allelic association may hold in practice is likely to be small (<2 cM) (Chapman and Wijsman 1998). This is an example of a fine mapping study, in which susceptibility loci are localized to small genomic regions.

2.7.3 Transmission disequilibrium test

A common problem with association studies is population admixture. This can be overcome by employing family-based controls. The haplotype relative risk (HRR) method (Falk and Rubinstein 1987) employs a set of simplex families (two parents plus one affected offspring). A modification of HRR is the transmission disequilibrium test (TDT) (Spielman *et al.* 1993). TDT uses the fact that transmitted and non-transmitted alleles from a given parent are paired observations, so in the case of a biallelic locus it examines preferential transmission of one identifiable allele over the other in all heterozygous parents. TDT probably tests both linkage and allelic association simultaneously (Schaid 1998). This approach has been applied to studies of diabetes (Spielman *et al.* 1993). In stroke patients, any parent control is unlikely to be available, except of course for juvenile stroke, and there is a test to compare affected and unaffected siblings, the sibling TDT (Spielman and Ewens 1998). However, although parent controls avoid overmatching, the use of sibs rather than parent controls is a less powerful test. In common with all linkage studies, TDT will still require substantive populations. For example, with a baseline allele frequency of 0.3, for an odds ratio of 1.50, a sample size of 947 (trios) would be required (Hassan and Markus 2000).

2.7.4 Alternative approaches

Other investigators have studied the heritability of an intermediate phenotype, such as carotid artery intimal medial thickness (IMT), a marker of subclinical atherosclerosis. Lange and colleagues hypothesize that in families with multiple members having diabetes, carotid IMT is likely to be associated with both inherited and environmental factors (Lange *et al.* 2002). The age-, sex-, and race-adjusted heritability estimate for carotid IMT was 0.32 and ethnicity was one of the strongest predictors of IMT. The use of this intermediate phenotype is covered in detail in Chapter 8.

Alternatively, 'model-based' linkage analysis can be applied to multifactorial disorders such as stroke, by fitting a range of different possible inheritance models at any given locus (Greenberg *et al.* 1996). Such an approach has the advantage that the asymptotic probability of a false positive is not increased by using an incorrect model, providing that the parameters of either the disease or marker model are known. Complex segregation analysis is being used to estimate the parameters of the genetic model prior to conducting a linkage analysis (Bonney 1984). The segregation models can then incorporate major gene and polygenic/residual factors. Alternatively, segregation and linkage analysis can be combined into a joint procedure (Bonney *et al.* 1988). This approach was applied to studies of the angiotensin converting enzyme (ACE) gene, ACE levels, and hypertension in Jamaican families (McKenzie *et al.* 1995).

2.7.5 Replication of linkage studies

The criteria by which linkage results will be judged are replication. However, it is important to consider that certain factors are likely to influence the findings. First, ascertainment differences will exist for the populations under study. There is also likely to be genetic heterogeneity between the populations. It is also unlikely that any single study would have sufficient statistical power to detect all of the susceptibility loci involved in a complex trait. Sampling variability is likely to affect the location estimates of contributing loci and it has been shown that such large effects are possible (Roberts *et al.* 1999).

2.7.6 Animal studies

Animal models have been employed to study quantitative trait loci, and have been used to investigate both stroke risk factors such as hypertension and stroke using the stroke-prone rat model. This approach is covered in detail in Chapter 5. Well-established mouse disease models have improved our understanding of the molecular basis of complex disorders. In spite of millions of years of evolutionary separation, there is close homology between many mouse and human gene sequences. Data sets of this mouse–human homology can be found in human and mouse databases and these are becoming even more comprehensive (*www.ncbi.nlm.nih.gov/Homology*; and *www.informatics.jax.org/menus/homology_menu.shtml*). Mouse models are characterized by short generation times and high breeding efficiency. They provide insights into disease gene identification, unequivocal proof that a mutation in that gene causes the disease, and rapid dissection of the molecular pathway in which the mutant protein acts. Positional cloning of a mouse disease gene is relatively straightforward, because of the possibility of controlled breeding and crossing of the mice. Suspected chromosomal regions can be genetically restricted to a section that is small enough to be sequenced, and then the mutated gene within this section can be identified. The mutated gene can be further analysed for functional variations in human study samples (Stoll *et al.* 2000). Transgenic and knockout mutant mice remove some of the difficulties associated with human disease where the genetic background is extremely heterogeneous. For example, transgenic mice have been used to study the contribution of nitric oxide to experimental ischaemic brain injury *in vivo* (Sampei *et al.* 2000). There is increasing use of *in vivo* gene transfer. For example, adenovirus-mediated gene transfer in hyperlipidaemic rabbits (Lund *et al.* 1999). It is plausible that in the future, gene transfer to the ischaemic brain may be a treatment for the ischaemic penumbra (Ooboshi *et al.* 2001).

2.8 **The candidate gene approach**

The application of techniques such as positional cloning has proved effective in identifying genes associated with simple (Mendelian) disorders. However each gene has only a small overall contribution to the phenotype and therefore is of low relative risk. These factors have resulted in researchers seeking other approaches to identifying genes implicated in complex disorders such as stroke. The majority of stroke genetic studies have employed the candidate gene approach. Candidate gene studies are in some respects limited, as they require an existing hypothesis or more substantive evidence linking the variant with a plausible pathological process in stroke pathogenesis.

Certain epidemiological criteria should be satisfied for gene association studies. Specifically, there must be biological plausibility of association. The investigator will be interested in establishing whether or not the candidate gene is likely to be involved in the outward stroke phenotype. It is also important to establish whether or not the polymorphism is likely to have any functional effects on the protein. Second, the strength of association between the risk factor and stroke disease is examined. When considering multiple SNPs in a candidate gene, those with the strongest association are most likely to be causally related. Third, there should be evidence of a dose–response relationship between possession of alleles and expression of the disease. Individuals with two copies of a variant might be at greater risk of disease than individuals with one copy of the variant. Fourth, there should be some historical consistency of association across previous and future studies. A frequently quoted example in stroke genetics is the relationship between the ACE insertion/deletion variant and risk of ischaemic stroke. In the mid-1990s there was a host of studies showing evidence both for (Markus *et al.* 1995) and against (Catto *et al.* 1996) risk of stroke with the I/D polymorphism. This particular variant was the subject of a meta-analysis by Sharma (1998), which found a weak relationship with risk of stroke. However, consistent replication across populations is a strong evidence of an association, although not necessarily causality. It is also important to recognize that a positive association does not imply a true causality but may simply indicate linkage disequilibrium resulting from close proximity to the locus under study and an undiscovered stroke susceptibility locus. For example, the recently described ACE/H homologue of ACE (Turner *et al.* 2002).

Lack of replication in itself does not refute association or causality, but might point to the need for more studies in certain populations, or more detailed study of a particular gene. There are also statistical considerations, as multiple sample tests will produce a positive result by chance for one in every 20 tests, and multiple comparison statistics should be used. For example, for a 10-marker system a *P*-value 0.005 is required for statistical significance, if a Bonferroni correction is applied. The difficulty with all association studies is how to interpret the data. Very few associations of sufficient magnitude have been discovered that are of practical value in risk estimation, although HLA-B27 allele is a good example of a stronger association, as individuals with this allele are about 100 times more likely to develop ankylosing spondylitis. Further information on the epidemiologic aspects of gene association studies may be found elsewhere (Ioannidis *et al.* 2001).

2.8.1 What are the problems with the candidate gene approach?

Certain variants have been fairly consistently associated with risk of stroke, such as in the fibrinogen gene (Carter *et al.* 1997). However non replication has been frequently observed in stroke–gene association studies. For example, the ACE I/D polymorphism (as referred to above), or the PAI-1 4G/5G promoter polymorphism (Catto *et al.* 1997, Margaglione *et al.* 1997). There is also evidence to suggest that the first study to report an association often indicates a stronger effect than subsequent studies (Ioannidis *et al.* 2001). Any lack of reproducibility may be due to study design and interpretation of the results. This is crucial in stroke genetics, where accurate phenotyping of the various subtypes of ischaemic and haemorrhagic stroke present particular research challenges. There is a multiplicity of clinical classifications (see Section 1.3) and no clear agreement exists as to what represents the gold standard. Classifications include TOAST (Adams *et al.* 1993), and the Oxfordshire Community Stroke Project (Bamford *et al.* 1991). This is at the heart of stroke genetic studies.

Marker systems may show dramatic differences in allele frequencies in closely related subpopulations. However, it is of equal importance to ensure close matching of stroke cases and controls, paying attention to matching for age, gender, socioeconomic class, domicile and risk factors. Additionally, mutation rates at both the marker locus and hypothetical disease susceptibility locus should be relatively low, as a genuine disease–gene association may be obscured. It should be remembered that differences in population substructure can induce spurious associations between gene and disease. This is a complex area and various statistical techniques such as genomic control or structured association can be used to control for population effects. This has been comprehensively reviewed by Devlin (2001).

There are multiple candidate genes for stroke and it is beyond the scope of this chapter to consider them all. However, they can broadly be considered in terms of their possible pathogenic effect. For example, candidate genes might contribute to those processes implicated in the development of stroke, for example, ischaemic heart disease (Luscher and Noll 1999), diabetes mellitus and atrial fibrillation (Brugada and Roberts 1999), and those that might influence the outcome following occlusion such as haemostatic factors (Catto 2001) or free radicals. However, it is highly likely that certain genes have an effect on both processes, for example, the renin–angiotensin system (Carluccio *et al.* 2001). Other processes for consideration include lipid (Vaughan and Delanty 1999), and homocysteine metabolism (Meiklejohn *et al.* 2001), and endothelial nitric oxide (Markus *et al.* 1998). The results of candidate gene studies of these systems in ischaemic stroke are discussed in Chapter 7. Given the complexity of stroke pathogenesis, the investigator will be required to consider the effect of a given candid-ate gene within the subtypes of ischaemic stroke. It is important not to neglect younger adults and children with stroke, as genetic processes are less likely to be the result of atherothromboembolism. For example, factor V Leiden is not a risk factor for stroke in older adults, but has been associated with juvenile stroke (Kenet *et al.* 2000).

Candidate gene studies are likely to continue informing knowledge of stroke genetics, but more attention will be needed in terms of phenotyping, improved match-ing of cases to controls and possibly younger subjects, where genetics may be playing a greater role. There may also be a role for prospective studies, and the collaborative United Kingdom BIOBANK study (a £48 million Department of Health, Medical Research Council and Wellcome Trust initiative) will aim to recruit 500,000 middle-aged volunteers, who will provide information about their diet and life-style, their medical history and a DNA sample. It is estimated that approximately 5000 strokes will occur in the life of the study, and this will provide insights into gene–environment interactions in the development of stroke (*http://www.wellcome.ac.uk/ en/1/ biovenpopfaq.html*).

2.9 **Human genome mapping project**

Two reports in February 2001 heralded the publication of the human genome mapping project (Lander *et al.* 2001, Venter *et al.* 2001). The project was undertaken by both the publicly funded National Institute for Health, and Celera, a company. Sequencing the three billion base pairs of the human genome required unique molecu-lar approaches. Celera conducted high-throughput sequencing (175,000 reads per day). By contrast, the Human Genome Project (HGP) divided the sequencing task among several large laboratories, subcloning the human genome into bacterial artifi-cial chromosomes, which were sequenced and arranged. Celera used 'shotgun' whole genome approach to sequencing, which involved generating small, random fragments of DNA for sequencing. For both projects, the genome was sequenced approximately five times to minimize errors and eliminate gaps in the final map. The completed map revealed that just 1.1 per cent of the genome coded for exons, 24 per cent is intronic, and 75 per cent is intergenic DNA. The average human gene spans 27,000 to 29,000 bases of DNA and consists of 7–9 exons. The mean coding sequence for a human gene is 1340 base pairs. Contrary to expectation, the human genome has between 26,500 and 39,000 genes, compared to about 13,000 genes in the fly. It does not follow that a relatively small number of genes will code for a small number of proteins. A single gene can undergo alternative splicing; messenger RNA has an average of 2.6–3.2 distinct transcripts per gene. Post-translational modifications of proteins can also change their function and activity.

In addition to identifying the genes, the physical map of the genome identified genetic markers throughout the genome (McPherson *et al.* 2001), the commonest of which is the SNP. The project identified approximately 2.1 million SNPs (Sachidanandam *et al.* 2001). These markers allow genetic linkage studies to be performed. A map with accurately mapped numerous markers will allow disease causing genes to be located to high precision. Genes that are close to the linked markers may provide clues for possible stroke candidate genes.

It is recognized that linkage analysis of complex disorders has yielded relatively little scientific gain. However, by identifying/scoring sequence variation there are a greater number of polymorphisms to study. Association studies could therefore be extended to include a systematic search through the entire human genome for single-nucleotide polymorphisms in linkage disequilibrium with a disease-causing allele (Risch and Merikangas 1996). A genome-wide association studies is likely to be more powerful than a whole-genome linkage study in detecting variants with small effects on disease risk. It is important to ensure that this resource is catalogued (Peltonen and McKusick 2001), for example, the use of SNPs from expressed sequence tags (ESTs). However, the concept of EST is not new, being first described in 1991 (Adams *et al.* 1991), although at that time it was thought that EST might be an alternative to genomic sequencing. It is hoped that future approaches arising from EST research might include differential display, random sequencing of subtracted and normalized cDNA libraries, and the use of microassay technologies (Hassan and Markus 2000). There is some evidence to suggest the benefits of this approach (Wang *et al.* 1998).

There is an abundance of internet-based resources and the reader is referred to sites for the EST database (*www.ncbi.nlm.nih.gov/dbEST/index.html*) and physical positions of the ESTs (*www.ncbi.nlm.nih.gov/genemap98*) and catalogues of sequence variation (*http://www.ncbi.nlm.nih.gov/SNP*). Other SNP databases are available (*http://snp.cshl.org/ and http://hgvbase.cgb.ki.se/*). Information regarding genetic loci can also be found at *http://www.ncbi.nlm.nih.gov/LocusLink/*. The ENSEMBL genome browser produces and maintains automatic annotation on eukaryotic genomes. ENSEMBL presents up-to-date sequence data and the best possible automatic annotation for eukaryotic genomes. For more information see *http://www.ensembl.org/*. The reader is referred to the OMIM, Online Mendelian Inheritance in Man. This NIH database is a catalogue of human genes and genetic disorders see *http://www.ncbi.nlm.nih.gov/Omim/*.

In time, the human genome project will provide us with a clearer understanding of those genes involved in the aetiology and pathogenesis of stroke. This should provide insights into protein function in novel and established metabolic pathways (Peltonen and McKusick 2001).

2.10 Genome-wide screening and gene transcript variations

Differential gene expression in cells and tissues has been revolutionized by oligo-nucleotide and cDNA microarrays. This has been applied to studies of cancer. Microarray techniques are sensitive enough to detect expression of a target gene among

50,000–300,000 transcripts (Lockhart and Winzeler 2000). It is probable that the transcription rate of virtually every gene from even modest amounts of tissue will be possible. Array techniques are under development to analyse protein and protein variants (Pandey and Mann 2000). The reader is also referred to Section 2.12.3 on microarrays in mutation detection.

Genome-wide profiling of gene transcription in tissue from patients has been used in the study of leukaemic disorders (Golub *et al.* 1999). However, there is a relative paucity of information concerning intra- and individual variations in gene expression, and profiling human traits presents considerable difficulties. Changes in transcription profiles with progression through the cell cycle and during tissue differentiation, as well as variations in expression profiles between individuals, create background noise. This disturbs the detection of 'real' signals signifying actual disease-related changes in gene expression.

2.11 Novel metabolic disease pathways

The majority of publications reporting genetic studies of complex diseases investigate candidate genes and known metabolic pathways. The major problem with any strategy for analysing a candidate gene or metabolic pathway is that we tend to study known candidates, and overlook other essential genes or pathways. Furthermore, only a fraction of protein networks have been identified and characterized through classical and structural biochemistry, and activity assays. A knowledge of the human genome should ultimately lead to the identification of all human metabolic pathways, irrespective of protein half-life. Biocomputing-based strategies are currently under development to construct genetic, and ultimately protein, networks (Eisenberg *et al.* 2000). This is employing technologies such as biocomputing-based motif searches and expression microarrays. Expression microarrays directly examine gene co-regulation under a variety of experimental conditions. The importance of animal models in this process should not be overlooked. For example, similar strategies have been applied to the study of the *Drosophila* insulin-signalling pathway (Bohni *et al.* 1999), with implications for insulin pathways in humans.

2.12 Methods for the identification of common polymorphic variants

Over the decades the methods available for identifying genetic variants have become more and more sophisticated. Initially, variants giving rise to a functional difference in the encoded protein could be detected by differences in electrophoretic analysis, which only provided information on molecular weight or charge. Subsequently, the identification of restriction fragment length polymorphisms (RFLP), where a polymorphism creates or destroys a recognition sequence for a restriction endonuclease, could be identified by Southern blotting. The dawn of the polymerase chain reaction (PCR) and dideoxysequencing revolutionized the field of molecular biology, providing a powerful tool for analysis of the human genome. Initially, PCR was used to detect VNTRs, insertions/deletions, SSRs, and provided a convenient method for RFLP analysis of gene fragments. Although dideoxysequencing is a high fidelity method for the detection of novel polymorphisms it is highly time consuming and can be problematic in identifying heterozygotes; therefore with the development of more sophisticated molecular biology techniques, a wide variety of methods are now employed for the detection of novel polymorphisms within genes of interest (Dianzani *et al.* 1993, Cotton 1997). A brief summary of the principles of each of these techniques follows.

2.12.1 **Single-strand conformational polymorphism**

Single-strand conformational polymorphism (SSCP) analysis is a relatively simple method of polymorphism detection (Fig. 2.1), which relies on the fact that, under non-denaturing conditions, single-stranded DNA has a folded structure, due to the formation of intra-strand interactions, which is highly sequence specific (Orita *et al.* 1989). The

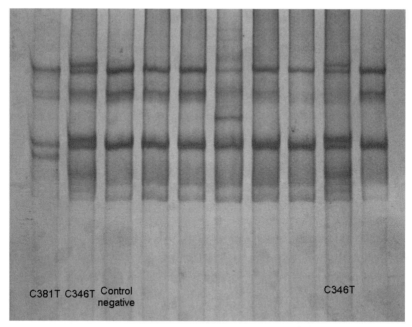

C381T C346T Control negative   C346T

Fig. 2.1 Single-strand conformational polymorphism. In this example exon 3 of the notch 3 gene (responsible for CADASIL) has been run. A normal control and three CADASIL cases with causative mutations are shown. Additional bands may be caused by causative mutations or polymorphisms, and differentiation between these requires DNA sequencing (courtesy of Kelly Gormley, St George's Hospital Medical School, London, UK, Copyright with Hugh Markus).

mobility of single-strands through a polyacrylamide gel matrix under non-denaturing conditions is dependent upon conformation and, therefore, any sequence variation within a particular region may be detected as a difference in band mobility (Orita *et al.* 1989). In order to increase the sensitivity of this method for detecting polymorphisms, several conditions are used, including different temperatures and gel compositions (Orita *et al.* 1989, Hayashi 1992, Hayashi and Yandell 1993). Although this is a relatively simple method of polymorphism detection and has the advantage that no expensive equipment is required, it has the disadvantage that its sensitivity decreases with increasing fragment size. It is therefore effective only for fragments of less than approximately 250 bp which makes it a rather time-consuming method for screening large regions (Hayashi and Yandell 1993).

2.12.2 Heteroduplex analysis

A heteroduplex is a double stranded DNA fragment which demonstrates incomplete complimentarity of bases. Heteroduplex analysis of candidate genes for polygenic disorders relies on the detection of polymorphisms in samples which are heterozygous for unknown sequence variants. The heteroduplexes are formed by denaturing PCR products by heating and then slowly cooling which promotes the annealing of the mismatched strands. There are a number of methods for detecting mismatches, including denaturing gradient gel electrophoresies (DGGE) (Myers *et al.* 1987), enzymatic cleavage mismatch detection (Youil *et al.* 1995, Deeble *et al.* 1997), chemical cleavage mismatch detection (Dianzani *et al.* 1991, Deeble *et al.* 1997) and temperature modulated heteroduplex analysis (TMHA) (Skopek *et al.* 1999, Cooksey *et al.* 2002). These methods are effective in the identification of novel polymorphisms, and although they confer the advantage of sensitivity they are still disadvantaged by being time consuming techniques for high-throughput screening of genes.

A recent advance in TMHA is denaturing high-performance liquid chromatography (dHPLC); this method combines temperature dependent denaturation of heteroduplexes with ion-paired reversed phase chromatography. Two automated systems designed specifically for dHPLC are currently available: the WAVE® from Transgenomic (Fig. 2.2) and the Helix™ from Varian (Klein *et al.* 2001). DNA is bound to a hydrophobic column by triethylammonium acetate and eluted from the column with an increasing gradient of acetonitrile at elevated temperatures; the retention time is dependent upon the melting characteristics of the DNA fragment (Cooksey *et al.* 2002). The technique is based on the principal that heteroduplexes have a lower melting temperature than corresponding homoduplexes and consequently denature at a lower concentration of acetonitrile; therefore, the presence of a polymorphism can be identified by a reduced retention time, leading to multiple elution peaks. The advantage of this method is that it is a high-throughput and sensitive means of detecting unknown polymorphisms, the main disadvantage being the cost of the dHPLC system.

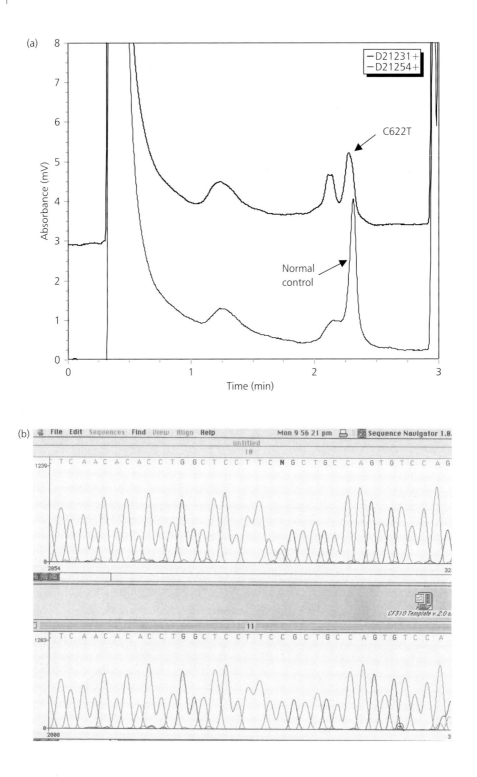

Fig. 2.2 (a) WAVE® heteroduplex analysis. This automated method combines temperature dependent denaturation of heteroduplexes with ion-paired reversed phase chromatography. DNA is bound to a hydrophobic column by triethylammonium acetate and eluted from the column with an increasing gradient of acetonitrile at elevated temperatures; the retention time is dependent upon the melting characteristics of the DNA fragment. The technique is based on the principal that heteroduplexes have a lower melting temperature than corresponding homoduplexes and consequently denature at a lower concentration of acetonitrile; therefore, the presence of a polymorphism can be identified by a reduced retention time, leading to multiple elution peaks. This tracing shows an example from a normal control and a patient with a C622T notch 3 exon 4 mutation. An additional peak can be seen in the CADASIL trace. The next stage is to sequence the PCR produce to confirm the mutation (see b). (b) Automated DNA sequencing using fluorescent primers from the same two samples. The CADASIL sample is shown in the upper trace and the control in the lower trace. Four different fluorescent dyes are used as labels for the base specific reactions. During the electrophoresis run, a laser beam is focused at a fixed position on the gel. As the DNA fragments pass this position the laser causes the dyes to fluoresce. Maximum fluorescence occurs at different wavelengths for the four dyes, and the information is recorded directly. onto a computer. It is presented as a series of dye-specific and (therefore base-specific) intensity profiles. In this example, indicated by 'N', a C is replaced by a T in the CADASIL patient (both images courtesy of Andrea Haworth, St George's Hospital Medical School, London, UK, Copyright with Hugh Markus).

2.12.3 DNA microarrays in mutation detection

A microarray is a tool for analysing gene expression that consists of a small membrane or glass slide containing samples of many genes arranged in a regular pattern. A microarray works by exploiting the ability of a given mRNA molecule to bind specifically to, or hybridize to, the DNA template from which it originated. By using an array containing many DNA samples, scientists can determine, in a single experiment, the expression levels of hundreds or thousands of genes within a cell by measuring the amount of mRNA bound to each site on the array. With the aid of a computer, the amount of mRNA bound to the spots on the microarray is precisely measured, generating a profile of gene expression in the cell. Microarrays are a significant advance both because they may contain a very large number of genes and because of their small size. Microarrays are therefore useful when one wants to survey a large number of genes quickly or when the sample to be studied is small. When researchers use microarrays to detect mutations or polymorphisms in a gene sequence, the target, or immobilized DNA, is usually that of a single gene. In this case, the target sequence placed on any given spot within the array will differ from that of other spots in the same microarray, sometimes by only one or a few specific nucleotides. This analysis allows the inclusion of SNPs. Another difference in mutation microarray analysis, as compared to expression or Comparative Genomic Hybridization microarrays, is that this type of experiment only requires genomic DNA derived from a normal sample for use in the hybridization mixture.

Once researchers have established that a SNP pattern is associated with a particular disease, they can use SNP microarray technology to test an individual for that disease expression pattern in order to determine if he or she is susceptible to, or at risk of developing, a particular disease. When genomic DNA from an individual is hybridized to an array loaded with various SNPs, the sample DNA will hybridize with greater frequency only to specific SNPs associated with that person. Those spots on the microarray will then fluoresce with greater intensity, demonstrating that the individual being tested may have, or is at risk for developing, that disease.

2.13 Conclusion

Studies of stroke genetics pose a major scientific challenge. There is good evidence from epidemiology, twin and animal studies to suggest a role for genetics in the pathogenesis of stroke. A raft of novel molecular biology technologies and bioinformatics will continue to improve our understanding of the genetics of stroke. However, even with the best molecular techniques, particular care is needed to ensure the high quality phenotyping, particularly in the subgroups of ischaemic stroke. It is unclear at this stage the precise benefits that will derive from an improved knowledge of stroke genetics, although genetic factors are likely to influence disease severity and outcome in terms of residual defect or mortality. Genetics may help define the different subtypes of stroke, which would assist in the design of new therapeutics targeted to specific subtypes of ischaemic stroke.

References

Adams, H.P., Jr., Bendixen, B.H., Kappelle, L.J., *et al.* (1993). Classification of subtype of acute ischemic stroke. Definitions for use in a multicenter clinical trial. TOAST. Trial of Org 10172 in Acute Stroke Treatment. *Stroke*, 24, 35–41.

Adams, M.D., Kelley, J.M., Gocayne, J.D., *et al.* (1991). Complementary DNA sequencing: expressed sequence tags and human genome project. *Science*, 252, 1651–6.

Bamford, J., Sandercock, P., Dennis, M., Burn, J., and Warlow, C. (1991). Classification and natural history of clinically identifiable subtypes of cerebral infarction. *Lancet*, 337, 1521–6.

Bohni, R., Riesgo-Escovar, J., Oldham, S., *et al.* (1999). Autonomous control of cell and organ size by CHICO, a Drosophila homolog of vertebrate IRS1-4. *Cell*, 97, 865–75.

Bonney, G.E. (1984). On the statistical determination of major gene mechanisms in continuous human traits: regressive models. *American Journal of Medical Genetics*, 18, 731–49.

Bonney, G.E., Lathrop, G.M., and Lalouel, J.M. (1988). Combined linkage and segregation analysis using regressive models. *American Journal of Human Genetics*, 43, 29–37.

Brugada, R. and Roberts, R. (1999). Molecular biology and atrial fibrillation. *Current Opinion Cardiology*, 14, 269–73.

Carluccio, M., Soccio, M., and De Caterina, R. (2001). Aspects of gene polymorphisms in cardiovascular disease: the renin–angiotensin system. *European Journal of Clinical Investigation*, 31, 476–88.

Carter, A.M., Catto, A.J., Bamford, J.M., and Grant, P.J. (1997). Gender-specific associations of the fibrinogen B beta 448 polymorphism, fibrinogen levels, and acute cerebrovascular disease. *Arteriosclerosis Thrombosis and Vascular Biology*, 17, 589–94.

Carter, A.M., Catto, A.J., and Grant, P.J. (1999). Association of the alpha-fibrinogen Thr312Ala polymorphism with poststroke mortality in subjects with atrial fibrillation. *Circulation*, **99**, 2423–6.

Catto, A.J. (2001). Genetic aspects of the hemostatic system in cerebrovascular disease. *Neurology*, **57**(5 Suppl. 2), S24–S30.

Catto, A.J., Carter, A.M., Barrett, J., *et al.* (1996). Angiotensin converting enzyme insertion/deletion polymorphism and cerebrovascular disease. *Stroke*, **27**, 435–40.

Catto, A.J., Carter, A.M., Ireland, H., *et al.* (1995). Factor V Leiden gene mutation and thrombin generation in relation to the development of acute stroke. *Arteriosclerosis, Thrombosis, and Vascular Biology*, **15**, 783–5.

Catto, A.J., Carter, A.M., Barrett, J.H., *et al.* (1997). Plasminogen activator inhibitor-1 (PAI-1), 4G/5G promoter polymorphism and levels in subjects with cerebrovascular disease. *Thrombosis and Haemostasis*, **77**, 730–4.

Caulfield, M., Lavender, P., Farrall, M., *et al.* (1994). Linkage of the angiotensinogen gene to essential hypertension. *New England Journal of Medicine*, **330**, 1629–33.

Chapman, N.H. and Wijsman, E.M. (1998). Genome screens using linkage disequilibrium tests: optimal marker characteristics and feasibility. *American Journal of Human Genetics*, **63**, 1872–85.

Cooksey, R.C., Morlock, G.P., Holloway, B.P., Limor, J., and Hepburn, M. (2002). Temperature-mediated heteroduplex analysis performed by using denaturing high-performance liquid chromatography to identify sequence polymorphisms in Mycobacterium tuberculosis complex organisms. *Journal of Clinical Microbiology*, **40**, 1610–16.

Cotton, R.G. (1997). Slowly but surely towards better scanning for mutations. *Trends in Genetics*, **13**, 43–6.

Deeble, V.J., Roberts, E., Robinson, M.D., Woods, C.G., Bishop, D.T., and Taylor, G.R. (1997). Comparison of enzyme mismatch cleavage and chemical cleavage of mismatch on a defined set of heteroduplexes. *Genetic Testing*, **1**, 253–9.

Devlin, B., Roeder, K., and Bacanu, S.A. (2001). Unbiased methods for population-based association studies. *Genetic Epidemiology*, **21**, 273–84.

Dianzani, I., Camaschella, C., Ponzone, A., and Cotton, R.G. (1993). Dilemmas and progress in mutation detection. *Trends in Genetics*, **9**, 403–5.

Dianzani, I., Forrest, S.M., Camaschella, C., Gottardi, E., and Cotton, R.G. (1991). Heterozygotes and homozygotes: discrimination by chemical cleavage of mismatch. *American Journal of Human Genetics*, **48**, 423–4.

Eisenberg, D., Marcotte, E.M., Xenarios, I., and Yeates, T.O. (2000). Protein function in the post-genomic era. *Nature*, **405**, 823–6.

Falk, C.T. and Rubinstein, P. (1987). Haplotype relative risks: an easy reliable way to construct a proper control sample for risk calculations. *Annals of Human Genetics*, **51**, 227–33.

Farrall, M. (1997). LOD wars: the affected-sib-pair paradigm strikes back! *American Journal of Human Genetics*, **60**, 735–8.

Golub, T.R., Slonim, D.K., Tamayo, P., *et al.* (1999). Molecular classification of cancer: class discovery and class prediction by gene expression monitoring. *Science*, **286**, 531–7.

Greenberg, D.A., Hodge, S.E., Vieland, V.J., and Spence, M.A. (1996). Affecteds-only linkage methods are not a panacea. *American Journal of Human Genetics*, **58**, 892–5.

Hardwick, L.J., Walsh, S., Butcher, S., *et al.* (1997). Genetic mapping of susceptibility loci in the genes involved in rheumatoid arthritis. *Journal of Rheumatology*, **24**, 197–8.

Haseman, J.K. and Elston, R.C. (1972). The investigation of linkage between a quantitative trait and a marker locus. *Behavioural Genetics*, **2**, 3–19.

Hassan, A. and Markus, H.S. (2000). Genetics and ischaemic stroke. *Brain*, **123**, 1784–812.

Hayashi, K. (1992). PCR-SSCP: a method for detection of mutations. *Genetic Analysis, Techniques and Applications*, 9, 73–9.

Hayashi, K. and Yandell, D.W. (1993). How sensitive is PCR-SSCP? *Human Mutation*, 2, 338–46.

Ioannidis, J.P., Ntzani, E.E., Trikalinos, T.A., and Contopoulos-Ioannidis, D.G. (2001). Replication validity of genetic association studies. *Nature Genetics*, 29, 306–9.

Jeunemaitre, X., Soubrier, F., Kotelevtsev, Y.V., *et al.* (1992). Molecular basis of human hypertension: role of angiotensinogen. *Cell*, 71, 169–80.

Kenet, G., Sadetzki, S., Murad, H., *et al.* (2000). Factor V Leiden and antiphospholipid antibodies are significant risk factors for ischemic stroke in children. *Stroke*, 31, 1283–8.

Klein, B., Weirich, G., and Brauch, H. (2001). DHPLC-based germline mutation screening in the analysis of the VHL tumor suppressor gene: usefulness and limitations. *Human Genetics*, 108, 376–84.

Kruglyak, L. (1997). What is significant in whole-genome linkage disequilibrium studies? *American Journal of Human Genetics*, 61, 810–12.

Kruglyak, L. and Lander, E.S. (1995). Complete multipoint sib-pair analysis of qualitative and quantitative traits. *American Journal of Human Genetics*, 57, 439–54.

Lander, E.S., Linton, L.M., Birren, B., *et al.* (2001). Initial sequencing and analysis of the human genome. *Nature*, 409, 860–921.

Lange, L.A., Bowden, D.W., Langefeld, C.D., *et al.* (2002). Heritability of carotid artery intima-medial thickness in type 2 diabetes. *Stroke*, 33, 1876–81.

Lockhart, D.J. and Winzeler, E.A. (2000). Genomics, gene expression and DNA arrays. *Nature*, 405, 827–36.

Lund, D.D., Faraci, F.M., Ooboshi, H., Davidson, B.L., and Heistad, D.D. (1999). Adenovirus-mediated gene transfer is augmented in basilar and carotid arteries of heritable hyperlipidemic rabbits. *Stroke*, 30, 120–5.

Luscher, T.F. and Noll, G. (1999). Is it all in the genes . . . ? Nitric oxide synthase and coronary vasospasm. *Circulation*, 99, 2855–7.

Margaglione, M., Grandone, E., Vecchione, G., *et al.* (1997). Plasminogen activator inhibitor-1 5G/5G genotype are associated with a lower occurrence of ischemic stroke. *Thrombosis and Haemostasis*, 78(Suppl. 1), 102.

Markus, H.S., Barley, J., Lunt, R., *et al.* (1995). Angiotensin-converting enzyme gene deletion polymorphism. A new risk factor for lacunar stroke but not carotid atheroma. *Stroke*, 26, 1329–33.

Markus, H.S., Ruigrok, Y., Ali, N., and Powell, J.F. (1998). Endothelial nitric oxide synthase exon 7 polymorphism, ischemic cerebrovascular disease, and carotid atheroma. *Stroke*, 29, 1908–11.

McCarthy, A. (2001). Pharmacogenetics. *British Medical Journal*, 322, 1007–8.

McKenzie, C.A., Julier, C., Forrester, T., *et al.* (1995). Segregation and linkage analysis of serum angiotensin I-converting enzyme levels: evidence for two quantitative-trait loci. *American Journal of Human Genetics*, 57, 1426–35.

McPherson, J.D., Marra, M., Hillier, L., *et al.* (2001). A physical map of the human genome. *Nature*, 409, 934–41.

Meiklejohn, D.J., Vickers, M.A., Dijkhuisen, R., and Greaves, M. (2001). Plasma homocysteine concentrations in the acute and convalescent periods of atherothrombotic stroke. *Stroke*, 32, 57–62.

Meschia, J.F., Brott, T.G., Chukwudelunzu, F.E., *et al.* (2000). Verifying the stroke-free phenotype by structured telephone interview. *Stroke*, 31, 1076–80.

Meschia, J.F., Brown, R.D., Jr., Brott, T.G., *et al.* (2001). Feasibility of an affected sibling pair study in ischemic stroke: results of a 2-center family history registry. *Stroke*, 32, 2939–41.

Meschia, J.F., Brown, R.D. Jr., Brott, T.G., Chukwudelunzu, F.E., Hardy, J., and Rich, S.S. (2002). The Siblings With Ischemic Stroke Study (SWISS) Protocol. *BioMed Central Medical Genetics*, 3, 1.

Myers, R.M., Maniatis, T., and Lerman, L.S. (1987). Detection and localization of single base changes by denaturing gradient gel electrophoresis. *Methods in Enzymology,* 155, 501–27.

Ooboshi, H., Ibayashi, S., Takada, J., *et al.* (2001). Adenovirus-mediated gene transfer to ischemic brain: ischemic flow threshold for transgene expression. *Stroke*, 32, 1043–7.

Orita, M., Iwahana, H., Kanazawa, H., Hayashi, K., and Sekiya, T. (1989). Detection of polymorphisms of human DNA by gel electrophoresis as single-strand conformation polymorphisms. *Proceedings of the National Academy of Science USA*, 86, 2766–70.

Pandey, A. and Mann, M. (2000). Proteomics to study genes and genomes. *Nature*, 405, 837–46.

Peltonen, L. and McKusick, V.A. (2001). Genomics and medicine. Dissecting human disease in the postgenomic era. *Science*, 291, 1224–9.

Ridker, P.M., Hennekens, C.H., Lindpaintner, K., *et al.* (1995). Mutation in the gene coding for coagulation factor V and the risk of myocardial infarction, stroke, and venous thrombosis in apparently healthy men. *New England Journal of Medicine*, 332, 912–17.

Risch, N. (1990). Linkage strategies for genetically complex traits. II. The power of affected relative pairs. *American Journal of Human Genetics*, 46, 229–41.

Risch, N. and Merikangas, K. (1996). The future of genetic studies of complex human diseases. *Science*, 273, 1516–17.

Roberts, S.B., MacLean, C.J., Neale, M.C., Eaves, L.J., and Kendler, K.S. (1999). Replication of linkage studies of complex traits: an examination of variation in location estimates. *American Journal of Human Genetics*, 65, 876–84.

Roses, A.D. (2000). Pharmacogenetics and the practice of medicine. *Nature*, 405, 857–65.

Sachidanandam, R., Weissman, D., Schmidt, S.C., *et al.* (2001). A map of human genome sequence variation containing 1.42 million single nucleotide polymorphisms. *Nature*, 409, 928–33.

Sampei, K., Mandir, A.S., Asano, Y., *et al.* (2000). Stroke outcome in double-mutant antioxidant transgenic mice. *Stroke*, 31, 2685–91.

Schaid, D.J. (1998). Transmission disequilibrium, family controls, and great expectations. *American Journal of Human Genetics*, 63, 935–41.

Schell, T., Kulozik, A.E., and Hentze, M.W. (2002). Integration of splicing, transport and translation to achieve mRNA quality control by the nonsense-mediated decay pathway. *Genome Biology*, 3, 1006 (Reviews).

Sharma, P. (1998). Meta-analysis of the ACE gene in ischaemic stroke. *Journal of Neurology Neurosurgery Psychiatry*, 64, 227–30.

Skopek, T.R., Glaab, W.E., Monroe, J.J., Kort, K.L., and Schaefer, W. (1999). Analysis of sequence alterations in a defined DNA region: comparison of temperature-modulated heteroduplex analysis and denaturing gradient gel electrophoresis. *Mutation Research*, 430, 13–21.

Spielman, R.S. and Ewens, W.J. (1998). A sibship test for linkage in the presence of association: the sib transmission/disequilibrium test. *American Journal of Human Genetics*, 62, 450–8.

Spielman, R.S., McGinnis, R.E., and Ewens, W.J. (1993). Transmission test for linkage disequilibrium: the insulin gene region and insulin-dependent diabetes mellitus (IDDM). *American Journal of Human Genetics*, 52, 506–16.

Strachan, T. and Read, A.P. (1999). *Human Molecular Genetics 2*, 2nd edn. BIOS Scientific Publishers, Oxford, UK.

Stoll, M., Kwitek-Black, A.E., Cowley, A.W., *et al.* (2000). New target regions for human hypertension via comparative genomics. *Genome Research*, 10, 473–82.

Turner, A.J., Tipnis, S.R., Guy, J.L., Rice, G., and Hooper, N.M. (2002). ACEH/ACE2 is a novel mammalian metallocarboxypeptidase and a homologue of angiotensin-converting enzyme insensitive to ACE inhibitors. *Canadian Journal of Physiology and Pharmacology*, **80**, 346–53.

Vaughan, C.J. and Delanty, N. (1999). Neuroprotective properties of statins in cerebral ischemia and stroke. *Stroke*, **30**, 1969–73.

Venter, J.C., Adams, M.D., Myers, E.W., *et al.* (2001). The sequence of the human genome. *Science*, **291**, 1304–51.

Wang, X., Barone, F.C., White, R.F., and Feuerstein, G.Z. (1998). Subtractive cloning identifies tissue inhibitor of matrix metalloproteinase-1 (TIMP-1) increased gene expression following focal stroke. *Stroke*, **29**, 516–20.

Whittemore, A.S. (1996). Genome scanning for linkage: an overview. *American Journal of Human Genetics*, **59**, 704–16.

Youil, R., Kemper, B.W., and Cotton, R.G. (1995). Screening for mutations by enzyme mismatch cleavage with T4 endonuclease VII. *Proceedings of the National Academy of Science USA*, **92**, 87–91.

Zoller, B. and Dahlback, B. (1994). Linkage between inherited resistance to activated protein C resistance and factor V mutation in venous thrombosis. *Lancet*, **343**, 1536–8.

Chapter 3

Genetic epidemiology of stroke

James F. Meschia and Robert D. Brown, Jr.

Stroke is rarely a manifestation of a single gene disorder. Much more commonly it is a multifactorial disease, but increasing evidence suggest that genetic predisposition is also important for this apparently 'sporadic' stroke. This chapter reviews this evidence, both for stroke in general and for particular subtypes of stroke, particularly ischaemic stroke subtypes and subarachnoid haemorrhage due to intracranial aneurysms.

3.1 Evidence for a genetic predisposition to multifactorial stroke

Evidence from both twin and family history studies, although not always entirely consistent, supports the role of genetic predisposition as a risk factor for stroke.

3.1.1 Twins studies of stroke

A surprisingly small number of twins studies have been performed to assess the heritability of stroke (Table 3.1). de Faire *et al.* (1975) studied cerebrovascular mortality in the Swedish Twin Registry, which consisted of 10,900 same-sex pairs born between 1886 and 1925 with both members alive when the registry was founded in 1961. Vital status and cause of death were assessed in December 1975. At that time, 259 male and 222 female twin pairs were concordant for death (both members of a pair had died). Of these, 85 male and 75 female pairs were concordant for cause of death. The concordance rate for cerebrovascular death did not differ significantly between monozygotic and dizygotic twins. One limitation of the study is that non-fatal stroke events were not assessed. Many strokes are disabling, but not fatal. This may have led to systematic underreporting of individuals affected by stroke. Another concern is that cerebrovascular disease was defined broadly, with no attempt made to distinguish ischaemic from haemorrhagic stroke.

The National Academy of Sciences–National Research Council (NAS–NRC) Twins Registry has been used to study the heritability of stroke. The NAS–NRC Twins Registry is a cohort of 15,924 twin pairs of white men who had served in the US Armed Services (Braun *et al.* 1994). In 1985, the cohort was surveyed for responses to the question: 'Have you ever been told by a doctor that you had a stroke?' About 24,000 members of the cohort were living at the time, and 9475 individuals responded to the

Table 3.1 Twins studies of stroke

Study	Population	Results
Stroke		
de Faire *et al.* (1975)	Male and female same-sex Swedish twins born between 1886 and 1925	No significant difference in concordance rates for fatal cerebrovascular disease in monozygotic and dizygotic twins
Brass *et al.* (1992)	White, male veterans of the US armed services born between 1917 and 1927	Monozygotic twins had a relative risk of self-reported stroke of 4.3 ($P < 0.05$)
Bak *et al.* (2002)	Over 32,000 male and female same-sex Danish twins born 1870–1952 and surviving 6 years	The age- and sex-matched relative risk of stroke death in monozygotic compared with dizygotic co-twins was 2.1 (95% CI, 1.3–3.3)
Carotid disease		
Haapanen *et al.* (1989)	49 male and female same-sex identical twins discordant for cigarette smoking	Smoking twins were significantly more likely to have stenotic carotid arteries. Degree of stenosis and inner layer arterial thickening were also greater in the smoking co-twin

survey. Prevalence of stroke for the entire cohort was 3.1 per cent. The proband concordance rates were 17.7 per cent for monozygotic twins and 3.6 per cent for dizygotic twins, corresponding to a relative risk of 4.3 ($P < 0.05$) (Brass *et al.* 1992). The study provided evidence that a genetic component of stroke risk exists, but the authors acknowledged that the study had certain limitations. In contrast to the Swedish Twin Registry, stroke end points were collected only on survivors. The diagnosis of stroke was not verified by examination or record review, and information on stroke types (haemorrhagic versus ischaemic) was not collected.

An updated analysis of the NAS–NRC registry was reported in abstract form in 1996 (Brass *et al.* 1996). Stroke was assessed using the previous survey data along with data from a telephone health screen in 1994 and review of mortality records. The proband concordance rates were 12.8 per cent for monozygotic twins and 8.08 per cent for dizygotic twins, corresponding to a relative risk of 1.63. Cohort members ranged in age from 67 to 77 years when the survey was taken. The latest follow-up study included telephone health screen data from 1997 and 1998 (Brass *et al.* 1999). The proband concordance rates for stroke were 17.0 per cent for monozygotic twin pairs and 18.4 per cent for dizygotic twin pairs. The authors concluded that genetic factors might account for a smaller proportion of stroke risk in older age groups than in younger age groups.

A recent analysis of the Danish Twin Registry further suggests that genetic factors increase the risk of stroke but the magnitude of the effect is moderate (Bak *et al.* 2002). Attempts were made to distinguish intracerebral haemorrhage from cerebral infarction, but diagnoses recorded in the registry were found to have inadequate predictive values. Long-term follow-up data were available from the Danish National Discharge Registry and the Registry of Causes of Death. The age- and sex-adjusted relative risk of stroke death in monozygotic compared with dizygotic co-twins was 2.0 (95% confidence interval [CI], 0.9–2.4). Because the relative risk for fatal stroke, which is likely to be haemorrhagic, was greater than that for fatal and non-fatal strokes combined, the authors hypothesized that the genetic component might be stronger for haemorrhagic stroke than for ischaemic stroke. The authors speculated that non-differential misclassification may have led to an underestimation of the genetic contribution to stroke risk.

Classical twins studies look for differences among a cohort of monozygotic twins and dizygotic twins. However, another important use of twins is to study identical twins discordant (or divergent) in a behaviour or an environmental exposure and to look for differences in disease state. The goal of such a study is to control for genetic differences so that environmental risk factors can be studied in isolation. A Finnish cohort study looked at identical twins with the highest discordance in cigarette smoking (Haapanen *et al.* 1989). The study looked at 49 pairs, with a mean age of 52 years, in which one twin smoked and the other did not. The mean lifelong smoking dose for the co-twins was 20 pack-years. Carotid artery stenosis, defined as >15 per cent luminal reduction as measured by carotid ultrasonography, was found in nine pairs;

in all nine twins who smoked and in two of their non-smoking co-twins ($P = 0.036$). Total area of carotid plaque was 3.2 times larger in the twins who smoked ($P < 0.001$). The thickness of the inner layer of carotid arteries was more pronounced among twins who smoked ($P < 0.001$). The findings remained significant after adjusting for age, total plasma cholesterol level, diastolic blood pressure, and body mass index in multivariate logistic regression analyses. The results suggested that cigarette smoking is a strong risk factor in the development of carotid atherosclerosis independent of genetic factors.

The basic assumption of twins studies is that the relatedness of monozygotic twins to each other is similar to that of dizygotic twins in all respects except genetic relatedness. However, this assumption is not always valid. There may be differences in environmental sharing according to zygosity (Kendler and Holm 1985). For example, dizygotic twins tend to have older siblings, and mothers of dizygotic twins tend to be older than mothers of monozygotic twins and are more likely to have taken fertility drugs (Brass *et al.* 1992).

3.1.2 Family history as a risk factor for stroke

If there are genetic variants that predispose to stroke, a positive family history of stroke should be a risk factor for stroke. Stated another way, stroke should cluster within pedigrees if genetic risk factors exist. Family history studies of stroke have been reported since at least the 1960s (Gifford 1966). However, these studies vary considerably in design, methodological rigor, and scope. Many studies rely on unconfirmed proband reports to diagnose stroke among family members. For example, in the Progetto 3A study, patients were asked about number of relatives, occurrence of stroke and myocardial infarction in their first-degree relatives, age at onset of stroke or myocardial infarction, and age at death (Vitullo *et al.* 1996). Similarly in an epidemiological study of stroke and myocardial infarction in women in the United Kingdom, family history of stroke was obtained by interview of the study participant or the participant's next-of-kin (Thompson *et al.* 1989). Such data gathering is one step removed from self-report, and clinical experience suggests that information derived in this manner is prone to error. The error rate in reporting stroke histories in first-degree relatives is likely to be influenced by characteristics of the historian, such as age, education, and whether the historian has had a stroke. Patients who have had a stroke may be more likely to recognize symptoms of stroke in their relatives. Alternatively, stroke patients may have impairment of language or memory that makes recounting a family history less reliable.

A more valid approach to characterizing disease status among all living pedigree members is by direct questioning of all members rather than relying on proband report alone. Direct questioning of every pedigree member was the method used in the Family Heart Study, a population-based, multicentre study of the genetic and non-genetic determinants of cardiovascular disease (Liao *et al.* 1997). History of stroke in the probands and their family members was based on response to a question on a standardized self-administered questionnaire. This method is similar to the way stroke was assessed in the NAS–NRC twins study (Brass *et al.* 1992).

Studies that rely only on responses to self-administered questionnaires are limited because they exclude fatal cases. Studies that rely only on data from death certificates are limited because they exclude non-fatal cases. For example, one study examined the prevalence of deaths certified as caused by cerebral haemorrhage, thrombosis, or embolism in relatives of male index patients with angiographic evidence of occlusive disease of extracranial or intracranial vessels. It found a barely significant excess of such deaths among mothers of the index patients (Marshall 1971). In addition to ignoring non-fatal events among controls and relatives of index patients, this type of study attempts to establish a relationship between non-fatal stroke in index cases and fatal stroke in relatives. One should consider the extent to which this approach is valid. Because ischaemic stroke carries a lower case fatality rate than haemorrhagic stroke, the proportion of strokes due to cerebral infarction would be expected to be greater for non-fatal stroke than for fatal stroke.

Many family history studies do not distinguish haemorrhagic from ischaemic stroke in early generations. There are complex reasons for this. Studies that rely on responses to standardized questionnaire items often do not require more than a 'yes/no' response to the question of whether the subject has experienced a stroke (Liao *et al.* 1997). At least one study attempted to differentiate cerebral haemorrhage, cerebral thrombosis, and cerebral embolism without using findings from head CT (Welin *et al.* 1987). This undoubtedly led to misclassification of the type of stroke, and perhaps compromised the investigators' ability to detect an inherited component of a specific type of stroke.

Some investigators have treated a history of stroke within families as a categorical variable. For example, in the study by Thompson *et al.* (1989), a positive family history of stroke was recorded if the proband's father, mother, or any brother or sister had suffered a fatal or non-fatal stroke. Dichotomizing family histories in this way ignores the fact that inheritance patterns, like autosomal-dominant and autosomal-recessive patterns, may differ depending on the risk factor genes involved.

Despite these methodological concerns, family history studies generally support a genetic component of stroke risk. A prospective cohort of 789 men living in Gothenburg, Sweden, was followed for up to 18.5 years (Welin *et al.* 1987). At the inception of the study, all subjects were 54 years of age (born in 1913). By the end of follow-up, 57 men (7.2%) had sustained a stroke. Causes of parental death were taken from death certificates. Medical records were not reviewed to verify death certificate coding. Stroke was the principal cause of death in 29.8 per cent of mothers of cohort members who had had a stroke, and in 11.2 per cent of mothers of members who had not ($P = 0.0005$). Stroke was either a principal or contributing cause of death in 29.8 per cent of mothers of cohort members who had had a stroke, and in 14.2 per cent mothers of unaffected members ($P = 0.002$). In the prospective component of the study, men whose mothers had died of stroke had a three-fold increased incidence in the risk of stroke compared with men without a maternal history of stroke. Maternal history of stroke remained a risk factor even after adjusting for blood pressure and abdominal obesity assessed by waist-to-hip ratio. Intriguingly, the study did not find paternal history of fatal stroke to be a risk factor for stroke in cohort members.

In the Family Heart Study, personal and family histories of stroke were assessed in 3168 individuals (probands) who were at least 45 years of age or older and 29,325 of their first-degree relatives (Liao et al. 1997). The age-, ethnicity-, and sex-adjusted odds ratios (OR) for stroke were 2.0 (95% CI, 1.13–3.54) for a positive paternal history of stroke and 1.41 (95% CI, 0.80–2.50) for a positive maternal history of stroke. The association was not altered by further adjustment for hyperlipidaemia, cigarette smoking, coronary disease, hypertension, and diabetes status in probands. The pattern seen for African Americans was comparable to that of European Americans.

A prospective study of a cohort of 14,371 middle-aged men and women in Finland found a risk ratio of stroke associated with a positive parental history of stroke of 1.89 in men ($P = 0.004$), and 1.80 in women ($P = 0.007$), after adjusting for age, smoking, blood pressure, cholesterol, diabetes, and education (Jousilahti et al. 1997). The association between parental history of stroke and risk of stroke was related to proband age, and was greatest for probands between the ages of 25 and 49 years. A parental history of coronary disease was not associated with risk of stroke in men, and a parental history of coronary disease had only a borderline significant association in women with regard to ischaemic stroke. This suggests that there may not be a one-to-one correlation between genetic risk factors for myocardial infarction and genetic risk factors for ischaemic stroke. Important stroke-specific genetic risk factors may be missed in studies that do not treat ischaemic stroke and myocardial infarction as distinct conditions.

Support for a genetic contribution to stroke risk also comes from the Framingham Offspring Study (Kiely et al. 1993). The cohort was evaluated initially in 1971 and consisted of 5124 descendants or spouses of descendants of the original cohort members from the Framingham Heart Study. Atherothrombotic brain infarction (ischaemic stroke) in siblings conferred a three-fold increased risk of atherothrombotic brain infarction on cohort members. After adjustment for age, sex, and sibship size, the relative risk fell to 2.52 (95% CI, 1.05–4.94) ($P = 0.04$). With multivariate adjustment, the relative risk fell to 1.83 (95% CI, 0.68–4.94). It should be noted, however, that there were only 35 stroke events in the study at the time of analysis.

Hassan et al. (2002) performed a large case-control family history study of 727 consecutive patients with ischaemic stroke or transient ischaemic attack (TIA) recruited from a single referral clinic in southeast London, compared with 623 age-, sex-, and ethnicity-matched controls recruited from the same geographical area. Detailed family histories were obtained from all participants by interview. On univariate analysis, a family history of any stroke was associated with both an increased risk of ischaemic stroke at any age (OR, 1.27; 95% CI, 1.00–1.60; $P = 0.046$), and an increased risk of 'young (at ≤65 years) ischaemic stroke' (OR, 1.29; 95% CI, 0.98–1.71; $P = 0.07$). A family history of any stroke at less than 65 years of age was a stronger risk factor, both for all types of ischaemic stroke (OR, 1.63; 95% CI, 1.15–2.31; $P = 0.0005$) and for young ischaemic stroke (OR, 2.15; 95% CI, 1.46–3.18; $P < 0.0001$). When age, sex, smoking, hypertension, diabetes mellitus, and number of siblings were controlled for, a family history of early-onset stroke remained a risk factor for both ischaemic stroke at all ages, and young ischaemic stroke.

An incidence-type, population-based, case–control study performed in Asturias, Spain, involved 470 cases and 477 controls (Caicoya *et al.* 1999). A family history of stroke in a first-degree relative was found to be an independent risk factor for cerebral infarction and intracerebral haemorrhage. The multivariate-adjusted OR for cerebral infarction was 1.79 (95% CI, 1.25–2.56). The multivariate-adjusted OR for intra-cerebral haemorrhage was 1.71 (95% CI, 0.91–3.71). Cerebral infarction was independently associated with both a positive paternal and a positive sibling history of stroke. An association with a positive maternal history of stroke had borderline significance. Intracerebral haemorrhage was not significantly associated with a positive paternal, maternal, or sibling history of stroke.

3.1.3 Family history studies of ischaemic stroke subtypes

As discussed above, stroke is generally viewed as a heterogeneous phenotype, and even ischaemic stroke itself is considered heterogeneous. One pragmatic way to address this heterogeneity is to classify ischaemic stroke into more homogeneous clinical entities or subtypes. Two studies have investigated whether different clinical subtypes of ischaemic stroke differ from each other in tendency to group within families.

In one study, family history of stroke was obtained by interviewing 421 consecutive stroke patients admitted to the neurology and internal medicine wards of the University Hospital of Patras, Greece (Polychronopoulos *et al.* 2002). Family history of stroke was also obtained from 266 age- and sex-matched stroke-free controls. Ischaemic stroke was subtyped in accordance with the Trial of ORG10172 in Acute Stroke Treatment (TOAST) criteria (Adams *et al.* 1993). As expected, diabetes mellitus and hypertension were significantly more common among cases than among controls. Of the 421 cases of stroke, 351 (83.4%) were ischaemic. Patients with ischaemic stroke were more likely to have a first-degree relative with a history of stroke than controls (48% vs 28%, $P < 0.0001$). The most common ischaemic stroke subtype was large-vessel (37%). The rates of positive first-degree relative history of stroke were significantly greater for the large-, small-vessel, and undetermined ischaemic stroke subtypes than for controls.

The second study was a two-centre, prospective family history registry to assess the feasibility of an affected sibling pair study in consecutive patients with stroke. For the different TOAST subtypes, the percentages of probands who had a sibling or parent with stroke were as follows: large-vessel, 42 per cent (95% CI, 30–53%); cardioembolic, 45 per cent (95% CI, 32–59%); small-vessel, 48 per cent (95% CI, 35–60%); other, 38 per cent (95% CI, 8–76%); and unknown subtype, 51 per cent (95% CI, 41–61%) (Meschia *et al.* 2001).

Both studies suggest that in ischaemic strokes of diverse clinical subtypes, inherited factors are involved to a comparable degree.

3.1.4 Population genomics: lessons from Iceland

The role of genetic predisposition as a risk factor for 'multifactorial' stroke is supported by the recent study from DeCODE Genetics, which mapped the first locus for common (sporadic) stroke. Gretarsdottir *et al.* (2002) cross-matched a population-based list of patients with stroke in Iceland with a database clustering 476 patients with stroke within 179 pedigrees. Linkage was detected between stroke and a locus designated STRK1 located on chromosomal region 5q12. STRK1 covers a 20-centimorgan (cM) region between markers D5S474 and D5S2046. The log-of-the-odds (LOD) score for STRK1 met criteria for genomewide significance (multipoint allele-sharing LOD score of 4.40, $P = 3.9 \times 10^{-6}$). Despite intense interest from the scientific community, the risk factor gene itself remains unreported to date.

To find the STRK1 locus, investigators crossed a list of 2000 Icelandic patients with stroke or transient ischaemic attacks with a computerized genealogy database that covers the entire Icelandic population. Patients were screened using hospital International Classification of Diseases, Ninth Revision (ICD-9) codes. Every patient had computed tomography of the head, and most had Doppler ultrasonography of the carotid arteries and echocardiography. Patients were excluded if they had subarachnoid haemorrhage or hereditary cerebral haemorrhage with amyloidosis of the Icelandic type. Patients were selected only if they were related to at least one other patient, that is, separated by no more than six meiotic events (second cousins are separated by six meiotic events). Ischaemic stroke or TIA was subtyped using a modification of the TOAST criteria (Adams *et al.* 1993) in which patients were classified as having symptomatic large-vessel atherosclerotic ischaemic stroke only if they had >70 per cent stenosis of the symptomatic artery.

The population of patients with stroke or TIA included in the study was clinically heterogeneous. Of the 476 patients, approximately 5 per cent had a diagnosis of haemorrhagic stroke. The remaining patients had ischaemic stroke or TIA, with cardioembolic stroke being the most common subtype for which a mechanism was identified. The distribution of subtypes was as follows: cardioembolic, 23 per cent; large-vessel, 13 per cent; small-vessel, 16 per cent; other cause, 4 per cent; and more than one subtype or unknown cause, 39 per cent. In a separate analysis of patients with ischaemic stroke (excluding the 22 patients with haemorrhagic stroke), the LOD score increased from 4.40 to 4.86.

Although the increase in LOD score was not significant ($P = 0.09$), this finding implies that STRK1 is primarily involved in increasing the risk of ischaemic stroke.

The DeCODE discovery vindicates those who have argued for a model-free linkage approach to discovering stroke risk factor genes. The DeCODE approach was model-free in that no mode of inheritance was assumed for the genetic risk factor. The DeCODE approach was also model-free in that no assumptions were made about the pathophysiology of stroke, and STRK1 did not correspond to known susceptibility loci for classical risk factors for stroke like diabetes mellitus or hypertension. In contrast, traditional linkage analysis requires an understanding of the mode of inheritance of a disease, which is deduced from the study of the pattern of disease-affected and disease-unaffected individuals in large pedigrees. This type of traditional linkage analysis led to the discovery of the mutations in the notch 3 gene that cause CADASIL. In case–control studies, it is usually best to select a candidate gene based on an understanding of the pathophysiology of the condition and an understanding of the biochemistry and biology of the gene product.

DeCODE was able to discover STRK1 efficiently because the company and the federal government of Iceland worked together to create a unique electronic database linking medical records generated by a national health care system, genetic data generated by DeCODE, and genealogical data compiled with the help of DeCODE. Data on about 80 per cent of the 270,000 population of Iceland are included in the database (Gulcher and Stefansson 1998). It is unlikely that a similar resource will be generated for any other large population in the near future. This is due in part to concerns about the potential for corporate or governmental abuses of the vast store of information gathered on individuals and to divergent views on the right to privacy and the right of self-determination regarding participation in research (Stefansson 2001). Although clearly less efficient, other means exist for assembling informative pedigrees for genomic research without having to resort to controversial research methods requiring community consent or an opt-out strategy for obtaining blanket consent (Annas 2000, Gulcher and Stefansson 2000). For example, proband-initiated contact can be used to identify and recruit siblings of probands, as in the National Institutes of Health-supported Siblings With Ischemic Stroke Study (SWISS) (Meschia *et al.* 2002).

3.2 Evidence for a genetic predisposition for intracranial aneurysms and subarachnoid haemorrhage

Subarachnoid haemorrhage (SAH) is a type of stroke in which bleeding occurs surrounding the brain tissue, under the lining of the brain. It accounts for approximately 5 per cent of all strokes and is most commonly caused by intracranial saccular aneurysms, which are small, berry-like projections that particularly occur at intracranial arterial bifurcations. Approximately 80–90 per cent of aneurysms occur in the anterior aspect of the circle of Willis. Intracranial aneurysms occasionally occur as part of monogenic connective tissue disorders (see Chapter 10) but these represent a minority. For apparently 'sporadic' aneurysms and subarachnoid haemorrhage, a number of studies have investigated the extent of genetic predisposition and the evidence from these is considered below.

The overall frequency of intracranial aneurysms in the population is between 0.2 and 9 per cent (Jellinger 1977, Jakubowski and Kendall 1978, Atkinson et al. 1989), with approximately 2 per cent of the population having an aneurysm. They are rarely noted in childhood and increase in frequency of detection with older age, similar to subarachnoid haemorrhage. There is a higher proportion of aneurysms in women than in men (ISUIA Investigators 1998). In childhood and adolescence, the opposite appears to be the case (Storrs et al. 1982, Meyer et al. 1989). The overall incidence of subarachnoid haemorrhage varies worldwide (Broderick et al. 1992, Fogelholm 1992, Brown et al. 1996, Ingall et al. 2000, Thrift et al. 2001), ranging from approximately 4 to 25 per 100,000 persons per year.

Because a high proportion of non-traumatic SAH is caused by intracranial saccular aneurysm (approximately 80%), the risk factors for both intracranial aneurysm and SAH are often considered as a combined entity. In addition to the effects of hemodynamic variables, numerous environmental factors appear to influence risk: cigarette smoking (Longstreth et al. 1985, Juvela 1996), binge drinking (Longstreth et al. 1985, Sankai et al. 2000), hormonal factors in women (Mhurchu et al. 2001), hypertension (Longstreth et al. 1985, Juvela 1996, Kissela et al. 2002), and seasonal factors (Chyatte et al. 1994, Gallerani et al. 1996, Feigin et al. 2001, Inagawa 2002).

The influence of genetic factors on the risk of SAH and intracranial aneurysm has also been explored. The overall risk of having a relative with intracranial aneurysm was investigated in a population-based case–control study in Rochester, MN (Schievink et al. 1995). All 81 patients with an aneurysmal SAH between 1970 and 1989 were evaluated by contact with either the patients themselves or their families. The observed number of SAHs in the families was compared with an expected number based on established age- and sex-specific incidence rates in the community. Of the 76 patients with complete family history data available, 15 (20%) had a first- or second-degree relative with aneurysmal SAH. Of the first-degree relatives, 11 had an aneurysmal SAH, with an expected number of 2.7, yielding a relative risk of 4.14 (95% CI, 2.06–7.40; $P < 0.001$).

A subsequent analysis of the literature before 1994 (Schievink et al. 1994) included 238 intracranial aneurysm families, with 560 affected members harbouring an intracranial aneurysm. Segregation analysis was performed for 73 of the families. Of these, 79 per cent had two affected members, 15 per cent had three, 3 per cent had four, and 3 per cent had five. Sibling relation was the most common familial association. In the 73 families, 75 per cent of 282 men were affected, compared with 37 per cent of 281 women. Daughters appeared to be more frequently affected than were sons, but the difference was not significant. Segregation analyses included likelihood models fit for a number of possibilities. The best-fitting model was an autosomal-dominant model with a very rare disease susceptibility allele and an autosomal-recessive model with a not so rare susceptibility allele.

In another study, 533 patients with intracranial aneurysm, residing in a geographically isolated area of Quebec, were compared with 1599 controls. Examination of genealogies showed that 48 patients (9.0%) were first-degree relatives compared with 1.9 per cent of controls. As defined by the presence of intracranial aneurysm in two or more first- to third-degree relatives, familial aggregation was higher for the patients with intracranial aneurysm (29.8%) than for controls (18.6%) (De Braekeleer *et al.* 1996).

In a population-based case–control study in King County, Washington, 149 patients with spontaneous SAH were compared with age- and sex-matched controls (Wang *et al.* 1995). Of the patients, 11.4 per cent had a first-degree relative with a history of SAH compared with 6.4 per cent of controls (OR, 1.8; 95% CI, 1.1–5.2).

A population-based case–control study in Cincinnati included 107 patients with SAH and 194 controls (Kissela *et al.* 2002). A history of SAH or intracranial aneurysm in first-degree relatives was reported for 9.4 per cent of patients with SAH versus 4.1 per cent of controls, in second-degree relatives for 14 per cent of patients versus 6.1 per cent of controls, and in any relative for 23.4 per cent of patients versus 8.6 per cent of controls. History of SAH or intracranial aneurysm in any family member was associated with SAH due to intracranial aneurysm in both univariate and multivariate analysis (multivariate analysis OR, 3.2; 95% CI, 1.5–6.9; $P = 0.003$). Other significant risk factors in the multivariate analysis included hypertension, current smoker, heavy alcohol use, and body mass index (lower values being protective). An increased OR was observed for the presence of either an S or a Z mutation of alpha-1 antitrypsin, but the effect was not significant (95% CI, 0.4–4.1; $P = 0.7$). The data suggest both a significant environmental and a significant genetic influence on the occurrence of SAH.

Limited data report potential alleles shared by affected relatives in SAH families. In a sibling-pair approach using 48 pairs from 24 families, two regions with multipoint LOD scores exceeding 2 were noted, including one on chromosome 19 associated with cerebrovascular and cardiovascular disorders (Olson *et al.* 1998).

3.3 Ethnic differences in distribution of cervicocephalic atherosclerosis

Several studies have consistently demonstrated ethnic (racial) differences in the distribution of cervicocephalic atherosclerosis.

Preliminary results of the Northern Manhattan Stroke Study (NOMASS), a prospective registry of stroke patients who reside in this region, demonstrated ethnic differences in intracranial atherosclerotic stenosis (Sacco *et al.* 1995). Atherosclerotic stroke accounted for 17 per cent of all index ischaemic strokes. Extracranial carotid atherosclerosis was assessed by duplex ultrasonography and conventional angiography. Intracranial atherosclerosis was assessed by transcranial Doppler and cerebral angiography. Cerebral angiography was performed in 48 per cent of those diagnosed with extracranial atherosclerotic stroke and 45 per cent of those with intracranial atherosclerotic stroke. Intracranial atherosclerotic stroke was significantly more common in blacks and Hispanics than in whites: 6 per cent of blacks, 11 per cent of Hispanics, and 1 per cent of whites ($P = 0.014$). The ratio of extracranial to intracranial disease was 1.2 in blacks, 0.9 in Hispanics, and 9.0 in whites. The greater prevalence of diabetes and hypercholesterolaemia among blacks and Hispanics accounted for much of the increased frequency of intracranial atherosclerotic stroke.

Inzitari *et al.* (1990) analysed the entry characteristics of 1367 patients enrolled in a multinational randomized trial of extracranial or intracranial bypass surgery. The study found that blacks were more often hypertensive, diabetic, or cigarette smokers, but whites had higher haemoglobin values. Asians had the lowest prevalence of vascular risk factors. Multivariate analysis showed ethnicity to be a strong independent predictor of the location of cerebrovascular atherosclerotic lesions. For example, a stenotic lesion in the middle cerebral artery was noted in 20 per cent of Asians, 10 per cent of blacks, and 5 per cent of whites in the study ($P < 0.001$). This study had the advantage of systematic recording of baseline risk factors in all patients and the results of conventional angiography in all patients. However, because this study represented an exploratory analysis of the clinical trials data set, its generalizability is limited by possible biases related to patient selection.

Several smaller case–control studies of angiographic findings among different ethnic groups have shown similar results. Feldmann *et al.* (1990) compared clinical and angiographic features of 24 white and 24 Chinese patients with symptomatic occlusive cerebrovascular disease. Severe vascular lesions tended to be extracranial in white patients and intracranial in Chinese patients. The difference in distribution of the lesions was not explained by differences in the incidence of transient ischaemia, hypertension, diabetes, or hypercholesterolaemia. In a case–control study involving 26 white and 45 black patients with symptomatic occlusive cerebrovascular disease, Gorelick *et al.* (1984) noted more severe disease of the middle cerebral artery stem and supraclinoid internal carotid artery among blacks than among whites. Again, angiographic differences were not explained by ethnic differences in the prevalence of hypertension, diabetes, hypercholesterolaemia, or ischaemic heart disease. A follow-up study by Gorelick *et al.* (1988) of 106 patients with symptomatic unilateral carotid territory occlusive disease showed more asymptomatic lesions of the supraclinoid internal carotid artery, anterior cerebral artery stem, and middle cerebral artery stem in black patients than in white patients. White patients had more asymptomatic disease at the extra-cranial carotid and vertebral artery sites.

Although some studies have attempted to adjust for differential rates of conventional risk factors through multivariate analyses, systematic differences in environmental factors might explain the differences in angiographic findings. Not only do many ethnic groups differ in environmental factors or habits, but they may also differ in their access to and utilization of health care. For example, some patient groups may use pharmacotherapies for hypertension more than others do. Despite these concerns, the most likely explanation for the observed differences is at least partly related to underlying genetic differences. There may be a systematic tendency for atherosclerosis to affect some segments of the arterial tree rather than others. Variations in endothelial cell function depend not only on the vascular bed of origin but also on the size of the vessel within the same vascular territory. Differences have been observed in phenotype, antigen expression, cell size and growth, secretory function, and G-protein expression in endothelial cells from different parts of the vascular system (Thorin and Shreeve 1998). Some of these regional differences in endothelial cell function may be genetically determined.

References

Adams, H.P. Jr., Bendixen, B.H., Kappelle, L.J., *et al.* (1993). Classification of subtype of acute ischemic stroke: definitions for use in a multicenter clinical trial. TOAST. Trial of Org 10172 in Acute Stroke Treatment. *Stroke*, 24, 35–41.

Annas, G.J. (2000). Rules for research on human genetic variation: lessons from Iceland. *New England Journal of Medicine*, 342, 1830–3.

Atkinson, J.L., Sundt, T.M. Jr., Houser, O.W., and Whisnant, J.P. (1989). Angiographic frequency of anterior circulation intracranial aneurysms. *Journal of Neurosurgery*, 70, 551–5.

Bak, S., Gaist, D., Sindrup, S.H., Skytthe, A., and Christensen, K. (2002). Genetic liability in stroke: a long-term follow-up study of Danish twins. *Stroke*, 33, 769–74.

Brass, L.M., Carrano, D., Hartigan, P.M., Concato, J., and Page, W.F. (1996). Genetic risk for stroke: a follow-up study of the National Academy of Sciences/Veterans Administration Twin Registry (abstract). *Neurology*, 46 (Suppl), A212.

Brass, L.M., Isaacsohn, J.L., Merikangas, K.R., and Robinette, C.D. (1992). A study of twins and stroke. *Stroke*, 23, 221–3.

Brass, L.M., Page, W.F., and Lichtman, J.H. (1999). Stroke in Twins III: a follow-up study (abstract). *Stroke*, 30, 256.

Braun, M.M., Haupt, R., and Caporaso, N.E. (1994). The National Academy of Sciences: National Research Council Veteran Twin Registry. *Acta Geneticae Medicae et Gemellologiae (Roma)*, 43, 89–94.

Broderick, J.P., Brott, T., Tomsick, T., Huster, G., and Miller, R. (1992). The risk of subarachnoid and intracerebral hemorrhages in blacks as compared with whites. *New England Journal of Medicine*, 326, 733–6.

Brown, R.D. Jr., Whisnant, J.P., Sicks, J.D., O'Fallon, W.M., Petty, G.W., and Wiebers, D.O. (2001). Subarachnoid hemorrhage and intracerebral hemorrhage: trends in incidence and survival in a population-based study (abstract). *Neurology*, 56 (Suppl), A86.

Brown, R.D., Whisnant, J.P., Sicks, J.D., O'Fallon, W.M., and Wiebers, D.O. (1996). Stroke incidence, prevalence, and survival: secular trends in Rochester, Minnesota, through 1989. *Stroke*, 27, 373–80.

Caicoya, M., Corrales, C., and Rodriguez, T. (1999). Family history and stroke: a community case–control study in Asturias, Spain. *Journal of Epidemiology and Biostatistics*, 4, 313–20.

Chyatte, D., Chen, T.L., Bronstein, K., and Brass, L.M. (1994). Seasonal fluctuation in the incidence of intracranial aneurysm rupture and its relationship to changing climatic conditions. *Journal of Neurosurgery*, **81**, 525–30.

De Braekeleer, M., Perusse, L., Cantin, L., Bouchard, J.M., and Mathieu, J. (1996). A study of inbreeding and kinship in intracranial aneurysms in the Saguenay Lac-Saint-Jean region (Quebec, Canada). *Annals of Human Genetics*, **60**, 99–104.

de Faire, U., Friberg, L., and Lundman, T. (1975). Concordance for mortality with special reference to ischaemic heart disease and cerebrovascular disease: a study on the Swedish Twin Registry. *Preventive Medicine*, **4**, 509–17.

Feigin, V.L., Anderson, C.S., Anderson, N.E., *et al.* (2001). Is there a temporal pattern in the occurrence of subarachnoid hemorrhage in the Southern Hemisphere? Pooled data from 3 large, population-based incidence studies in Australasia, 1981 to 1997. *Stroke*, **32**, 613–19.

Feldmann, E., Daneault, N., Kwan, E., *et al.* (1990). Chinese-white differences in the distribution of occlusive cerebrovascular disease. *Neurology*, **40**, 1541–5.

Fogelholm, R. (1992). Subarachnoid hemorrhage in Finland (letter). *Stroke*, **23**, 437.

Gallerani, M., Portaluppi, F., Maida, G., *et al.* (1996). Circadian and circannual rhythmicity in the occurrence of subarachnoid hemorrhage. *Stroke*, **27**, 1793–7.

Gifford, A.J. (1966). An epidemiological study of cerebrovascular disease. *American Journal of Public Health and the Nation's Health*, **56**, 452–61.

Gorelick, P.B., Caplan, L.R., Hier, D.B., Parker, S.L., and Patel, D. (1984). Racial differences in the distribution of anterior circulation occlusive disease. *Neurology*, **34**, 54–9.

Gorelick, P.B., Caplan, L.R., Langenberg, P., *et al.* (1988). Clinical and angiographic comparison of asymptomatic occlusive cerebrovascular disease. *Neurology*, **38**, 852–8.

Gretarsdottir, S., Sveinbjornsdottir, S., Jonsson, H.H., *et al.* (2002). Localization of a susceptibility gene for common forms of stroke to 5q12. *American Journal of Human Genetics*, **70**, 593–603.

Gulcher, J. and Stefansson, K. (1998). Population genomics: laying the groundwork for genetic disease modeling and targeting. *Clinical Chemistry and Laboratory Medicine*, **36**, 523–7.

Gulcher, J.R. and Stefansson, K. (2000). The Icelandic Healthcare Database and informed consent. *New England Journal of Medicine*, **342**, 1827–30.

Haapanen, A., Koskenvuo, M., Kaprio, J., Kesaniemi, Y.A., and Heikkila, K. (1989). Carotid arteriosclerosis in identical twins discordant for cigarette smoking. *Circulation*, **80**, 10–16.

Hassan, A., Sham, P.C., and Markus, H.S. (2002). Planning genetic studies in human stroke: sample size estimates based on family history data. *Neurology*, **58**, 1483–8.

Inagawa, T. (2002). Seasonal variation in the incidence of aneurysmal subarachnoid hemorrhage in hospital- and community-based studies. *Journal of Neurosurgery*, **96**, 497–509.

Ingall, T., Asplund, K., Mahonen, M., and Bonita, R. (2000). A multinational comparison of subarachnoid hemorrhage epidemiology in the WHO MONICA stroke study. *Stroke*, **31**, 1054–61.

Inzitari, D., Hachinski, V.C., Taylor, D.W., and Barnett, H.J. (1990). Racial differences in the anterior circulation in cerebrovascular disease: how much can be explained by risk factors? *Archives of Neurology*, **47**, 1080–84.

Jakubowski, J. and Kendall, B. (1978). Coincidental aneurysms with tumours of pituitary origin. *Journal of Neurology, Neurosurgery, and Psychiatry*, **41**, 972–9.

Jellinger, K. (1977). Pathology of intracerebral hemorrhage. *Zentralblatt für Neurochirurgie*, **38**, 29–42.

Jousilahti, P., Rastenyte, D., Tuomilehto, J., Sarti, C., and Vartiainen, E. (1997). Parental history of cardiovascular disease and risk of stroke: a prospective follow-up of 14371 middle-aged men and women in Finland. *Stroke*, **28**, 1361–6.

Juvela, S. (1996). Prevalence of risk factors in spontaneous intracerebral hemorrhage and aneurysmal subarachnoid hemorrhage. *Archives of Neurology*, 53, 734–40.

Kendler, K.S. and Holm, N.V. (1985). Differential enrollment in twin registries: its effect on prevalence and concordance rates and estimates of genetic parameters. *Acta Geneticae Medicae et Gemellologiae (Roma)*, 34, 125–40.

Kiely, D.K., Wolf, P.A., Cupples, L.A., Beiser, A.S., and Myers, R.H. (1993). Familial aggregation of stroke: the Framingham Study. *Stroke*, 24, 1366–71.

Kissela, B.M., Sauerbeck, L., Woo, D., *et al.* (2002). Subarachnoid hemorrhage: a preventable disease with a heritable component. *Stroke*, 33, 1321–6.

Liao, D., Myers, R., Hunt, S., *et al.* (1997). Familial history of stroke and stroke risk: the Family Heart Study. *Stroke*, 28, 1908–12.

Longstreth, W.T. Jr., Koepsell, T.D., Yerby, M.S., and van Belle, G. (1985). Risk factors for subarachnoid hemorrhage. *Stroke*, 16, 377–85.

Marshall, J. (1971). Familial incidence of cerebrovascular disease. *Journal of Medical Genetics*, 8, 84–9.

McKusick, V.A. (2001). The anatomy of the human genome: a neo-Vesalian basis for medicine in the 21st century. *Journal of the American Medical Association*, 286, 2289–95.

Meschia, J.F., Brown, R.D. Jr., Brott, T.G., Chukwudelunzu, F.E., Hardy, J., and Rich, S.S. (2002). The Siblings With Ischemic Stroke Study (SWISS) Protocol. *BioMed Central Medical Genetics*, 3, 1.

Meyer, F.B., Sundt, T.M. Jr., Fode, N.C., Morgan, M.K., Forbes, G.S., and Mellinger, J.F. (1989). Cerebral aneurysms in childhood and adolescence. *Journal of Neurosurgery*, 70, 420–5.

Mhurchu C.N., Anderson, C., Jamrozik, K., Hankey, G., Dunbabin, D. (2001). Hormonal factors and risk of aneurysmal subarachnoid haemorrhage: an international population-based, case-control study. *Stroke*, 32, 606–12.

Olson, J., Vongpunsawad, S., Kuivaniemi, H., *et al.* (1998). Genome scan for intracranial aneurysm susceptibility loci using Finnish families (abstract). *American Journal of Human Genetics*, 63, A17.

Polychronopoulos, P., Gioldasis, G., Ellul, J., *et al.* (2002). Family history of stroke in stroke types and subtypes. *Journal of Neurologic Sciences*, 195, 117–22.

Sacco, R.L., Kargman, D.E., Gu, Q., and Zamanillo, M.C. (1995). Race-ethnicity and determinants of intracranial atherosclerotic cerebral infarction: the Northern Manhattan Stroke Study. *Stroke*, 26, 14–20.

Sankai, T., Iso, H., Shimamoto, T., *et al.* (2000). Prospective study on alcohol intakes and risk of subarachnoid haemorrhage among Japanese men and women. Alcoholism, clinical and experimental research, 24, 386–9.

Schievink, W.I., Schaid, D.J., Michels, V.V., and Piepgras, D.G. (1995). Familial aneurysmal subarachnoid hemorrhage: a community-based study. *Journal of Neurosurgery*, 83, 426–9.

Schievink, W.I., Schaid, D.J., Rogers, H.M., Piepgras, D.G., and Michels, V.V. (1994). On the inheritance of intracranial aneurysms. *Stroke*, 25, 2028–37.

Stefansson, K. (2001). Health care and privacy: an interview with Kari Stefansson, founder and CEO of deCODE Genetics in Reykjavik, Iceland. *EMBO Reports*, 2, 964–7.

Storrs, B.B., Humphreys, R.P., Hendrick, E.B., and Hoffman, H.J. (1982). Intracranial aneurysms in the pediatric age-group. *Childs Brain*, 9, 358–61.

Thompson, S.G., Greenberg, G., and Meade, T.W. (1989). Risk factors for stroke and myocardial infarction in women in the United Kingdom as assessed in general practice: a case–control study. *British Heart Journal*, 61, 403–9.

Thorin, E., and Shreeve, S.M. (1998). Heterogeneity of vascular endothelial cells in normal and disease states. *Pharmacology and Therapeutics*, 78, 155–66.

Thrift, A.G., Dewey, H.M., Macdonell, R.A., McNeil, J.J., and Donnan, G.A. (2001). Incidence of the major stroke subtypes: initial findings from the North East Melbourne Stroke Incidence Study (NEMESIS). *Stroke*, **32**, 1732–8.

Vitullo, F., Marchioli, R., Di Mascio, R., Cavasinni, L., Pasquale, A.D., and Tognoni, G. (1996). Family history and socioeconomic factors as predictors of myocardial infarction, unstable angina and stroke in an Italian population: PROGETTO 3A Investigators. *European Journal of Epidemiology*, **12**, 177–85.

Wang, P.S., Longstreth, W.T. Jr., and Koepsell, T.D. (1995). Subarachnoid hemorrhage and family history: a population-based case–control study. *Archives of Neurology*, **52**, 202–4.

Welin, L., Svardsudd, K., Wilhelmsen, L., Larsson, B., and Tibblin, G. (1987). Analysis of risk factors for stroke in a cohort of men born in 1913. *New England Journal of Medicine*, **317**, 521–6.

Chapter 4

Genetics of conventional stroke risk factors

Giuseppe A. Sagnella

Several of the major risk factors for stroke have long been recognized and include hypertension, vessel wall abnormalities, dyslipidemia, defects in haemostasis, diabetes and life-style factors such as smoking. This chapter focuses on the genetics of three major classical risk factors, namely hypertension, diabetes and dyslipidaemia.

4.1 Principles of the genetic investigation of stroke risk factors

Given that these conditions are defined by reference to an arbitrarily defined upper range of the underlying trait, namely blood pressure, plasma glucose and measures of plasma cholesterol, genetic analysis of these conditions relates essentially to the genetic analysis of the corresponding quantitative traits (QTs). With these characteristics there is no clear discontinuity between the phenotypes; the range of appearance (or values) amongst individuals often overlaps extensively giving the appearance of a continuous distribution. The continuous distribution of QTs does not exclude the possibility that only one gene is involved in any particular instance, as any one gene may have many allelic states. In reality, however, it is likely that for continuous biological variables such as blood pressure and plasma glucose, and plasma cholesterol several, and possibly very many genes, are involved. In this case, phenotypic variation arises from allelic variation in several genes, each with a relatively small effect on the phenotype. The overall additive effects of many such variants contributes to the unimodal distribution of a quantitative trait. Accordingly QTs are referred to as polygenic traits. More recently the term QT loci (QTL) has been introduced to define polygenic traits and the genes that control them.

The key questions in any attempt to investigate the genetic basis of these quantitative traits are:

- Is there a single gene with a major effect (a single gene with multiple allelic variants)?
- Can the variation be explained by only a few (2–6) genes (an oligogenic trait) or are a large number of genes involved (a polygenic trait)?
- Is there locus heterogeneity and epistasis?
- Is phenotype also dependent on a complex interaction between genes and environment factors (a multifactorial trait)?

As the distribution of these quantitative traits is continuous and largely unimodal, the concepts of classical genetics describing dominant (heterozygous) and recessive (homozygous) modes of inheritance are too limited. The concept of genetic susceptibility or genetic risk factor becomes more appropriate. One way to estimate the magnitude of the potential effect of a gene variant is by calculating the relative risk. This can be derived from case–control comparisons as an odd ratio (OR)—an index of how many times more frequently the disease is found in those positive for the risk (gene variant) compared with those without the risk factor (gene variant). The relevance of a particular risk factor in the population depends not only on its individual relative risk but also on its prevalence within the community. This is quantified by the population attributable risk, a measure of the proportion of the trait/disease which can be attributed to that particular risk factor (Jekel *et al.* 1996).

Several approaches have been used to understand the genetic basis of hypertension, diabetes and dyslipidaemia. These have included biometrical approaches, association studies with candidate genes, and more recently genome-wide scans with anonymous markers (Table 4.1). Biometrical methods are fundamental in defining the extent of the genetic contribution to these traits. Key indices for the assessment of the genetic contribution have relied on analysis of familial aggregation. One approach to assessing familial aggregation has relied on the estimation of intra-family correlations of the quantitative trait. The estimation of the relative risk for siblings (λs) is another measure of the strength of genetic contribution for a complex trait. This is defined as the ratio of the risk of the trait (disease) in the sibling of an affected individual, divided by the risk that an unrelated individual from the same population has the trait (i.e. population prevalence of the trait). λs reflects the net effect of genes of varying penetrance,

Table 4.1 Approaches to investigate genetic determinants of polygenic traits in humans

Biometrical approaches
Complex segregation analysis
Whole genome mapping for quantitative trait loci
Family pedigrees
Affected sib-pairs
Discordant sib-pairs
Linkage disequilibrium mapping
Association studies with Candidate genes
Cases versus controls in unrelated individuals
Intra-family case (affected) versus control (unaffected sib)
Intra-familial association studies
Transmission disequilibrium test (TDT)
Sibling transmission disequilibrium test (sTDT)

For further reading on these approaches see: Boehnke (2000), Cardon and Bell (2001), Falconer and Mackay (1996), Ghosh and Collins (1996), Hilgers and Schmieder (2002), Kruglyak (1999), Lander and Skork (1994), Risch and Zhang (1995), Tabor (2002), Thomson and Esposito (1999), and Weiss and Clark (2002).

shared environment and gene–environment interactions. It is important in planning genetics studies, as the magnitude of familial clustering expressed by λs provides a direct reflection of the ease of mapping susceptibility loci (Risch 1990). In general, the higher the λs, the stronger the genetic component and the easier the mapping. The values of λs for traits contributing to cardiovascular disease such as hypertension and diabetes are relatively low (~3–15), when compared with those for highly penetrant monogenic conditions such as cystic fibrosis which display a λs > 500 (Risch 1990).

The candidate gene approach has been used mainly within the context of association studies to test the hypothesis of whether specific DNA variant(s) are more prevalent in unrelated cases with a given trait than in unrelated controls. This is a very powerful way to assess the contribution of a specific variant to a trait as it provides estimates of relative risk. Because association studies are relatively easy to carry out they have become increasingly common. However, several design issues are important. Of these, particular attention should be given to validation of protocols for defining cases and controls. Selection of appropriate controls can be problematic for conditions developing in later life especially when based on an arbitrary classification of a continuous variable. For instance, blood pressure increases with age and clearly a 'normotensive' classification even in an adult does not exclude the possibility that the individual will develop 'hypertension' at a later date. Ideally, cases and controls should also have comparable environmental exposure, especially when dealing with multifactorial conditions such hypertension and diabetes (Fig. 4.1). Moreover, it is also important to note that any positive association between a specific gene variant and disease may not necessarily indicate a causative relationship. A positive association may also arise from other reasons and especially from linkage disequilibrium and population stratification.

The high risk of false positives is of particular relevance in case–control association studies. The availability of sufficient statistical power is an essential requirement since the relative risk from a single candidate gene is likely to be relatively small. When testing hypotheses for multiple alleles, the likelihood of false positives is further compounded by setting a significance level at the customary 5 per cent level. A significance level at 5 per cent implies that 1 in 20 of all comparisons carried out may give rise to positive associations purely by chance. One way to overcome this problem is to reduce the level of significance according to the number of comparisons (Cardon and Bell 2001). A further disadvantage of the candidate gene approach is that it only allows association with known genes to be identified and does not enable the detection of novel genes.

When assessing the potential role of a candidate gene in association studies several major questions should be considered: is the selection of the controls appropriate for the cases? Can the results be replicated in comparable populations? What is the functional significance of the gene variant(s) as a causative mechanism?

Linkage analysis with anonymous markers to identify QTLs makes no assumptions about the functional significance of the products of gene loci. Linkage analysis depends on the co-segregation of a trait with genetic markers in families with multiply affected

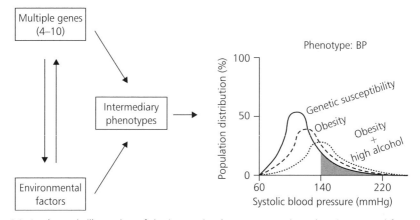

Fig. 4.1 A schematic illustration of the interaction between genetic and environmental factors in the development of hypertension. The left side of the figure shows how environmental factors and multiple genes responsible for high blood pressure (BP) interact and affect intermediate phenotypes. The result of these intermediate phenotypes is BP with a normal distribution skewed to the right. The continuous line in the graph indicates the theoretical BP distribution in a population that is not exposed to environmental hypertension factors. The shaded area indicates a systolic blood pressure in the hypertensive range. The broken lines and dotted lines indicated populations in which one (obesity), or two (obesity and high alcohol intake), environmental factors have been added. (Adapted from Carretero O.A. and Oparil S. 2000).

relatives. It is based on the principle that alleles at loci close together will tend to be inherited jointly. If a marker allele and a locus for a specific trait are close together on the same chromosome they are unlikely to be separated by cross-overs during meiosis. Linkage analysis can therefore be used to map quantitative trait loci by geno-typing of anonymous DNA markers scattered throughout the genome. A measure of linkage is given by the calculation of the log-of-the-odds (LOD) score: a measure of the likelihood of linkage compared with no linkage. Conventionally, acceptance of significant genome-wide linkage requires a LOD score of >3.6 but a lower score of at least 2.2 is usually taken to indicate the presence of suggestive linkage (Lander and Kruglyak 1995).

This approach contrasts with the candidate gene approach, in that the variants being genotyped are not themselves biological determinants, but if they are close enough to a real susceptibility locus both will co-segregate within a family pedigree. The use of markers selected to be evenly spaced through the genome is now being used to search the whole genome for the identification of susceptibility loci. The power of positional cloning with anonymous markers has been confirmed in the identification of gene variants responsible for monogenic diseases with classical Mendelian inheritance. To a large extent this has been aided by the fact that monogenic conditions are usually characterized by high penetrance, low number of phenocopies, and little genetic heterogeneity, and by the availability of informative family pedigrees. In general, however, the family-based approach does not lend itself well to identification of the genetic basis of QTL and of multifactorial traits with late onset. Conditions such as hypertension and type 2 diabetes develop late in life at a time when not all family members may still be alive; moreover the inheritance pattern is generally not known. Another problem with the family-based linkage approach is that it requires making certain, and at times unverifiable, assumptions about the genetic model (e.g. gene frequency, degree of penetrance, number of phenocopies). The derived LOD scores can be very sensitive to even small changes in these assumptions.

In addition, genetic heterogeneity can become a problem as mutations in any one of several genes may result in identical phenotypes, or a chromosomal region may co-segregate with the disease in some families but not in others. Because of these issues, non-parametric allele-sharing methods have become particularly popular for the identifications of the genetic background of QTL. These approaches require no prior knowledge of the mode of inheritance of the disease, the disease allele (gene) frequencies, or the penetrance.

A commonly used non-parametric genetic mapping approach is the affected sib-pair (ASP) method based on randomly spaced polymorphic markers (usually every 5–10 cM). The basis of the ASP method is that individuals concordant for a trait (e.g. high blood pressure) would share marker alleles close to the susceptibility locus more often than would be expected by chance. As linkage is a long-range phenomenon, as few as 300–400 highly polymorphic markers may be sufficient for genome-wide mapping for a specified trait. However, this approach generally requires large numbers of ASPs to obtain sufficient power for detecting linkage for loci having relatively small effect in relation to the total familial aggregation (Gosh and Collins 1996). Many hundreds or even thousands of sib-pairs may be required to map loci of relatively small effect ($\lambda s < 4$).

To avoid the likelihood of linkage arising from random chance events, it is essential that regions of proposed linkage should reach at least the minimum LOD score of suggestive linkage for genome-wide scans (LOD score >2.2). Moreover, statistically significant replication of linkage in independent populations is essential to provide further support for a putative susceptibility locus. The localization of a QTL for a complex trait needs to be followed up by the identification of individual gene variants within the regions of significant linkage (Boerwinkle et al. 2000). Ultimately, association studies will be needed to obtain estimates of relative importance of each gene variant(s). Again, this will entail questions about biological plausibility and the pathophysiological significance of any new candidate gene variants identified by the genome-wide approach. The steps in following up a genome-wide linkage scan are summarized in Fig. 4.2.

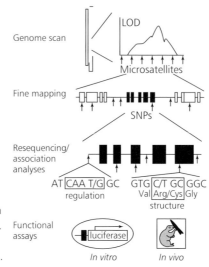

Fig. 4.2 Steps for following up a genome-wide linkage scan. Once a locus has been identified these can include fine mapping, gene re-sequencing and association studies, and functional assays. (Adapted from Boerwinkle E., Hixson J.E., Hanis C.L. (2000)).

4.2 **Blood pressure and hypertension**

Hypertension is common in the western world and is also becoming increasingly common in the developing countries. The distribution of blood pressure within a population is essentially continuous and unimodal and hence hypertension is clearly an arbitrary definition. Given its arbitrary definition, prevalence rates necessarily depend on the cut-off values used to define hypertension. Using the generally recognized definition (systolic >140 mmHg and/or diastolic >90 mmHg), prevalence rates in most industrialized countries are of the order of 10–25 per cent, and usually range from 4 per cent in young adults (18–29 years) to more than 60 per cent in those older than 80 years (Whelton 1994). The presence of chronic hypertension is important as it is associated with several complications and is a major risk factor for:

◆ stroke

◆ coronary heart disease

◆ left ventricular hypertrophy

◆ heart failure

◆ large vessel disease

◆ renal damage and renal failure

◆ retinopathy.

More generally, the higher the blood pressure the worse the severity of the complications. There is no apparent dividing line between pressures that carry a low risk and those associated with a higher risks. This is clearly illustrated by the direct association between the actual level of blood pressure and risk of stroke or coronary heart disease (MacMahon *et al.* 1990).

It has long been known that high blood pressure tends to cluster in families. This is clearly confirmed by measuring the degree of blood pressure association within family members (Ward 1990). The blood pressure correlations between parents and their biological children and those between biological sibs are much stronger when compared with those between parents and those between parents and their adopted children (Ward 1990). Moreover, there is a higher concordance of blood pressure between monozygotic twins (correlation coefficients: 0.55–0.58) compared with diazygotic twins (correlation coefficients: 0.25–0.27). Further evidence for a genetic component is supported by the fact that the risk of hypertension is much higher in individuals with one or two hypertensive parents compared with those with two normotensive parents. Overall, it has been estimated that heritability can account for about 60–70 per cent of the familial aggregation of blood pressure (Ward 1990). However, environmental factors are also important. These include demographic characteristics, ethnic origin, life-style and diet, in particular sodium and potassium intake (Beevers and MacGregor 1995, Kaplan 2002).

Despite substantial research efforts, there is still considerable debate about the patho-physiology of hypertension. Distinct causes can be traced in only a small proportion (about 5%). In these the development of hypertension is secondary to known causes (Table 4.2). In the vast majority, however, there is no apparent cause. In this case, the presence of high blood pressure is known as 'essential' or 'primary' hypertension.

The maintenance of systemic blood pressure depends on the balance between cardiac output and peripheral vascular resistance. Therefore factors that modulate cardiac output and peripheral resistance can have profound effects on blood pressure. In general, cardiac output is not raised in established essential hypertension. By contrast, it is generally agreed that high blood pressure in the majority of individuals with essential hypertension is due to an increase in peripheral resistance (Beevers and MacGregor 1995, Kaplan 2002). Many interacting mechanisms are known to influence

Table 4.2 Some secondary causes of hypertension

- Renal diseases (volume overload, activation of pressor systems)
- Vascular causes (renal artery stenosis)
- Hormonal abnormalities (phaechromocytomas)
- Drugs (contraceptive pill; liquorice)
- Pregnancy (pre-eclampsia)
- Rare familial monogenic syndromes

Secondary forms of hypertension account for <5 per cent of cases with high blood pressure.

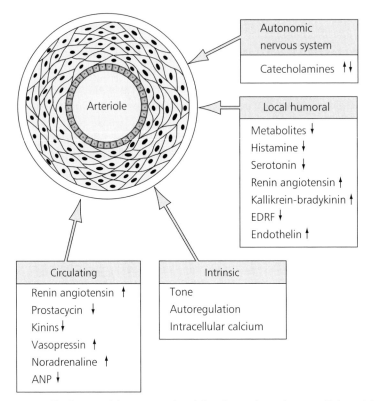

Fig. 4.3 Factors affecting arteriolar tone and peripheral vascular resistance. (Adapted from Beevers D.G. and MacGregor G. (1995)).

peripheral resistance and abnormalities in several of these have been suggested as causative mechanisms (Fig. 4.3).

Although, the presence of intrinsic defects in vascular smooth muscle contraction cannot be ruled out, there is considerable support for the view that essential hypertension may arise from a defect in renal excretion of sodium in susceptible people exposed to a high sodium intake. There is a strong link between a high sodium intake and high blood pressure. Blood pressure does not increase with age in human societies whose sodium intake is low. Furthermore the Intersalt study clearly demonstrated a positive association between increasing sodium intake and increasing blood pressure in 52 different populations (Stamler 1997). At the same time, numerous interventional studies have demonstrated that sodium restriction leads to significant reductions in blood pressure (Law *et al.* 1991).

However, it is also apparent that essential hypertension is not associated with overt sodium retention and volume overload. This has led to the hypothesis that the development of high blood pressure could be a consequence of the need to maintain sodium balance in the face of a high intake of sodium. The exact mechanisms linking a high sodium intake with the development of hypertension are still unclear. One intriguing

Table 4.3 Monogenic syndromes associated with high blood pressure

Syndrome	Gene defect/consequences
Apparent mineralocorticoid excess	Deficiency of 11-beta hydroxy steroid dehydrogenase (type 2). Allows activation of renal mineralocortocoid receptors by cortisol.
Glucocorticoid-remediable hyperaldosteronism	Hybrid gene of aldosterone synthase and 11-beta hydroxylase. High aldosterone production under ACTH control
Hypertensive forms of congenital adrenal hyperplasia	Deficiency of 11-beta hydroxylase or 17-alpha hydroxylase. Excessive synthesis of deoxycorticosterone and corticosterone.
Liddle's syndrome (pseudo-hypoaldosteronism type 1)	Several mutations within the renal epithelial sodium channel. Excessive sodium reabsorption

For further reading see Lifton *et al.* (2001) and Ferrari (2002).

hypothesis suggests that increased levels of an ouabain-like factor may provide the link between high salt intake and hypertension in genetically susceptible individuals (Beevers and MacGregor 1995). Nonetheless, the potential importance of renal sodium handling for blood pressure is now clearly highlighted by the identification of rare monogenic syndromes linked with mutations within genes important in the control of renal sodium excretion (Table 4.3). For example, the genetic defect in Liddle's syndrome leads to an overactive renal epithelial sodium channel, which in turn leads to increased sodium reabsorption and to high blood pressure. Conversely the genetic abnormalities in Bartter's and in Gilteman's syndromes, which limit the ability of the kidney to maintain sodium reabsorption, are generally associated with lower blood pressures (Simon and Lifton 1996).

4.2.1 Genetics of essential hypertension

The dissection of the molecular mechanisms underlying monogenic syndromes associated with high blood pressure (Table 4.3) has encouraged further research on the genetics of essential hypertension. Although these syndromes are extremely rare even in those referred for secondary hypertension, it is also likely that they may be under-diagnosed in the general population.

The recognition that these rare conditions are associated with defects in the control of sodium balance has led to renewed interest in the importance of genes involved in the control of sodium excretion as candidate genes for essential hypertension. This has raised the possibility of the existence of common variants in these genes displaying more moderate effects. Such effects, although small, could be amplified in the presence

Table 4.4 Selected candidate genes for essential hypertension

Renin–angiotensin–aldosterone system
Angiotensinogen
Renin
Angiotensin converting enzyme
Angiotensin 2 receptor
Aldosterone synthase
Atrial natriuretic peptides and
Natriuretic peptide receptors
Epithelial sodium channel
Intracellular modulators of sodium transport
Adducin
G protein beta3 subunit
Mediators of vascular and endothelial function
ENOS
Endothelin
Beta adrenergic receptors

For further reading on candidate genes for hypertension see, Siffert (1998), Manunta *et al.* (1998), Corvol *et al.* (1999), Lifton *et al.* (2001), Melander (2001) and Luft (2002).

of a consistently long-term exposure to a high salt diet thereby leading to the development of high blood pressure.

The majority of studies to date using candidate genes have relied on examining possible associations between variants in selected genes and essential hypertension in case–control designs, or in population-based studies. Selected candidate genes have included those important in the control of renal sodium excretion and those believed to be important modulators of smooth muscle function (Table 4.4). In general, however, the contribution of most of these investigations to our understanding of hypertension and its genetic determinants has been modest. A major problem has been a lack of replication. To some extent this lack of replication is probably due to (i) differences in selection criteria for the cases and the controls; (ii) inadequate power to detect small effects; and (iii) the presence of variable degree of linkage disequilibrium between candidate alleles. Some of the problems and achievements of research with candidate genes for essential hypertension can be illustrated with reference to two promising candidate genes, namely the angiotensinogen gene and the genes coding for the epithelial sodium channel.

4.2.2 The angiotensinogen gene and essential hypertension

The renin–angiotensin–aldosterone system is of fundamental importance in the control of sodium balance and of cardiovascular homeostasis. Although this system is an important component of the control of sodium balance and thereby of blood pressure in response to changes in sodium intake, raised levels of the components of the system are not usually associated with essential hypertension. Indeed, plasma renin activity is low in a substantial proportion of individuals with essential hypertension. Nevertheless, there is evidence suggesting that raised levels of angiotensinogen (ANG) may be important in the development of high blood pressure, in subgroups at least, of individuals with essential hypertension.

Angiotensinogen is the immediate precursor of angiotensin I and hence a key factor in the activity of the renin–angiotensin–aldosterone system. The potential importance of ANG is underscored by the observation of (i) a strong correlation between plasma ANG and blood pressure; (ii) plasma levels of ANG appear to co-segregate within families and offsprings of hypertensive individuals have raised levels of plasma ANG; and (iii) positive linkage between the ANG gene locus (or a nearby region) and hypertension (Corvol et al. 1999). This is supported by experimental work in trangenic animals demonstrating that ANG gene over-expression is associated with higher blood pressures; moreover in these animals, the blood pressure achieved was related to the number of ANG gene copies over-expressed (Kim et al. 1995).

The human ANG gene is relatively large and examination of the gene sequence in different individuals has revealed several polymorphisms. Importantly, one of these variants located in exon 2 (M235T) is associated with raised plasma levels of ANG. However, this polymorphism does not alter the affinity of ANG for renin. As increased levels could be due to increased expression, further work led to the identification of another variant, A(-6), located within the promotor region of the ANG gene. Functional analysis demonstrated that this variant increases the transcription rate of ANG. The A(-6) variant is in tight linkage disequilibrium with the 235T allele, and this seems to account for the increased expression in those with the 235T allele (Corvol et al. 1999, Jeunemaitre et al. 1999).

A large number of studies have reported a positive association between the M235T polymorphism and hypertension, but there has been some controversy as to the magnitude of the effect. Kunz et al. (1997) carried out a meta-analysis on the association between the M235T polymorphism and essential hypertension in white people. The results were consistent with a weak but statistically significant association (pooled odds ratio (OR) of 1.2 with a 95% CI of 1.1–1.29). However, the association appeared to be stronger in the presence of a positive family history of hypertension. The impact at the population level depends not only on the OR but also on the frequency of the risk factor. Assuming a causative link for the 235T (or the A(-6) allele) with an allele frequency of 0.42 in white people, an OR of 1.2 translates into a modest population attributable risk of 8 per cent. The research work on the ANG gene demonstrates that a single gene can contribute to hypertension even though the effect is relatively small. It also highlights the importance of linkage disequilibrium and cautions against making inferential conclusions about causality based on association studies involving single polymorphic variants.

4.2.3 The epithelial Na⁺ channel and hypertension in blacks

The principal pathways and disorders altering renal sodium reabsorption are illustrated in Fig. 4.4. The renal epithelial sodium channel, located within the collecting duct, accounts for only a small proportion of renal sodium reabsorption (~5%). Nevertheless it is one of the most important sodium transport mechanisms in the overall control of sodium balance, being responsible for the final adjustments in the amount of sodium excreted. The potential importance of abnormal renal tubular sodium reabsorption as a determinant of sodium balance and blood pressure has been highlighted by genetic studies of renal sodium transporters in rare familial conditions such as Liddle's syndrome (Fig 4.5; Lifton *et al.* 2001).

Liddle's syndrome is an autosomal dominant form of hypertension characterized by hypokalemia and suppressed plasma renin and aldosterone. It had long been known that hypertension in individuals with Liddle's syndrome is sensitive to a low sodium diet, and to treatment with the sodium channel inhibitor amiloride. This, in conjunction with the observation that hypertension could be 'cured' by kidney transplant, led to the hypothesis that this syndrome was due to increased activity of the renal epithelial

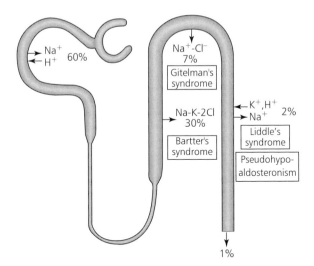

Fig. 4.4 The principal pathways and disorders altering renal sodium reabsorption. Plasma is filtered at the glomerulus, and sodium is reabsorbed as the filtrate passes along the nephron. The sites of sodium reabsorption and the proportion of sodium reabsorption usually occurring at each site are shown. The principal components are: Na⁺–H⁺ exchange in the proximal tubule; Na–K–2Cl co-transport in the ascending loop of Henle; Na–Cl co-transport in the distal convoluted tubule; electrogenic sodium reabsorption via the epithelial sodium channel which is composed of by at least three different subunits. Disorders resulting from single gene defects affecting specific components of the system are shown in the boxes. (Adapted from Simon D.B., Karet F.E., Hamdan J.M., Di Pietro A., Sanjad S.A., and Lifton R.P. (1996)).

sodium channel in the distal nephron. A specific genetic basis for this condition was suggested by the observation of a strong linkage to a site on chromosome 16 close to the genes coding for the beta and gamma subunits of the epithelial sodium channel. At the molecular level, this channel consists of three subunits and the gene for the alpha subunit is located on chromosome 12. Subsequently, analysis of DNA sequences of the three subunits from affected individuals led to the identification of mutations located in the cytosolic carboxy-terminal part of the ß-subunit of the epithelial sodium channel in families with Liddle's syndrome (Lifton *et al.* 2001).

Several mutations have now been described in Liddle's pedigrees. Some are in the ß-subunit while others have been found in the γ-subunit (Hansson 1995). The presence of these mutations leads to a reduction in intracellular turn-over of the sodium channel and to an increase in the number of active channels exposed at the apical membrane. The overall effect of these mutations is to increase sodium channel activity thereby reducing the amount of sodium excreted by the kidney. In turn this leads to the volume-dependent hypertension characteristic of Liddle's syndrome.

The hormonal features of Liddle's syndrome, low plasma renin and low/normal aldosterone, have also been described in a subset of hypertensive patients, especially those of black African origin. Hypertension is common in blacks living within industrial-based societies, and especially in African Americans in the USA (Burt *et al.* 1995). Blacks have suppressed plasma renin activity and angiotensin II levels compared with whites and, in general, black hypertensives are more responsive to salt restriction and to diuretic therapy (Sagnella 2001). These observations suggested the possibility that other mutations in subunits of the epithelial sodium channel, possibly leading to less drastic disruption of channel activity, could provide a genetic basis for high blood pressure in subgroups of black people. Several variants are known within the genes coding for the epithelial sodium channel, and some of these are much more common in black people than in white people. The T594M polymorphism within the sodium channel ß-subunit is of particular relevance in blacks. This polymorphism is extremely rare in whites but the frequency of the 594M mutation is about 5 per cent in blacks. One study in blacks living in London found that this variant was significantly higher in black subjects with essential hypertension (8.3% in hypertensive blacks compared with 2.1% in normotensive blacks; Baker *et al.* 1998). An association with increasing blood pressure was also found in a population-based study of black people (Dong *et al.* 2001). This polymorphism affects the regulatory carboxy-terminal region of the sodium channel ß-subunit, and could influence channel activity leading to an increase in sodium reabsorption and thereby to an increase in blood pressure. This possibility is reinforced by a recent study which demonstrated that the sodium channel inhibitor amiloride alone effectively controlled blood pressure in black hypertensives with the T594M polymorphism (Baker *et al.* 2002).

However, despite the possibility that the presence of the T549M polymorphism may be a major secondary cause of hypertension in about 5 per cent of black

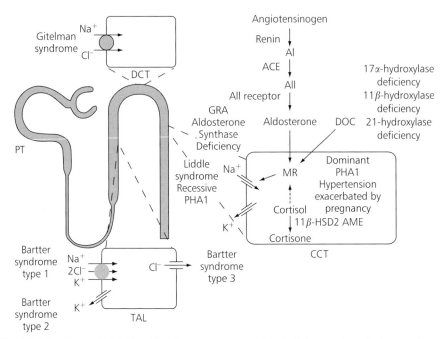

Fig. 4.5 Mutations which affect blood pressure in man. On the left a nephron is shown. The molecular pathways mediating sodium reabsorption in the thick ascending limb of the loop of Henle (TAL), the distal convoluted tubule (DCT), and the cortical collecting tubule (CCT) are shown. The renin–angiotensin system, the major regulator of renal salt reabsorption, is also illustrated. Inherited diseases affecting these pathways are indicated. Abbreviations: AI angiotensin, I., ACE angiotensin converting enzyme, AII angiotensin II, MR mineralocorticoid receptor, GRA glucocorticoid-remediable aldosteronism, PHA1 pseudohypoaldosteronism type 1, AME apparent mineralocorticoid excess, 11 βHSD2 11β-hydroxysteroid dehydrogenase-2, DOC deoxycorticosterone, PT proximal tubule. (Adapted from Lifton, R.P., Gharavi, A.G., and Geller, D.S. (2001) Molecular mechanisms of human hypertension. *Cell*, 104, 545–56.

hypertensives, this particular mutation cannot provide a basis for the high blood pressure in the remaining and much larger proportion of black hypertensives or in white hypertensives.

4.2.4 Genome-wide scans for blood pressure QTL and for essential hypertension

In view of the realization that single genes may have relatively small effects there is now increasing interest in the influence of variation in multiple genes (haplotypes) as determinants of high blood pressure. More importantly, over the past few years several groups have completed genome-wide scans to identify chromosomal regions harbouring genes likely to influence blood pressure.

Two studies were based on the discordant sib-pair approach. Using a highly discordant sib-pair design, Kruskal *et al.* (1999) reported suggestive linkage with blood pressure on chromosome 2p, 5q, 6q, and 15q. Xu *et al.* (1999*a*) in a Chinese population also examined discordant sib-pairs. Although no regions achieved a LOD score >3, suggestive linkage (maximum LOD scores >2) was achieved on chromosomes 3, 11, 15, 16, and 17. The region on chromosome 15q was promising as by refining the trait definition and genotyping additional markers, in a subsequent study significant linkage with a maximum LOD score of 3.77 was detected near D15S203 in sibling pairs with lower extreme diastolic blood pressure. This was marginally replicated (Xu *et al.* 1999*b*) in a second independent data set from the same geographical area, suggesting that this locus may be involved in the regulation of diastolic blood pressure.

Several other studies have used family-based resources and/or affected sib-pairs with essential hypertension (Table 4.5). A number of points are apparent from these studies. Linkage has been observed on several chromosomes. However, few regions gave strong linkage signals and at best most can be classified as suggestive of linkage. Although, overall, there appears little agreement amongst the different studies, nonetheless some regions have been replicated in different studies. Strong linkage (LOD score >4) with systolic blood pressure has been reported for chromosome region 17q (Baima *et al.* 1999). Evidence for linkage between this blood pressure QTL has also been found in French/UK hypertensive sib-pairs (Julier *et al.* 1997). In addition, this region has been reported to be linked in several families with a rare form of hypertension (pseudohypoaldosteronism type IIB; or Gordon's syndrome) characterized by hyperkalaemia and normal renal glomerular filtration rate (Mansfield *et al.* 1997, O'Shaughnessy *et al.* 1998).

Moreover, there is evidence that linkage zones may be population-dependent. For instance, Kristjansson *et al.* (2002) examined 120 extended Icelandic families with 490

Table 4.5 Chromosomal regions linked with blood pressure QTL and hypertension from recent genome-wide scans

Author	Population	Chromosome(s)
Rice *et al.* (2000)	Quebec Family Study	1p, 2p, 5p, 7q, 8q, 19p
Hsueh *et al.* (2000)	Old Order Amish families	2q31
Levy *et al.* (2000)	Framingham Heart Study	17, 18
Perola *et al.* (2000)	Finnish affect sib-pairs	2q, 3q21, 22q, Xp
Sharma *et al.* (2000)	UK Affected sib-pairs	11q
Atwood *et al.* (2001)	Mexican Americans	2, 8, 18, 21
Allayee *et al.* (2001)	Dutch dyslipidemic families	4p
Zhu *et al.* (2001)	Chinese Affected sib-pairs	2q14
Rice *et al.* (2002)	HERITAGE Family Study	2p, 3p, 12q
Kristjanson (2002)	Icelandic affected sib-pairs	18q
Hunt *et al.* (2002)	NHLBI Family Study	1, 6, 7, 12, 15

individuals with essential hypertension and confirmed suggestive linkage on chromosomes 2, 11, and 17. More interestingly they identified strong linkage on chromosome 18. Pankow *et al.* (2000) also mapped chromosome 18q as a QTL for postural blood pressure response, and Destefano *et al.* (1998) identified chromosome 18 in autosomal dominant orthostatic hypotension suggesting that this region may accommodate genes involved in the regulation of blood pressure.

None of these regions however overlap with those reported by Hunt *et al.* (2002) who carried out genome scans for hypertension and blood pressure based on 2959 individuals in 500 white families from the NHL and Blood Institute Family Heart study. Five regions with suggestive linkage to hypertension were identified; these include chromosomes 1, 7, 12, and 15 (Table 4.5) but only chromosome 6 displayed linkage with blood pressure with a LOD score >3.0. They concluded that promising linkage with hypertension appeared to be mainly on chromosomes 1 and 6. Linkage on chromosome 1 is of particular interest as this region contains potentially relevant candidate genes, and in particular the gene for ANG.

In another recent whole genome scan, Rice *et al.* (2002) searched for genomic regions likely to influence systolic and diastolic blood pressure in white Americans and in African Americans. A genome-wide scan was conducted on 317 black individuals from 114 families, and 519 white individuals from 99 families using a multipoint variance-components linkage model and a panel of 509 markers. Promising results were primarily, but not exclusively, found in the black families. Linkage evidence with baseline systolic blood pressure was observed on 2p14, 3p26.3, and 12q21.33, and provided new evidence on 3q28, 11q21, and 19p12. This study clearly provides promising leads for further investigation of genetic determinants of high blood pressure. Of note, the region on 2p14 replicates at least three other studies (Kruskal *et al.* 1999, Rice *et al.* 2000, Atwood *et al.* 2001).

The blood pressure QTL on chromosome 2q31 is also of interest because of its close proximity to a locus for primary pulmonary hypertension, a very rare condition (Morse *et al.* 1997). The locus for this condition has not been cloned yet, but the region contains genes that could influence vascular wall function such as parathyroid receptor 2 and insulin growth factor binding proteins 2 and 5 (Hsueh *et al.* 2000).

These results are of considerable interest and provide a basis for future work. But it is also clear that there is considerable genetic heterogeneity. The heterogeneity observed in whole genome scans may arise from differences in study design in relation to phenotype, in that some examined blood pressure as a QTL and others were based on affected hypertensive sib-pairs. Although weak linkage may arise from purely random chance, some regions such as those on chromosome 2, chromosome 6, chromosome 17, and chromosome 18 appear promising. The hunt is now on to identify specific gene variants within these regions, but whether any of these will turn out to be important new candidate genes for essential hypertension remains to be seen.

4.3 **Hyperglycaemia and diabetes mellitus**

Diabetes mellitus has become a major health problem worldwide. Collectively, it is one of the most common chronic diseases afflicting up to 5–10 per cent of individuals in the Western world. Globally, about 125 million people are currently affected and it has been projected that by the year 2010, the number of persons with diabetes will double although most of the increase will result from changing demographic trends, especially in the developing countries (Day 2001). Although the symptoms of overt diabetes are well recognized, mild hyperglycaemia, and dyslipedaemia may be present in the absence of significant symptoms. This leads to a number of complications developing over a long-term period and typically include:

- microangiopathy
- retinopathy
- nephropathy
- neuropathy.

The development of atheroscerosis and microvascular complications underscore the importance of diabetes as a major risk factor for cardiovascular disease and stroke. In addition, hyperglycaemia in the acute phase of stroke may exacerbate the degree of ischaemic damage. The presence of the chronic hyperglycaemia makes a major contribution to the development of such a diversity of micro- and macrovascular damage. The damaging effects of chronic hyperglycaemia appear to be mediated primarily by the associated increase in advanced glycation-end-products (AGE). Advanced glycation of proteins can alter the normal function of intracellular proteins. Modified extracellular matrix proteins can interact abnormally with other matrix components and with cellular receptors for matrix proteins (intergrins). Plasma proteins modified by AGE precursors bind to AGE receptors on endothelial cells, mesangial cells, and macrophages, inducing receptor-mediated overproduction of damaging oxygen free radicals. Moreover, the presence of AGE modified proteins also activates the pleiotropic transcription factor NF-κB leading to pathological changes in gene expression (Brownlee 2001).

Diabetes mellitus is a heterogeneous clinical disorder with numerous causes, however the measurement of plasma glucose is of fundamental importance in the diagnosis of diabetes (Lamb and Day 2000). On the basis of observed clinical and biochemical phenotype, several aetiological forms of diabetes are recognized (Table 4.6). This classification takes into account of the different aetiological mechanisms which lead to hyperglycaemia. For instance, secondary diabetes can arise from any pathological process that damages pancreatic beta-cells leading to a reduction in insulin secretion. In addition, diabetes mellitus can also develop from any process which impairs the cellular response to insulin leading to a state of insulin resistance. Primary diabetes, further classified into type 1 or 2 diabetes, however, accounts for the vast majority of cases (>90%).

Table 4.6 Aetiological classification of diabetes mellitus

Type 1
(beta-cell destruction, usually leading to absolute insulin deficiency)
    Autoimmune
    Idiopathic

Type 2
(may range from predominantly insulin resistance with
relative insulin deficiency to a predominantly secretory defect
with or without insulin resistance)

Other specific types
    Genetic defects in beta-cell function
    Genetic defects in insulin action
    Diseases of the exocrine pancreas
    Endocrinopathies
    Drug- or chemical-induced
    Infections
    Uncommon forms of immune-mediated diabetes
    Other genetic syndromes sometimes associated with diabetes

Gestational diabetes

From: World Health Organization. Definition, diagnosis and classification of diabetes mellitus and its complications: Report of a WHO consultation. Part 1: Diagnosis and classification of Diabetes Mellitus. Geneva: World Health Organization, 1999.

Type 1 diabetes most often manifests in childhood (hence previously known as juvenile onset diabetes) and describes the majority of cases where the basic pathology involves pancreatic beta-cell destruction as a consequence of an autoimmune process. This eventually leads to insulin deficiency, and the associated ketoacidosis, coma and death in the absence of insulin replacement. The presence of an autoimmune condition is confirmed by the presence of anti-GAD, islet cells or insulin antibodies (Atkinson and Eisnbarth 2001).

By contrast type 2—the more common form of diabetes—accounting for about 90 per cent of all cases, is characterized by either a diminished insulin secretion (i.e. an islet defect), or an increase in resistance to the actions of insulin (decreased peripheral glucose uptake in insulin-sensitive tissues or increased hepatic glucose output). Type 2 diabetes generally—but not always—manifests after 40 years of age; it is characterized by milder hyperglycaemia and rarely leads to ketoacidosis and seems to be consequent to a genetic predisposition that causes a variable expression of insulin resistance and insulin deficiency.

4.3.1 Genetic basis of diabetes mellitus

Plasma levels of glucose are kept within normal limits by a multiplicity of mechanisms. Insulin is of fundamental importance in the maintenance of glucose homeostasis. Insulin increases glucose transport at insulin-sensitive tissues, mainly muscle and adipose tissue. Insulin also inhibits glucose production by the liver, lipolysis in adipose tissue, and proteolysis in muscle. At the same time it promotes synthesis of glycogen and triglycerides by the liver and inhibits liver ketogenesis. Not surprisingly, lack of insulin and/or resistance to the actions of insulin leads not only to abnormalities of carbohydrate metabolism, but also of lipid and protein metabolism.

The metabolic actions of insulin at the cellular level depend on its interaction with the insulin receptor at the cellular membrane. The binding of insulin to its receptor activates a cascade of intracellular biochemical events which mediate the various effects of insulin (Saltiel and Kahn 2001). Molecular variation in the insulin receptor therefore is clearly potentially relevant for insulin resistance. This is supported by the identification of genetically determined abnormalities in the insulin receptor in very rare and unusual cases of diabetes. Metabolic abnormalities associated with mutations of the insulin receptor range from hyperinsulinaemia to moderate hyperglycaemia to overt symptomatic diabetes. Some mutations in the insulin receptor are associated with Leprechaunism and Rabson–Mendenhal syndromes. These paediatric syndromes display extreme forms of insulin resistance. Other affected individuals have acanthosis nigricans and women may have virilization and enlarged cystic ovaries.

Several forms of diabetic states associated with monogenic defects in pancreatic beta-cell function leading to impairment in insulin secretion, but with minimal or no defect in insulin action, are also known. These are usually autosomal dominant, highly penetrant, and are frequently characterized by early onset of mild hyperglycemia before 25 years of age. Genetic analysis of these conditions collectively known as maturity onset diabetes of the young (MODY) has demonstrated a number of mutations in a variety of genes (Hattersley 1998).

One of the first variants to be identified was in the gene for the enzyme glucokinase (MODY2). This was an obvious candidate gene as glucokinase had been identified as a crucial glucose sensor—controlling the rate of glucose metabolism—in both the pancreatic beta-cell and the liver hepatocyte. Because of the defect in the glucokinase gene, higher levels of glucose are necessary to elicit normal insulin secretion. The other four MODY genes encode transcription factors—proteins that regulate the activity of other genes. These play a critical role in the development of the beta-cells and thereby in the regulation of insulin secretion. For instance, MODY4 is associated with a gene variant in the transcription factor IPF-1; in its homozygous form it leads to total pancreatic agenesis (Stoffers et al. 1997). Other gene defects affecting beta-cell function arise from point mutations in mitochondrial DNA, and are often associated with other phenotypic abnormalities such as deafness and have a maternal mode of inheritance (Maassen and Kadawaki 1996).

These conditions possibly account for 5–10 per cent of all those with diabetes and clearly do not provide a basis for the genetic background of the common forms of diabetes mellitus. Although both types 1 and 2 diabetes have a strong genetic component, their aetiology is fundamentally different, and different genes are likely to be involved. Moreover environmental background is also an important aetiological factor in the development of types 1 and of 2 diabetes.

4.3.2 Type 1 diabetes mellitus

The incidence of type 1 diabetes varies widely across the world and amongst different ethnic groups ranging from the lowest rates of 0.1/100,000 in rural China, to more than 40/100,000 per year, representing more than a 400-fold variation. In the West, the prevalence of type 1 diabetes is about 0.3 per cent and unlike many other auto-immune diseases it has no gender preference (Karvonen *et al.* 2000, Atkinson and Eisnbarth 2001).

Genetic susceptibility is a major risk factor for type 1 diabetes. However, it is also recognized that a large number of cases with type 1 diabetes appear to be sporadic and have no family history. In most Caucasian populations, the risk to the sibling of an affected individual is of the order of 5–10 per cent and this is about 15-fold compared with the prevalence in the general population. Type 1 diabetes exhibits 30–50 per cent concordance in monozygotic twins, compared with 5–27 per cent in dizygotic twins (5–27%), suggesting that the disorder is dependent on environmental factors as well as genetic susceptibility (Kumar *et al.* 1993, Kyvik *et al.* 1995).

Despite much research, no environmental agent(s) responsible for triggering type 1 diabetes have been uncovered. Nonetheless, several are suspected (Atkinson and Eisenbarth 2001). These include viral infections (e.g. coxsackie virus and cytomegalovirus), early infant diet (e.g. breast feeding versus early introduction of cow's milk components), and toxins (e.g. N-nitroso derivatives). However, it is proved difficult to confirm the importance of these agents in the development of type 1 diabetes. One major difficulty is that the pathological process leading to insulin deficiency may predate clinical presentation by many years.

Although the exact role of environmental agents remains to be established, genes for type 1 diabetes provide both susceptibility towards to, and protection from, the disease. The most important genes identified to date for type 1 diabetes are located within the major histocompatibility complex (MHC) HLA class II region on chromosome 6p21 (She 1996, Atkinson and Eisenbarth 2001). This region, formally termed IDDMl, contains at least three genetic loci (HLA-DR, HL-DQ and HLA-DP). These are highly polymorphic and the genes encode MHC type II glycoproteins. The function of these genes in terms of an immune response is well known (i.e. presentation of antigenic peptides to T lymphocytes), yet their specific contribution to the pathogenesis of type 1 diabetes remains unclear. Only certain MHC variants can bind fragments from beta-cell proteins, so an autoimmune reaction against those proteins will occur only in those people whose genes encode such variants.

The importance of the class II haplotypes depends not only on the well-known risk for disease associated with HLA-DR3 and HLA-DR4, but also on additional susceptibility associated with DQ-chains and DQß-chains. Type 1 diabetes seems atypical among autoimmune diseases in that in addition to inducing susceptibility, certain MHC haplotypes provide significant protection (e.g. HLA-DR2 alleles), with protection dominant over susceptibility (Atkinson and Eisenbarth 2001). Several studies also suggest that differences in distribution of these alleles may account to some extent for differences in the prevalence of type 1 diabetes in different populations. This is demonstrated by several investigations on the association between selected HLA alleles and type 1 diabetes in different populations (Dorman *et al.* 1990, Park *et al.* 2000).

Although the HLA component has a major genetic impact on the development of diabetes accounting for possibly 25–45 per cent of type 1 diabetes, it is clear that the MHC genes are not the only determinants of disease. Fifty five per cent of the general population also carries the risk haplotypes, but only 0.4 per cent of the population develops type 1 diabetes.

Type 1 diabetes represents a heterogeneous and polygenic disorder, and a number (about 20) of non-HLA loci contributing to disease susceptibility have been suggested. One obvious candidate was the insulin gene itself. In the mid-1980s, it had been suggested that there was a type 1 diabetes locus close to the insulin gene. This locus (also known as IDDM2) on chromosome 11p5.5 contributes about 10 per cent towards susceptibility to type 1 diabetes. The IDDM2 locus contains a polymorphic region in the 5' flanking region of the insulin gene (INS) consisting of a variable number of tandemly repeated (VNTR) 14-base-pair sequences. This polymorphism has been found to be associated with type 1 diabetes in several populations (She and Marron 1998, Atkinson and Eisenbarth 2001).

In Europeans, there are two main categories of VNTR alleles: those with fewer than 50 repeats (short class I VNTR), and those with more than 200 repeats (longer class III alleles). People with only the low number repeats, and the necessary MHC polymorphisms, are more likely to have type 1 diabetes while the longer class III alleles provides a dominant protective effect. Carrying a protective allele seems to provide at least 50 per cent protection from the disease. The variability in the length of the repeat is important in the way autoimmunity arises or is prevented. The VNTR polymorphism plays a role in regulating the expression of the insulin gene in the thymus. The long alleles (class III VNTRs) seem to be associated with increased thymic expression and decreased pancreatic expression of insulin (She and Marron 1998). Such increased expression of insulin in the thymus may lead to deletion of autoreactive T-cells or to the generation of a suppressor population, while the short alleles with lower levels of thymic expression may be less efficient in deletion of autoreactive cells. Thus, the long VNTR may offer protection against autoimmunity by stimulating insulin expression in the thymus and increasing the body's awareness that insulin is one of its own proteins.

Although around 20 other loci have been suggested, linkage data implicating these other disease susceptibility loci for type I diabetes are conflicting. This is likely due to

(1) the limited power for detection of additional susceptibility loci of relatively small effects; (2) factors such as genetic heterogeneity between populations; and (3) potential gene–gene and gene–environment interactions. To circumvent some of these problems, the European Consortium for IDDM Genome Studies (Nerup and Pociot 2001) conducted a genome-wide linkage analysis for type I diabetes mellitus-susceptibility loci in 408 multiplex families from Scandinavia, a population expected to be homogeneous for genetic and environmental factors. In addition to verifying the HLA and INS susceptibility loci, this study confirmed an additional locus on chromosome 6q21. Suggestive evidence of additional susceptibility loci was found on chromosome 2p, 5q, and 16p. For some loci, the support for linkage increased substantially when families were stratified on the basis of HLA or INS genotypes. These data support both the existence of non-HLA genes of significance for type I diabetes mellitus, and the interaction between HLA and non-HLA loci in the determination of the type I diabetes mellitus phenotype.

In order to increase the power to identify loci with relatively small effects, Cox *et al.* (2001) reported a genome scan using a new collection of 225 multiplex families with type I diabetes combined with the data from previous genome-wide investigations. Three chromosomal regions were identified which showed significant evidence of linkage with LOD scores greater than 4. Two of these coincided with the well-established regions, the HLA region (IDDM1 at 6p21), and the INS locus (IDDM2 at 11p15). A third region, which also displayed strong linkage, was on chromosome 16 at 16q22–q24. Several other regions showing suggestive evidence of linkage with LOD scores >2.2, were on chromosomes 10 (10p11), 2(2q31), 6 (6q21), and 1 (1q42).

Taken together these results clearly demonstrate that several loci scattered throughout the genome provide genetic susceptibility for type 1 diabetes. However, these are overshadowed by the major genetic components residing on chromosome 6 (HLA complex NIDDM1 locus) and chromosome 11 (INS gene VNTR polymorphism locus). These two account for up to 50–60 per cent of the genetic contribution; the NIDDM1 locus alone is estimated to account for 30–50 per cent of the siblings' recurrence risk for type 1 diabetes (Mein *et al.* 1998, She and Marron 1998).

4.3.3 Type 2 diabetes mellitus

Type 2 diabetes is the more common form of diabetes mellitus, accounting for 80–90 per cent of all diabetes in most countries. The actual prevalence is difficult to determine due to the mild onset of the disease in some individuals leading to a high proportion of undiagnosed cases. It is likely that type 2 diabetes is present in about 3–5 per cent of the Western population aged 20, and possibly an additional 4–11 per cent have impaired glucose tolerance (Day 2001). However there is a wide range in different populations, and to some extent this reflects the diversity of genetic background and differences in environmental risk factors among the different populations.

This is clearly illustrated by epidemiological studies that have examined the prevalence of type 2 diabetes in different populations.

Prevalence rates of type 2 diabetes range from low levels of less than 0.1 per cent among Eskimos, Japanese, Chinese, and Indonesians living in their original or rural environments, to the extremely high prevalences of nearly 50 per cent in the North American Pima Indians (Day 2001). To some extent, apart from genetic differences intrinsic in the different populations, the higher rates in North American Indians seem to be due to the their recent changes in life-style and diet and in particular a high energy intake coupled with low physical activity. This view is further supported by longitudinal observation of the development of type 2 diabetes in the two major populations of Samoans in the western Pacific. Over recent years, the prevalence of diabetes increased markedly in both the rural and urban Samoan populations, but the higher rates in the more urban populations suggest a major contribution from the changing environment (Hodge *et al.* 1994). Diabetes is now an increasingly important problem in populations shifting from a rural to an urban-based life style, and in particular in people of Asian or of African origin (Day 2001). Collectively, these observations indicate that apart from genetic factors, age, obesity, increase in abdominal fat, lack of physical exercise, and ethnic origin are also important in the development of type 2 diabetes.

Unlike patients with type 1 diabetes, those with type 2 have detectable levels of circulating insulin indicating that these individuals are resistant to the action of insulin. In the progression from impaired glucose tolerance to diabetes mellitus the level of insulin declines indicating that patients with NIDDM have decreased insulin secretion. However, there is still controversy about the relative importance of insulin resistance against impaired insulin secretion (Gerich 1998). In fact there is evidence suggesting that insulin resistance may be largely an acquired problem, as life-style changes such as exercise and weight reduction which reduce insulin resistance or increase insulin sensitivity have major beneficial effects in people with type 2 diabetes (Gerich 1998).

A strong argument for the importance of genetic factors in the development of type 2 diabetes comes from twin studies, family studies, and investigations of different ethnic groups living in the same environment. Type 2 diabetes shows familial aggregation in all populations investigated. The prevalence of type 2 diabetes is higher among offspring when either or both of their parents have diabetes (Weijnen *et al.* 2002). The concordance rate for Type 2 diabetes in older monozygotic twins can reach more than 80 per cent in some populations (Kaprio *et al.* 1992, Matsuda and Kuzuya 1994, Medici *et al.* 1999, Poulsen *et al.* 1999); these rates are much higher than the concordance rates seen in non-identical twins, but the relative risk to siblings (λs) is much less than that for type 1 diabetes (3.5 vs 15, respectively) (Rich 1990, Kahn *et al.* 1996). Other evidence for genetic components in the development of type 2 diabetes derives from studies of populations of mixed heritage, where the founding populations have different risks of developing the disease. Genetically-admixed groups having native American ancestry, such as Mexican Americans, have been shown to have rates of diabetes that are proportional to the degree of American Indian ancestry (Gardner *et al.* 1984).

A large number of genes involved in insulin secretion, insulin action, and in particular those involved in glucose homeostasis and adipose tissue metabolism have been examined as potential candidate genes for susceptibility for type 2 diabetes but the majority of these studies have not been able to identify consistent associations with type 2 diabetes (Kahn *et al.* 1996, Elbein 1997, Busch and Hegele 2001). Moreover, there has also been considerable interest in genes known to be associated with rare genetic forms of diabetes, specifically the insulin receptor substrate and nuclear transcription factors, but again no major genetic determinant have been identified for type 2 diabetes (Almind *et al.* 1998, Baier *et al.* 2000).

This aside, recent research on the insulin promoter factor-1 (IPF-1) and the peroxisome proliferator-activated receptor-γ (PPARγ) is of particular interest. The homeodomain-containing protein, IPF-1 (also known as STF1, IDX1, and PDX1), is a transcription factor critically required for the embryonic development of the pancreas and for the transcriptional regulation of endocrine pancreas-specific genes in adults, such as insulin, glucose transporter-2 (GLUT2) and glucokinase in ß-cells, and somatostatin in δ-cells (Habener and Stoffers 1998). Homozygosity for a base deletion mutation in IPF-1 was reported to cause pancreatic agenesis in a child and individuals who are heterozygous carriers of this mutation develop a rare form of MODY (Stoffers *et al.* 1997). Recently, Hani *et al.* (1999) described three common novel variants in the IPF-1 gene and found that these mutations were found in up to 6.2 per cent of French families with late-onset type 2 diabetes. These authors also provide evidence that, depending on the mutation impairing effect, IPF-1 mutations were associated with diabetes either through a monogenic-like mode of inheritance or in a polygenic context of disease susceptibility.

PPARγ is a member of the nuclear hormone receptor family. It is found in the nucleus of many cells and adipose cells in particular. PPARγ is a target for thiazolidinedione drugs, a relatively new class of drugs used to increase the sensitivity of the body to insulin. PPARγ is also a transcription factor and, when activated, binds to another transcription factor known as the retinoid X receptor (Kersten 2002). In turn this leads to increased transcription of specific genes whose products are important determinants of insulin response. Barroso *et al.* (1999) reported two loss-of-function mutations in the PPARγ that were associated with severe insulin resistance and type 2 diabetes. Although it is still unclear how impaired PPARγ signalling can affect the sensitivity of the body to insulin this work highlight the importance of variation in intracellular signalling mechanisms as potential determinants of insulin action. In this context the identification of a common PPARγ polymorphism associated with the development of diabetes is of interest. This particular polymorphism (Pro12Ala) is very common (frequency of the Pro allele = 83–87%), and several investigations have confirmed its association with type 2 diabetes. Although the estimated individual risk is relatively small with a relative risk of 1.25, its high frequency suggests that it can influence up to 25 per cent of the general European population (Altshuler *et al.* 2000).

4.3.4 Genome-wide scans for type 2 diabetes

Several genome-wide scans for type 2 diabetes have relied mainly on family-based linkage and the affected sib-pair approach. Evidence for significant linkage with the type 2 diabetes phenotype has been found on several chromosomal regions. A genome-wide scans in four American populations pointed to suggestive linkage to type 2 diabetes mellitus or impaired glucose homeostasis on chromosomes 5, 12, and X in whites, on chromosome 3 in Mexican Americans, and chromosome 10 in Afro-Americans (Ehm *et al.* 2000). In contrast Luo *et al.* (2001), in an eastern and south eastern Chinese Han population, found two loci in a region on chromosome 9 with suggestive evidence for linkage to type 2 diabetes.

Two more genome-wide scans for type 2 diabetes, one from the United Kingdom and one from Finland have also been reported recently. As in the previous reports, both studies also observed several regions linked with type 2 diabetes (Table 4.7). In the UK population, Wiltshire *et al.* (2001) found strong evidence for linkage on chromosome 8p, 10q, and 5q. This confirms previous reports of linkage to these regions in European populations. Additionally, this study demonstrated evidence for linkage on chromosome 1q24–25; linkage to this region has also been found in Utah, French and Pima families (Wiltshire *et al.* 2001). By contrast, the genome-wide data from the Finnish families (Lindgren *et al.* 2002) provided evidence for linkage with type 2 diabetes at a different set of chromosomes (Table 4.7) and in particular on chromosome 9p13–q21 and 12q24.

This widespread distribution of multiple loci certainly suggest a polygenic trait but may also reflect issues related to study-design including the phenotype investigated (insulin secretion vs. insulin resistance), the statistical analysis to derive the LOD scores, or may reflect true population differences. Despite such considerable variability, there is some consensus that loci at 2q37.3, 9p13–q21, and 12q24 could harbour strong candidate genes. Further investigation of the locus on 2q37.3 (also known as NIDDM1)

Table 4.7 Chromosomal regions linked with type 2 diabetes in selected genome-wide scans for type 2 diabetes in different populations

Author(s)	Population	Chromosomal localization
Hanson *et al.* (1998)	Pima Indians	1q, 7q, 11q
Wiltshire *et al.* (2001)	UK families	1q, 5q, 7p, 8p, 10q
Luo *et al.* (2001)	Chinese Hans	9, 20
Lindgren *et al.* (2002)	Finnish families	2p, 3p, 4q, 9p, 12q, 16p, 17p
Mori *et al.* (2002)	Japanese ASP	3q, 7p, 11p, 15q, 20q

led, rather surprisingly, to the identification of calpain-10 as a new candidate gene for type 2 diabetes (Horikawa *et al.* 2000).

Calpain-10 (CAPN10) was identified by positional cloning within the NIDDM1 region on chromosome 2 in Mexican Americans. Three gene variants of the CAPN10 gene were identified. Genetic susceptibility, however, appears to be due to the presence of multiple polymorphisms rather than a single polymorphism or allelic variant. Haplotype analysis demonstrated that the 112/121 haplotype combination was associated with a greater risk of diabetes with an odds ratio of 3.02 in Mexican Americans. This haplotype combination was also associated with an approximate 3-fold higher risk of diabetes in European populations. Despite such a high individual relative risk, the 112/121 haplotype accounted for 14 per cent of diabetes at the population level in Mexican Americans and only 4 per cent in Europeans.

Nonetheless, these observations suggest a novel pathway that may contribute to the development of type 2 diabetes mellitus. However, the exact mechanism whereby CAPN10, a member of the calpain-like cysteine protease family, may influence the development of diabetes remains puzzling, especially since the variants were within intronic regions. The enzyme is expressed in pancreatic cells, muscle cells and liver. It is possible that changes in expression of this protease may influence insulin secretion, insulin action or even hepatic glucose uptake, Indeed, mutations in other proteolytic enzymes known to influence pro-hormone processing such as carboxypeptidase E are associated with rare forms of diabetes and obesity (Jackson *et al.* 1997).

Despite these advances there is concern about the population specificity for CAPN10 as a genetic risk factor for type 2 diabetes. Recent investigations have not confirmed an association between the CAPN10 polymorphisms either singly or as haplotypes in a Samoan population (Tsai *et al.* 2001), and in a Caucasian population (Elbein *et al.* 2002). Similarly, Evans *et al.* (2001) in UK also did not confirm a significant association between the haplotype identified by Horikawa *et al.* (2000) and type 2 diabetes. However, in the UK group, Evans *et al.* (2001) did observe an increase in transmission of the SNP-44 polymorphism in a 'trios' group (two parents plus one affected offspring) of young and obese diabetic subjects. The C allele at this polymorphism was associated with a 1.5–2.0 fold increased risk of diabetes in both family-based and case–control comparisons. These results suggest that there may be the presence of multiple susceptibility alleles at CAP10 and/or different patterns of linkage disequilibrium between these polymorphisms and a common causal variant (Evans *et al.* 2001).

Taken together the results from the individual candidate genes and from the whole-genome scans clearly suggest that type 2 diabetes is genetically heterogenous. Several genes are likely to be involved, and epistatic (gene–gene) and gene–environment interactions may turn out to be of fundamental importance. Genetically predisposed subjects may not necessarily develop overt diabetes unless they are exposed to particular environmental factors. These additional layers of complexity makes the task identifying the genetic basis of type 2 diabetes a formidable challenge.

4.4 **Cholesterol and lipoproteins**

Cholesterol is an important lipid component. Amongst its many functions, it is essential for cellular membrane integrity, the synthesis of vitamin D, and the generation of many steroid hormones. Most of the cholesterol within the body is synthesized endogenously, mainly within the liver, rather than absorbed from the diet. Endogenous cholesterol is synthesized from acetate and the rate limiting step in the synthesis of cholesterol is catalysed by the enzyme HMG coA reductase—the key target for the statins class of drugs.

Cholesterol and triglycerides are the major plasma lipids. Because lipids are not soluble in the aqueous plasma, cholesterol, triglycerides and other lipids are transported within spherical particles known as lipoproteins. Structurally lipoproteins are characterized by a lipid core of triglycerides and cholesterol esters and an amphipathic surface coat. The coat consists mainly of phospholipids, cholesterol, and proteins (apoproteins). Apoproteins provide plasma lipoproteins with structural stability and solubility. They also serve as ligands for receptors and/or activators of enzymes involved in metabolism of lipoproteins. Each class contains varying proportion of cholesterol and triglycerides and apoproteins. The plasma levels of these lipoproteins are determined by a complex network of biochemical processes operating within the intestine, liver and peripheral cells.

Numerous investigations have demonstrated that the risk of developing coronary heart disease increases with increasing level of total cholesterol. The risk is graded and continuous without a threshold. A rise in total plasma cholesterol from 5.2 to 6.2 mmol (200–240 mg/dl) is associated with a 3-fold increase in risk of death from coronary heart disease (Stamler *et al.* 2000). When the lipoprotein profile is taken into account, it is now well established that coronary heart disease is also related directly with LDL-cholesterol and inversely with HDL-cholesterol (Rubins *et al.* 1995, Stamler *et al.* 2000).

LDL is responsible mainly for cholesterol transport into peripheral tissue. However excess LDL is atherogenic, because entrapped lipids can become oxidised generating toxic free-radical intermediates. These in turn can lead to stimulation of cytokines and to inflammatory activation. Chronic excess of LDL-cholesterol can also lead to the conversion of macrophages within arterial wall into foam cells, a key feature of the atherogenic process (Ross 1993).

Although the mechanisms by which HDL-lipoproteins protects against coronary heart disease are still not fully resolved, several possibilities have been suggested. High-density lipoproteins may increase the reverse transport of LDL-cholesterol from peripheral tissues to the liver for degradation. Another mechanism involves transfer of antioxidants from HDL to LDL, making these less susceptible to oxidation within the endothelium and vascular wall (MacKness *et al.* 1993). The potential role of HDL is further underscored by the observation that low levels of HDL-cholesterol without high levels of LDL-Cholesterol characterizes 20–30 per cent of patients with coronary heart disease in the United States (Rubins *et al.* 1995).

The relationship between abnormalities of serum lipids and stroke has been less clear than for coronary heart disease. Some prospective cohort studies including the Framingham Heart Study found no association between total serum cholesterol or HDL-cholesterol level and cerebral infarction but other investigations found a modest relationship (Knuiman *et al.* 1996, Gorelick *et al.* 1997, Elkind and Sacco 1998). The lack of a consistent relationship between total cholesterol levels and stroke may be partially explained by the heterogeneity of stroke. Most initial studies failed to differentiate cerebral haemorrhage from infarction. It appears that high cholesterol is probably a risk factor for the latter, perhaps particularly for large vessel disease stroke. The results of large scale trials with statins which significantly lower lipid levels by inhibiting 3-hydroxy-3-methylglutaryl coenzyme A (HMG-CoA) reductase have provided evidence for a strong beneficial effect not only for coronary heart disease but also for stroke (Hebert *et al.* 1997, Rosenson *et al.* 1998). However these agents do have possible effects other than cholesterol-lowering including up-regulation of endothelial nitric oxide synthase and plaque stabilization, and they could also contribute the stroke reduction.

Nevertheless the benefits of statins for stroke reduction have reinitiated discussions of the role of lipids as a stroke risk factor. Some researchers have suggested that the improvement in cardio- and cerebrovascular end points with statin agents cannot be completely explained by the baseline or treated LDL-cholesterol levels alone. Given the potential importance of the lipoprotein pattern, several studies have focused on the association between stroke and HDL-cholesterol. A few case–control studies have found the concentration of HDL-cholesterol to be lower in persons who had a stroke, even after controlling for other stroke risk factors; this is supported by the recent Northern Manhattan Stroke study (Sacco *et al.* 2001). This population-study confirmed that increased HDL-cholesterol levels were associated with reduced risk of ischaemic stroke in the elderly and among different racial or ethnic groups. These data add to the evidence relating lipids to stroke and support HDL-cholesterol as an important modifiable risk factor not only for coronary heart disease, but also for stroke. Exercise, weight reduction, moderate alcohol consumption, smoking cessation and statin agents have all been shown to increase plasma levels of HDL-cholesterol. However, there is also a substantial genetic element.

4.4.1 Genetic basis of plasma lipoprotein levels

Several monogenic syndromes associated with dyslipidaemia are known. These are associated with genetic variants in a number of the genes controlling pathways of lipoprotein metabolism. The presence of some of these variants can have substantial effects on the lipoprotein phenotype, and those that lead to raised levels of LDL-cholesterol are invariably associated with early coronary heart disease (Hegele 2001). Autosomal dominant familial hypercholesterolaemia is the classic example of a major gene defect which leads to an excess of LDL-cholesterol and premature coronary heart disease. The frequency of the heterozygotes is one in 500, and that of the homozygote is about one in a million. Familial hypercholesterolaemia is an inherited disorder comprising four different classes of mutation in the LDL receptor gene leading to reductions in uptake of LDL-cholesterol. The cellular uptake of cholesterol from LDLs occurs following the interaction of LDLs with the LDL receptor, also known as the apo-B-100 receptor. The class 1 defect is the most common and is associated with a complete loss of receptor synthesis. Familial hypercholesterolaemia sufferers may be either heterozygous or homologous for a particular mutation in the receptor gene. Homozygotes are more severely affected and exhibit grossly elevated serum cholesterol, primarily in LDL-cholesterol (Hegele 2001).

Several monogenic disorders are characterized by HDL-cholesterol deficiency or excess (Hegele 2001). Conditions associated with low-HDL display a profound disturbance in lipid metabolism and early coronary heart disease. Tangier Disease is associated with a lack of HDL which has been linked to the ABCA1 transporter (Rust *et al.* 1999). These diseases are extremely rare and unlikely to make a major contribution to the plasma levels of HDL-cholesterol in the population in general.

Numerous common polymorphisms in some of the genes encoding enzymes and structural components involved in lipoprotein metabolism have been identified. The impact of most on plasma cholesterol and lipoproteins is relatively weak. However there is considerable interest in polymorphic variants of a number of genes including LPL (Talmud and Humphries 2001), LIPC (Cohen *et al.* 1999), APOC3 (Shachter 2001) and Apoliprotein E.

Apoprotein E (APOE) is of particular interest as a common polymorphism of the APOE gene, which is associated with high plasma levels of LDL-cholesterol. APOE is produced mainly by the liver and is a constituent of chylomicron remnants and liver-derived very low-density lipoproteins (VLDL) and their remnants, and is also a component of HDL. APOE is a key factor in the cholesterol cycle and in the clearance of the highly atherogenic apoB-containing lipoproteins, in that it is a ligand for the apo B, E-receptor and the LDL-receptor related protein (Beisiegel 1989). The gene for APOE has three major alleles designated as $\varepsilon 2$, $\varepsilon 3$, and $\varepsilon 4$ with frequencies of about 7, 78, and 15 per cent, respectively in most populations. These code for three isoforms E2, E3, and E4 respectively which differ from each other by a single amino acid substitution (Mahley and Rall 2000). These differences appear to be sufficient to alter binding to the clearance receptor and thereby influence plasma cholesterol. In many populations, plasma levels of cholesterol are significantly higher in those with the $\varepsilon 4$ allele. On average, a single $\varepsilon 4$ allele *raises* total cholesterol level by about 7 mg/100 ml whereas the e2 allele *lowers* it by about 14 mg/100 ml. It has been estimated that this polymorphism can account for as much as 7–9 per cent of the total variation in plasma cholesterol, and numerous investigations have confirmed a positive association between the cholesterol raising allele ($\varepsilon 4$) and increased rate of mortality from ischaemic heart disease (Luc *et al.* 1994, Wilson *et al.* 1994). Such a deleterious effect is also consistent with the observation that the highest $\varepsilon 4$ allele frequency (0.23) is observed in Finland, a population with very high cholesterol levels and coronary heart disease (Stengard *et al.* 1995). The APOE polymorphism is potentially important as it may help to reassign individuals to a higher-risk group than those predicted by traditional risk factors.

The apoliprotein E polymorphism has also been shown to be an important risk factor for late onset familial cases of Alzheimer disease (Higgins *et al.* 1997). The association between Alzheimer disease and APOE $\varepsilon 4$ has been confirmed in many clinic- and population-based studies of patients from North America and Europe. Mounting evidence indicates that disease risk increases, and the age of onset decreases, with the number of APOE $\varepsilon 4$ alleles; in one study, $\varepsilon 4$ heterozygotes had a three-fold increase in risk of developing FAD and the $\varepsilon 4$ homozygotes had an 8-fold increase in risk of developing the disease to a near certainty by the age of 75 years 77–81 (Corder *et al.* 1993). However there appears to be variability in the strength and type of association between Alzheimer's disease and the APOE polymorphisms in different ethnic groups (Maestre *et al.* 1995, Kukull and Martin 1998).

Although there is general consensus that APOE $\varepsilon 4$ is strongly associated with AD, and that when present may represent an important risk factor for the disease, at the present time it is not recommended for use in routine clinical diagnosis (Tsuang *et al.* 1999). This is because the APOE genotype alone does not provide sufficient sensitivity or specificity—AD also develops in the absence of APOE $\varepsilon 4$ and many with APOE $\varepsilon 4$ seem to escape the disease.

4.4.2 Whole-genome scans for plasma lipoproteins

A genetic component for plasma lipoproteins is strongly supported by segregation analyses to identify major genes for plasma lipids and lipoproteins. Twin and family studies indicate that at least 50 per cent of the overall variation in LDL-cholesterol is genetically determined and several studies have reported heritability estimates for HDL-cholesterol of 40–60 per cent (Hamsten *et al.* 1986, O'Connel 1988, Heller *et al.* 1993, Perusse *et al.* 1997). Using family-based segregation analysis, some investigators reported evidence for a major locus for LDL-cholesterol (Coon *et al.* 1999). This statistically-inferred major gene accounted for 24 per cent of the variation in LDL-cholesterol, with the polygenic component accounting for another 28 per cent of the variation. Similarly, Mahaney *et al.* (1995) also provided evidence for a major gene locus for HLD-cholesterol accounting for about 20 per cent of the variation in plasma HDL-cholesterol. These observations have prompted the initiation of whole-genome scans based on anonymous markers to identify chromosomal regions linked to quantitative variation for plasma lipoproteins and HDL-cholesterol in particular.

In one investigation, Rainwater *et al.* (1999) performed a genome-wide screen for cholesterol concentrations in four LDL size subfractions (LDL-1 to LDL-4). Samples from 470 members of randomly ascertained families were typed for 331 microsatellite markers spaced at approximately 15 cM intervals. Linkage analyses used variance component methods that exploited all of the genotypic and phenotypic information in the large extended pedigrees. In multipoint linkage analyses with quantitative trait loci for the four fraction sizes, only LDL-3, a fraction containing small LDL particles, gave a peak with a LOD score that exceeded 3.0. The highest LOD scores for LDL-3 were found on chromosomes 3 (LOD = 4.1), 4 (LOD = 4.1), and 6 (LOD = 2.9). In oligogenic analyses, the 2-locus LOD score for chromosomes 3 and 4 increased significantly to 6.1, but including the third locus on chromosome 6 did not significantly improve the LOD score. These two quantitative trait loci on chromosomes 3 and 4 are located in regions that contain the genes for apolipoprotein D, and the large subunit of the microsomal triglyceride transfer protein, respectively. In the Hypergen study (Coon *et al.* 2001), full genome scans were carried out for quantitative lipid measurements in 622 African Americans and 649 white sib-pairs not taking lipid lowering medications. In this study, no major locus for LDL-cholesterol was found but evidence of linkage was observed for HDL-cholesterol on several chromosomal loci with a highest LOD score of 2.74 in white sibling pairs on chromosome 5.

Several other recent investigations confirm linkage of HDL-cholesterol with multiple chromosomal regions (Table 4.8). Peacock *et al.* (2001) conducted a genome-wide linkage scan for quantitative trait loci influencing total HDL-cholesterol concentration in a sample of 1027 whites from 101 families participating in the NHLBI Family Heart Study. Evidence for linkage of residual HDL-cholesterol was detected near marker D5S1470 at a location 39.9 cM from the p-terminal of chromosome 5 (LOD = 3.64). Suggestive linkage was detected near marker D13S1493 at location 27.5 cM on chromosome 13 (LOD = 2.36). These results suggest that there is at least one major genomic region containing genes that influences inter-individual variation in HDL cholesterol, but no new candidate genes were identified.

In a more recent linkage study of plasma HDL lipoprotein-cholesterol, Araya *et al.* (2002) used a multipoint variance components linkage approach to identify loci likely to influence plasma levels of HDL-cholesterol in Mexican Americans. A strong signal reaching standard levels of statistical significance was observed on chromosome 9

Table 4.8 Chromosomal regions linked with HDL-cholesterol in recent whole-genome scans for HDL-cholesterol

Population	Design	Location
Peacock *et al.* (2001)	White Americans	1,4,5,6,8,13
Coon *et al.* (2001)	White Americans	1,5,8,12,15
Coon *et al.* (2001)	African Americans	3,4,6
Almasy *et al.* (1999)	Mexican Americans	2,4,5,8,12,15
Arya *et al.* (2002)	Mexican Americans	2,3,7,8,9,11,20

between markers D9S925 and D9S741 (LOD = 3.4). Any causative genes are as yet unknown as this region does not contain any obvious candidate genes. However it is of interest to note that several of the genes involved in lipid metabolism during infection are close to this region. Additionally, the gene for the low-density lipoprotein receptor is also located on the short arm of chromosome 9. Interestingly, a smaller peak (LOD score = 1.4) was also found on chromosome 9q. This is close to the Tangier disease locus, a condition characterized by low HDL-cholesterol.

More generally, however, these genome-wide scans appear to exclude a large number of candidate genes known to be involved in lipoprotein metabolism. Thus Almasy *et al.* (1999) examined 477 individuals in 10 large pedigrees in a sub-sample of the San Antonio Family Heart Study for linkage with sub-fractions of HDL. The use of sub-fractions certainly has advantages in reducing the complexity of the HDL phenotype. Two major loci were identified, one on chromosome 8 and another on chromosome 15. The data suggested that the action of the locus on chromosome 8 is specific to unesterified cholesterol, whereas that on chromosome 15 appears to influence both HDL-concentration and the distribution of cholesterol among the different HDL sub-fractions. However, with the exception of that for the hepatic lipase locus on chromosome 15, Almasy *et al.* (1999) did not see any significant linkage near several HDL-related candidate genes, namely apolipoproteins (APOA1, APOA2, APOA4, APOCII and APOB), and selected enzymes involved in lipoprotein metabolism (LCAT, CETP and LPL).

Taken together, the results of all of these genome scans indicate that plasma levels of lipoproteins are influenced by many loci, which is perhaps not surprising given the intricacy of the lipoprotein trait. Indeed, the diversity of loci identified by the different investigations may, to some extent, be due to differences in the lipoprotein phenotype ascertained (e.g. total lipoprotein vs. lipoprotein subfractions). Although the QTL identified in different studies may not be the same, the use of genome-wide methods in combination with more refined phenotypic assessment may make it possible to identify multiple-component QTLs that contribute to the polygenic basis of plasma lipoproteins. This may lead to the identification of new mechanisms that influence variability in plasma lipoproteins and cholesterol.

4.5 **Perspectives and future directions**

Most of the traits now known to contribute to the development of hypertension, diabetes and dyslipedaemia in particular can be defined as complex traits. For these, there is no simple one-to-one relationship between genotype and phenotype. An individual's phenotype is likely to arise from the outcome of a constellation of polygenic alleles each displaying a relatively small effect. Variability at the population level is determined by the segregation of specific combinations of common allelic variants, possibly further modified by the environmental exposure. This genetic complexity is certainly not surprising when one considers the multiplicity of physiological mechanisms which maintain these variables within physiologically 'normal' limits.

Because of such multiplicity of genes and environmental factors, genetic studies aimed to identify gene variants contributing to these traits in human populations remain challenging. Nonetheless, and in view of the substantial health and economic burden arising as a consequence of the cardiovascular disease and stroke, there has been a substantial effort to understand the genetic basis of these traits. The genetic approach offers great potential. Identification of susceptibility loci promises to:

- advance our understanding of pathophysiological mechanisms,
- lead to further dissection of heterogeneity of multifactorial diseases,
- allow more targeted pharmacological treatment,
- develop tests for early identification of individual at risk,
- provide a basis for identification of relevant gene-environment interactions.

This chapter has provided a broad overview of the different approaches and outlined some of the major results obtained in relation to hypertension, diabetes, and dyslipidaemia. Several questions are pertinent. What has been achieved so far? Can any of the scientific information gained be translated into clinical practice? Does research to date point to the development of genetic tests which could be used to identify individuals at risk of developing cardiovascular disease?

Research into the genetic background of these traits has certainly contributed to a more detailed understanding of fundamental biochemical and pathophysiological events underlying the development of hypertension and the control of glucose and lipid metabolism. This is clearly exemplified by the elucidation of molecular mechanism of monogenic syndromes associated with hypertension (Table 4.3). Genetic analysis of Liddle's syndrome has stimulated new research into the epithelial sodium channel and on a more novel basis on the accessory factors involved in the control of the activity of this channel. At the same time, the effectiveness of the sodium channel inhibitor amiloride in Liddle's syndrome demonstrates the potential for a pharmacological treatment targeting an identified molecular defect (Lifton *et al.* 2001). New insights have also been gained on the cellular events relevant to the development of insulin resistance as highlighted by the identification of novel genetic variants in nuclear receptors activated by insulin (Kersten 2002).

Although these monogenic conditions are a great burden on those affected they are rare and contribute little to the population of the more common forms of hypertension, diabetes and raised plasma cholesterol. A large number of common candidate gene variants have been identified and investigated but promising results have been obtained with only a few of these. The ANG gene (Kunz *et al.* 1997) and the renal epithelial sodium channel (Baker *et al.* 1998) have been associated with essential hypertension. Two common variants in transcription factors critical to the actions of insulin, one in the PPARγ nuclear receptor (Altshuler *et al.* 2000) and the other in the IPF-1 gene (Hani *et al.* 1999), have been associated with type 2 diabetes. While variants in the IPF-1 gene influenced only about 6 per cent of the population (Hani *et al.* 1999), the Pro12Ala polymorphism of the PPARγ gene could influence as much as 25 per cent of type 2 diabetes in some populations (Stumvoll and Haring 2002). Common polymorphic variants have also been identified for plasma cholesterol and lipoproteins. In particular, the ε polymorphism of Apolipoprotein E provides a basis to reassign individuals to a higher risk level of cardiovascular disease. This polymorphism makes a substantial contribution to plasma levels of cholesterol and the E4 variant has consistently been associated with higher levels of plasma LDL-cholesterol (Larson *et al.* 2000). Moreover, recent investigations have demonstrated that the presence of the E4 allele was associated with a worse outcome in people with aneurysmal subarachnoid hemorrhage (Leung *et al.* 2002).

This aside, with the exception of the defined monogenic diseases it is perhaps too early to address the issue of genetic testing for the common forms of hypertension, diabetes and dyslipidaemias as none of candidate variants investigated as yet, meets the criteria for an ideal test in terms of sensitivity, specificity and predictive power. But a number of general conclusions can be derived from investigation of candidate genes:

◆ there can be substantial geographical/ethnic differences in allelic frequencies;

◆ causal relationships between molecular variants and phenotypic traits are difficult to establish;

◆ most molecular variants in candidate gene have minor effects;

◆ interpretation of associations can be distorted by linkage disequilibrium between putative alleles;

◆ the population attributable risk of specific candidate genes is generally low, but can be substantial (>20%) for common risk-conferring variants.

On the other hand, the identification of the HLA complex and the INS locus for type 1 diabetes is without doubt a substantial achievement in the elucidation of a major genetic background for polygenic diseases. The HLA complex and the INS loci clearly provides a strong genetic background accounting for up to 50 per cent of the genetic variability and their association with type 1 diabetes has repeatedly been confirmed (She and Marron 1998). By contrast there has been considerable controversy as to the relative importance of the numerous other loci also claimed to be linked with type 1 diabetes. Substantial attempts have also been made on trying to resolve genetic factors for essential hypertension and for type 2 diabetes using linkage analyses in whole-genome scans. For both of these, several chromosomal sites have been suggested as potential loci harbouring putative candidate genes. Unfortunately, not every region shows strong linkage and replicates in independent studies. To some extent this reflects the difficulties of identifying genetic components arising from relatively small effects of many individual loci (i.e. polygenic inheritance). The failure of replication within the same population has been attributed to some extent to inadequately powered studies. But as only weak linkages were also noted in large-scale investigations, the lack of consistency also questions the value of searching for such relatively weak genetic components.

The difficulties intrinsic in any attempts to discover genes for complex traits have been further highlighted in a recent review by Altmuller *et al.* (2001). The authors examined 101 recently reported studies of genome-wide scans of complex human diseases. They concluded that the application of linkage analysis to complex disorders without obvious Mendelian inheritance has had limited success thus far. In short, they felt that evidence of 'true linkage' was hard to find. Whether further work will overturn such a negative sentiment remains to be seen.

As genetic heterogeneity is a major problem in the mapping of human susceptibility loci for complex traits in human populations several ways to 'enrich the genetic background' have been proposed. Two approaches are relevant: selection on a defined intermediate phenotype, and the use of isolated populations or defined ethnic groups. Selection for a particular biochemical phenotype known to provide a mechanistic link between genes and the corresponding trait is of particular relevance, but selection could be also for other characteristics. For instance, potentially important intermediate phenotypes for essential hypertension could include 'salt sensitive' hypertension or 'low renin' hypertension (Gavras *et al.* 1999). For type 2 diabetes a corresponding intermediate phenotype could be achieved by selecting for insulin resistance or impaired pancreatic beta cell function (Gerich 1998). Other intermediate phenotypes to enhance the genetic background and increase the power to detect significant genetic linkage could include focus on individuals with early onset form of the trait. There is also renewed interest in the use of monozygotic and dizygotic twins. In conjuction with recent developments in biometrics and molecular biology, the study of twins now provides a unique opportunity to explore not only genetic basis of quantitative traits but also the complex interactions between genes and environment (MacGregor *et al.* 2000).

The value of isolated populations, or of defined ethnic groups, for genetic studies is potentially important but still controversial. One suggested benefit of this strategy is that populations isolated from historical, demographic, or geographical reasons might have a greatest proportion of individuals who carry risk alleles inherited from a common founder. These are likely to share considerable stretches of DNA around susceptibility genes as adjacent markers on a chromosome are often trasmitted together thereby increasing the likelihood of identifying significant linkage. It is also possible that genetic differences between populations might have arisen from evolutionary adaptation to a changing environment. This is highlighted by the 'thrifty genes' hypothesis as a potential basis to account for the widely different rates of type 2 diabetes in populations that have undergone rapid alterations in life-style such as Australian Aborigines, native American Indians, and people of Asian origin (Chukwuma and Tuomilehto 1998). The central features of this hypothesis is that early in the history of these people there has been positive selection for genetic variation which was associated with enhanced chance of survival. Such a genetic background could have facilitated efficient storage of fat during periods of plenty; on the other hand this adaptation might have helped to preserve blood glucose, for essential tissue functioning, during conditions of food scarcity. The transition of these populations to conditions of abundant and continuous energy supply, without a cycle of plenty followed by famine, now negates the beneficial effects of the 'thrifty genes' and simply predisposes them to obesity and insulin resistance. A similar argument could also be considered for the high prevalence of 'salt-sensitive hypertension' in black people who have made the transition from a low sodium rural environment to urban settings and the associated higher sodium intake. Despite the biological attractiveness of this concept, it is worth recalling that the putative genetic patterns have not, as yet, been identified.

Although it is likely that the use of an intermediate phenotype may increase the chances of finding regions of strong linkage, the task of identifying new genes within these regions is certainly not trivial and will require further fine-mapping. Given the use of genetic markers typically spaced at 5–10 cM, any regions showing significant linkage represent relative large stretches of DNA. Even a 1 cM region may contain more than 30 genes. Identification of specific putative genes within these regions may be a major hurdle to homing in on functionally relevant gene variants. High-density polymorphic markers to narrow down the existing QTL to ~1 cM may be required before physical mapping of the QTL can be undertaken. However, the completion of the Human Genome Project will undoubtly make the task much easier. Indeed, this is increasingly being exploited. For example, by reference to the NCBI RefSeq and Unigene Human sequence collection data bases, in their genome-wide scan for hypertension in Iceland, Kristjansson *et al.* (2002) provide a list of more than 30 genes under the peak on chromosome 18 which displayed strong linkage with essential hypertension. However, identifying putative causative gene variants from such lists is a much more difficult task.

The identification of the CALP genes within the NIDDM1 locus for type 2 diabetes illustrates a number of these points (Horikawa *et al.* 2000). First, this work endorsed the value of positional cloning for pinpointing genes not otherwise suspected to have a role in a disease (rather than the usual candidates), and generated new hypotheses for diabetes research. However, and despite the success in identifying associated haplotypes, answers to key questions remain uncertain. Does the association with CAPN10 account for linkage to NIDDM1? Is CAPN10 itself a gene for susceptibility to type 2 diabetes? What specific polymorphism(s) is directly responsible for altering risk of diabetes, and what is the functional link?

There is now considerable interest in the use of linkage disequilibrium mapping to narrow the search for individual genes. Although this would facilitate association studies of either positional or functional candidates it entails genotyping a truly large number of single nucleotide polymorphisms (SNPs). Theoretical calculations suggest that the use of linkage disequilibrium for whole genome mapping would require about 500,000 SNPs (Kruglyak 1999), but this could be an overestimate and others suggest that about 100,000 may be sufficient (Boehnke 2000). However, linkage disequilibrium mapping for more localized QTL is a more feasible approach and this has been used extensively for type 1 diabetes (She and Marron 1998). The technology for large scale genotyping is now becoming available. However, recent work on the patterns of linkage disequilibrium in one gene, lipoprotein lipase, points to complex patterns of associations (Clark *et al.* 1998). Understanding the real connection between genetic variants and phenotype in the presence uncertain patterns of linkage disequilibrium may not be as straight forward as anticipated.

New and improved technologies, such as microarrays that allow the genotyping of thousands of SNPs in a single assay, are likely to become of great importance in understanding genetic variation. This new technology in conjunction with transgenic experiments in animals designed to elucidate functional significance of genes will provide novel and exciting avenues of investigation for the genetic mechanisms of complex traits.

The impact that this massive expansion of knowledge will have on diagnosis, treatment and prevention of diseases arising from polygenic traits is difficult to predict at this time. Much still remains to be discovered and rationalized. But judging from the remarkable efforts and technical progress in molecular technology there is no doubt that inevitably this knowledge will influence clinical practice. However, it is also clear that understanding such a complex web of causative and interactive processess will require a deeper appreciation of the functional diversity arising from variability in genetic haplotypes.

References

Allayee, H., de Bruin, T.W., Michelle Dominguez, K., *et al.* (2001). Genome scan for blood pressure in Dutch dyslipidemic families reveals linkage to a locus on chromosome 4p. *Hypertension*, 38, 773–8.

Almasy, L., Hixson, J.E., Rainwater, D.L., *et al.* (1999). Human pedigree-based quantitative-trait-locus mapping: localization of two genes influencing HDL-cholesterol metabolism. *American Journal of Human Genetics*, 64, 1686–93.

Almind, K., Frederiksen, S.K., Ahlgren, M.G., *et al.* (1998). Common amino acid substitutions in insulin receptor substrate-4 are not associated with Type II diabetes mellitus or insulin resistance. *Diabetologia*, 41, 969–74.

Altmuller, J., Palmer, L.J., Fischer, G., Scherb, H., and Wjst, M. (2001). Genomewide scans of complex human diseases: true linkage is hard to find. *American Journal of Human Genetics*, 69, 936–50.

Altshuler, D., Hirschhorn, J.N., Klannemark, M., *et al.* (2000). The common PPARgamma Pro12Ala polymorphism is associated with decreased risk of type 2 diabetes. *Nature Genetics*, 26, 76–80.

Arya, R., Duggirala, R., Almasy, L., *et al.* (2002). Linkage of high-density lipoprotein–cholesterol concentrations to a locus on chromosome 9p in Mexican Americans. *Nature Genetics*, 30, 102–5.

Atkinson, M.A. and Eisenbarth, G.S. (2001). Type 1 diabetes: new perspectives on disease pathogenesis and treatment. *Lancet*, 358, 221–9.

Atwood, L.D., Samollow, P.B., Hixson, J.E., Stern, M.P., and MacCluer, J.W. (2001). Genome-wide linkage analysis of blood pressure in Mexican Americans. *Genetic Epidemiology*, 20, 373–82.

Baier, L.J., Permana, P.A., Traurig, M., *et al.* (2000). Mutations in the genes for hepatocyte nuclear factor (HNF)-1alpha, -4alpha, -1beta, and -3beta; the dimerization cofactor of HNF-1; and insulin promoter factor 1 are not common causes of early-onset type 2 diabetes in Pima Indians. *Diabetes Care*, **23**, 302–4.

Baima, J., Nicolaou, M., Schwartz, F., *et al.* (1999). Evidence for linkage between essential hypertension and a putative locus on human chromosome 17. *Hypertension*, **34**, 4–7.

Baker, E.H., Dong, Y.B., Sagnella, G.A., *et al.* (1998). Association of hypertension with T594M mutation in beta subunit of epithelial sodium channels in black people resident in London. *Lancet*, **351**, 1388–92.

Baker, E.H., Duggal, A., Dong, Y., *et al.* (2002). Amiloride, a specific drug for hypertension in black people with T594M variant? *Hypertension*, **40**, 13–17.

Barroso, I., Gurnell, M., Crowley, V.E., *et al.* (1999). Dominant negative mutations in human PPARgamma associated with severe insulin resistance, diabetes mellitus and hypertension. *Nature*, **402**, 880–3.

Beevers, D.G. and MacGregor, G. (1995). Factors controlling blood pressure. In *Hypertension in practice*, pp. 45–54. Martin Dunitz.

Beisiegel, U., Weber, W., Ihrke, G., Herz, J., and Stanley, K.K. (1989). The LDL-receptor-related protein, LRP, is an apolipoprotein E-binding protein. *Nature*, **341**, 162–4.

Boehnke, M. (2000). A look at linkage disequilibrium. *Nature Genetics*, **25**, 246–7.

Boerwinkle, E., Hixson, J.E., and Hanis, C.L. (2000). Peeking under the peaks: following up genome-wide linkage analyses. *Circulation*, **102**, 1877–8.

Brownlee, M. (2001). Biochemistry and molecular cell biology of diabetic complications. *Nature*, **414**, 813–20.

Burt, V.L., Cutler, J.A., Higgins, M., *et al.* (1995). Trends in the prevalence, awareness, treatment, and control of hypertension in the adult US population. Data from the health examination surveys, 1960 to 1991. *Hypertension*, **26**, 60–9.

Busch, C.P. and Hegele, R.A. (2001). Genetic determinants of type 2 diabetes mellitus. *Clinical Genetics*, **60**, 243–54.

Cardon, L.R. and Bell, J.I. (2001). Association study designs for complex diseases. *Nature Reviews Genetics*, **2**, 91–9.

Carretero, O.A. and Oparil, S. (2000). Essential hypertension. *Circulation*, **101**, 329–35.

Chukwuma, C. and Tuomilehto, J. (1998). The 'thrifty' hypotheses: clinical and epidemiological significance for non-insulin-dependent diabetes mellitus and cardiovascular disease risk factors. *Journal of Cardiovascular Risk*, **5**, 11–23.

Clark, A.G., Weiss, K.M., Nickerson, D.A., *et al.* (1998). Haplotype structure and population genetic inferences from nucleotide-sequence variation in human lipoprotein lipase. *American Journal of Human Genetics*, **63**, 595–612.

Cohen, J.C., Vega, G.L., and Grundy, S.M. (1999). Hepatic lipase: new insights from genetic and metabolic studies. *Current Opinion Lipidology*, **10**, 259–67.

Coon, H., Leppert, M.F., Kronenberg, F., *et al.* (1999). Evidence for a major gene accounting for mild elevation in LDL cholesterol: the NHLBI Family Heart Study. *Annals of Human Genetics*, **63**, 401–12.

Coon, H., Leppert, M.F., Eckfeldt, J.H., *et al.* (2001). Genome-wide linkage analysis of lipids in the Hypertension Genetic Epidemiology Network (HyperGEN) Blood Pressure Study. *Arteriosclerosis Thrombosis and Vascular Biology*, **21**, 1969–76.

Corder, E.H., Saunders, A.M., Strittmatter, W.J., *et al.* (1993). Gene dose of apolipoprotein E type 4 allele and the risk of Alzheimer's disease in late onset families. *Science*, **261**, 921–3.

Corvol, P., Persu, A., Gimenez-Roqueplo, A.P., and Jeunemaitre, X. (1999). Seven lessons from two candidate genes in human essential hypertension: angiotensinogen and epithelial sodium channel. *Hypertension*, **33**, 1324–31.

Cox, N.J., Wapelhorst, B., Morrison, V.A., *et al.* (2001). Seven regions of the genome show evidence of linkage to type 1 diabetes in a consensus analysis of 767 multiplex families. *American Journal of Human Genetics*, **69**, 820–30.

Day, C. (2001). The rising tide of type 2 diabetes. *British Journal of Diabetes and Vascular Disease*, **1**, 37–43.

DeStefano, A.L., Baldwin, C.T., Burzstyn, M., *et al.* (1998). Autosomal dominant orthostatic hypotensive disorder maps to chromosome 18q. *American Journal of Human Genetics*, **63**, 1425–30.

Dong, Y.B., Zhu, H.D., Baker, E.H., *et al.* (2001). T594M and G442V polymorphisms of the sodium channel beta subunit and hypertension in a black population. *Journal of Human Hypertension*, **15**, 425–30.

Dorman, J.S., LaPorte, R.E., Stone, R.A., and Trucco, M. (1990). Worldwide differences in the incidence of type I diabetes are associated with amino acid variation at position 57 of the HLA-DQ beta chain. *Proceedings of the National Academy Science USA*, **87**, 7370–4.

Ehm, M.G., Karnoub, M.C., Sakul, H., *et al.* (2000). Genomewide search for type 2 diabetes susceptibility genes in four American populations. *American Journal of Human Genetics*, **66**, 1871–81.

Elbein, S.C. (1997). The genetics of human non insulin-dependent (type 2) diabetes mellitus. *Journal Nutrition*, **127**, 1891S–6S.

Elbein, S.C., Chu, W., Ren, Q., *et al.* (2002). Role of calpain-10 gene variants in familial type 2 diabetes in Caucasians. *Journal Clinical Endocrinology and Metabolism*, **87**, 650–4.

Elkind, M.S. and Sacco, R.L. (1998). Stroke risk factors and stroke prevention. *Seminars in Neurology*, **18**, 429–40.

Evans, J.C., Frayling, T.M., Cassell, P.G., *et al.* (2001). Studies of association between the gene for calpain-10 and type 2 diabetes mellitus in the United Kingdom. *American Journal of Human Genetics*, **69**, 544–52.

Falconer, D.S. and Mackay, F.C. (1996). Quantitative trait loci. In *Introduction to quantitative genetics*, 4th edn. pp. 356–78.

Ferrari, P. (2002). Genetics of the mineralocorticoid system in primary hypertension. *Current Hypertenstion Reports*, **4**, 18–24.

Gardner, L.I., Jr., Stern, M.P., Haffner, S.M., *et al.* (1984). Prevalence of diabetes in Mexican Americans. Relationship to percent of gene pool derived from native American sources. *Diabetes*, **33**, 86–92.

Gavras, I., Manolis, A., and Gavras, H. (1999). Genetic epidemiology of essential hypertension. *Journal Human Hypertension*, **13**, 225–9.

Gerich, J.E. (1998). The genetic basis of type 2 diabetes mellitus: impaired insulin secretion versus impaired insulin sensitivity. *Endocrine Research*, **19**, 491–503.

Ghosh, S. and Collins, F.S. (1996). The geneticist's approach to complex disease. *Annual Reviews Medicine*, **47**, 333–53.

Gorelick, P.B., Schneck, M., Berglund, L.F., Feinberg, W., and Goldstone, J. (1997). Status of lipids as a risk factor for stroke. *Neuroepidemiology*, **16**, 107–15.

Habener, J.F. and Stoffers, D.A. (1998). A newly discovered role of transcription factors involved in pancreas development and the pathogenesis of diabetes mellitus. *Proceedings of the Association of American Physicians*, **110**, 12–21.

Hamsten, A., Iselius, L., Dahlen, G., and de Faire, U. (1986). Genetic and cultural inheritance of serum lipids, low and high density lipoprotein cholesterol and serum apolipoproteins A-I, A-II and B. *Atherosclerosis*, **60**, 199–208.

Hani, E.H., Stoffers, D.A., Chevre, J.C., *et al.* (1999). Defective mutations in the insulin promoter factor-1 (IPF-1) gene in late-onset type 2 diabetes mellitus. *Journal of Clinical Investigation*, **104**, R41–8.

Hanson, R.L., Ehm, M.G., Pettitt, D.J., *et al.* (1998). An autosomal genomic scan for loci linked to type II diabetes mellitus and body-mass index in Pima Indians. *American Journal of Human Genetics*, **63**, 1130–8.

Hansson, J.H., Nelson-Williams, C., *et al.* (1995). Hypertension caused by a truncated epithelial sodium channel gamma subunit: genetic heterogeneity of Liddle syndrome. *Nature Genetics* **11**, 76–82.

Hattersley, A.T. (1998). Maturity-onset diabetes of the young: clinical heterogeneity explained by genetic heterogeneity. *Diabetes Medicine*, **15**, 15–24.

Hebert, P.R., Gaziano, J.M., Chan, K.S., and Hennekens, C.H. (1997). Cholesterol lowering with statin drugs, risk of stroke, and total mortality. An overview of randomized trials. *Journal of American Medical Association*, **278**, 313–21.

Hegele, R.A. (2001). Monogenic dyslipidemias: window on determinants of plasma lipoprotein metabolism. *American Journal of Human Genetics*, **69**, 1161–77.

Heller, D.A., de Faire, U., Pedersen, N.L., Dahlen, G., and McClearn G.E. (1993). Genetic and environmental influences on serum lipid levels in twins. *New England Journal of Medicine*, **328**, 1150–6.

Higgins, G.A., Large, C.H., Rupniak, H.T., and Barnes, J.C. (1997). Apolipoprotein E and Alzheimer's disease: a review of recent studies. *Pharmacology, Biochemistry and Behavior*, **56**, 675–85.

Hilgers, K.F. and Schmieder, R.E. (2002). Association studies in cardiovascular medicine. *Journal of Hypertension*, **20**, 173–6.

Hodge, A.M., Dowse, G.K., Toelupe, P., Collins, V.R., Imo, T., and Zimmet, P.Z. (1994). Dramatic increase in the prevalence of obesity in western Samoa over the 13 year period 1978–1991. *International Journal of Obesesity and Relatated Metabolic Disorderders*, **18**, 419–28.

Horikawa, Y., Oda, N., Cox, N.J., *et al.* (2000). Genetic variation in the gene encoding calpain-10 is associated with type 2 diabetes mellitus. *Nature Genetics*, **26**, 163–75.

Hsueh, W.C., Mitchell, B.D., Schneider, J.L., *et al.* (2000). QTL influencing blood pressure maps to the region of PPH1 on chromosome 2q31–34 in Old Order Amish. *Circulation*, **101**, 2810–16.

Hunt, S.C., Ellison, R.C., Atwood, L.D., Pankow, J.S., Province, M.A., and Leppert, M.F. (2002). Genome scans for blood pressure and hypertension: the National Heart, Lung, and Blood Institute Family Heart Study. *Hypertension*, **40**, 1–6.

Jackson, R.S., Creemers, J.W., Ohagi, S., *et al.* (1997). Obesity and impaired prohormone processing associated with mutations in the human prohormone convertase 1 gene. *Nature Genetics*, **16**, 303–6.

Jekel, J.F., Elmore, J.G., and Katz, D.L. (1996). Assessment of risk in epidemiologic studies. In *Epidemiology biostatistics and preventitive medicine*, pp. 74–82. WB Saunders Company.

Jeunemaitre, X., Gimenez-Roqueplo, A.P., Celerier, J., and Corvol, P. (1999). Angiotensinogen variants and human hypertension. *Current Hypertension Reports*, **1**, 31–41.

Julier, C., Delepine, M., Keavney, B., *et al.* (1997). Genetic susceptibility for human familial essential hypertension in a region of homology with blood pressure linkage on rat chromosome 10. *Human Molecular Genetics*, **6**, 2077–85.

Kahn, C.R., Vicent, D., and Doria, A. (1996). Genetics of non-insulin-dependent (type-II) diabetes mellitus. *Annual Review Medicine*, **47**, 509–31.

Kaplan, N. (2002). Primary hypertension: pathogenesis. In *Kaplan's clinical hypertension*, 8th edn. Lippincot, Williams and Wilkins.

Kaprio, J., Tuomilehto, J., Koskenvuo, M., *et al.* (1992). Concordance for type 1 (insulin-dependent) and type 2 (non-insulin-dependent) diabetes mellitus in a population-based cohort of twins in Finland. *Diabetologia*, 35, 1060–7.

Karvonen, M., Viik-Kajander, M., Moltchanova, E., Libman, I., LaPorte, R., and Tuomilehto, J. (2000). Incidence of childhood type 1 diabetes worldwide. Diabetes Mondiale (DiaMond) Project Group. *Diabetes Care*, 23, 1516–26.

Kersten, S. (2002). Peroxisome proliferator activated receptors and obesity. *European Journal of Pharmacology*, 440, 223–34.

Kim, H.S., Krege, J.H., Kluckman, K.D., *et al.* (1995). Genetic control of blood pressure and the angiotensinogen locus. *Proceedings National Academy Sciences USA*, 92, 2735–9.

Knuiman, M.W. and Vu, H.T. (1996). Risk factors for stroke mortality in men and women: the Busselton study. *Journal of Cardiovascular Risk*, 3, 447–52.

Kristjansson, K., Manolescu, A., Kristinsson, A., *et al.* (2002). Linkage of essential hypertension to chromosome 18q. *Hypertension*, 39, 1044–9.

Kruglyak, L. (1999). Prospects for whole-genome linkage disequilibrium mapping of common disease genes. *Nature Genetics*, 22, 139–44.

Krushkal, J., Ferrell, R., Mockrin, S.C., Turner, S.T., Sing, C.F., and Boerwinkle, E. (1999). Genome-wide linkage analyses of systolic blood pressure using highly discordant siblings. *Circulation*, 99, 1407–10.

Kukull, W.A. and Martin, G.M. (1998). APOE polymorphisms and late-onset Alzheimer disease: the importance of ethnicity. *Journal of American Medical Association*, 279, 788–9.

Kumar, D., Gemayel, N.S., Deapen, D., *et al.* (1993). North-American twins with IDDM. Genetic, etiological, and clinical significance of disease concordance according to age, zygosity, and the interval after diagnosis in first twin. *Diabetes*, 42, 1351–63.

Kunz, R., Kreutz, R., Beige, J., Distler, A., and Sharma, A.M. (1997). Association between the angiotensinogen 235T-variant and essential hypertension in whites: a systematic review and methodological appraisal. *Hypertension*, 30, 1331–7.

Kyvik, K.O., Green, A., and Beck-Nielsen, H. (1995). Concordance rates of insulin dependent diabetes mellitus: a population based study of young Danish twins. *British Medical Journal*, 311, 913–7.

Lamb, E.J. and Day, A.P. (2000). New diagnostic criteria for diabetes mellitus: are we any further forward? *Annals Clinical Biochemisry*, 37, 588–92.

Lander, E.S. and Schork, N.J. (1994). Genetic dissection of complex traits. *Science*, 265, 2037–48.

Lander, E. and Kruglyak, L. (1995). Genetic dissection of complex traits: guidelines for interpreting and reporting linkage results. *Nature Genetics*, 11, 241–7.

Larson, I.A., Ordovas, J.M., DeLuca, C., Barnard, J.R., Feussner, G., and Schaefer, E.J. (2000). Association of apolipoprotein (Apo)E genotype with plasma apo E levels. *Atherosclerosis*, 148, 327–35.

Law, M.R., Frost, C.D., and Wald, N.J. (1991) By how much does dietary salt reduction lower blood pressure? III—Analysis of data from trials of salt reduction. *British Medical Journal*, 302, 819–24.

Leung, C.H., Poon, W.S., Yu, L.M., Wong, G.K., and Ng, H.K. (2002). Apolipoprotein E genotype and outcome in aneurysmal subarachnoid hemorrhage. *Stroke*, 33, 548–52.

Levy, D., DeStefano, A.L., Larson, M.G., *et al.* (2000). Evidence for a gene influencing blood pressure on chromosome 17. Genome scan linkage results for longitudinal blood pressure phenotypes in subjects from the Framingham heart study. *Hypertension*, 36, 477–83.

Lifton, R.P., Gharavi, A.G., and Geller, D.S. (2001). Molecular mechanisms of human hypertension. *Cell*, **104**, 545–56.

Lindgren, C.M., Mahtani, M.M., Widen, E., *et al.* (2002). Genomewide search for type 2 diabetes mellitus susceptibility loci in Finnish families: the Botnia study. *American Journal of Human Genetics*, **70**, 509–16.

Luc, G., Bard, J.M., Arveiler, D., *et al.* (1994). Impact of apolipoprotein E polymorphism on lipoproteins and risk of myocardial infarction. The ECTIM Study. *Arteriosclerosis and Thrombosis*, **14**, 1412–19.

Luft, F.C. (2002). Hypertension as a complex genetic trait. *Seminars in Nephrology*, **22**, 115–26.

Luo, T.H., Zhao, Y., Li, G., *et al.* (2001). A genome-wide search for type II diabetes susceptibility genes in Chinese Hans. *Diabetologia*, **44**, 501–6.

Maassen, J.A. and Kadowaki, T. (1996). Maternally inherited diabetes and deafness: a new diabetes subtype. *Diabetologia*, **39**, 375–82.

MacGregor, A.J., Snieder, H., Schork, N.J., and Spector, T.D. (2000). Twins. Novel uses to study complex traits and genetic diseases. *Trends Genetics*, **16**, 131–4.

Mackness, M.I., Abbott, C., Arrol, S., and Durrington, P.N. (1993). The role of high-density lipoprotein and lipid-soluble antioxidant vitamins in inhibiting low-density lipoprotein oxidation. *Biochemical Journal*, **294**, 829–34.

MacMahon, S., Peto, R., Cutler, J., *et al.* (1990). Blood pressure, stroke, and coronary heart disease. Part 1, Prolonged differences in blood pressure: prospective observational studies corrected for the regression dilution bias. *Lancet*, **335**, 765–74.

Maestre, G., Ottman, R., Stern, Y., *et al.* (1995). Apolipoprotein E and Alzheimer's disease: ethnic variation in genotypic risks. *Annals Neurology*, **37**, 254–9.

Mahaney, M.C., Blangero, J., Rainwater, D.L., *et al.* (1995). A major locus influencing plasma high-density lipoprotein cholesterol levels in the San Antonio Family Heart Study. Segregation and linkage analyses. *Arteriosclerosis Thrombosis and Vascular Biology*, **15**, 1730–9.

Mahley, R.W. and Rall, S.C. Jr. (2000). Apolipoprotein E: far more than a lipid transport protein. *Annual Review of Genomics and Human Genetics*, **1**, 507–37.

Mansfield, T.A., Simon, D.B., Farfel, Z., *et al.* (1997). Multilocus linkage of familial hyperkalaemia and hypertension, pseudohypoaldosteronism type II, to chromosomes 1q31–42 and 17p11–q21. *Nature Genetics*, **16**, 202–5.

Manunta, P., Barlassina, C., and Bianchi, G. (1998). Adducin in essential hypertension. *FEBS Letters*, **430**, 41–4.

Matsuda, A. and Kuzuya, T. (1994). Diabetic twins in Japan. *Diabetes Research and Clinical Practice*, **24**, S63–7.

Medici, F., Hawa, M., Ianari, A., Pyke, D.A., and Leslie, R.D. (1999). Concordance rate for type II diabetes mellitus in monozygotic twins: actuarial analysis. *Diabetologia*, **42**, 146–50.

Mein, C.A., Esposito, L., Dunn, M.G., *et al.* (1998). A search for type 1 diabetes susceptibility genes in families from the United Kingdom. *Nature Genetics*, **19**, 297–300.

Melander, O. (2001). Genetic factors in hypertension—what is known and what does it mean? *Blood Pressure*, **10**, 254–70.

Mori, Y., Otabe, S., Dina, C., *et al.* (2002). Genome-wide search for type 2 diabetes in Japanese affected sib-pairs confirms susceptibility genes on 3q, 15q, and 20q and identifies two new candidate Loci on 7p and 11p. *Diabetes*, **51**, 1247–55.

Morse, J.H., Jones, A.C., Barst, R.J., Hodge, S.E., Wilhelmsen, K.C., and Nygaard, T.G. (1998). Familial primary pulmonary hypertension locus mapped to chromosome 2q31–q32. *Chest*, 114, 57S–58S.

Nerup, J. and Pociot, F. (2001). A genome wide scan for type 1-diabetes susceptibility in Scandinavian families: identification of new loci with evidence of interactions. *American Journal of Human Genetics*, 69, 1301–13.

O'Connell, D.L., Heller, R.F., Roberts, D.C., *et al.* (1988). Twin study of genetic and environmental effects on lipid levels. *Genetic Epidemiology*, 5, 323–41.

O'Shaughnessy, K.M., Fu, B., Johnson, A., and Gordon, R.D. (1998). Linkage of Gordon's syndrome to the long arm of chromosome 17 in a region recently linked to familial essential hypertension. *Journal of Human Hypertension*, 12, 675–8.

Pankow, J.S., Rose, K.M., Oberman, A., *et al.* (2000). Possible locus on chromosome 18q influencing postural systolic blood pressure changes. *Hypertension*, 36, 471–6.

Park, Y., She, J.X., Wang, C.Y., *et al.* (2000). Common susceptibility and transmission pattern of human leukocyte antigen DRB1-DQB1 haplotypes to Korean and Caucasian patients with type 1 diabetes. *Journal Clinical Endocrinology Metabolism*, 85, 4538–42.

Peacock, J.M., Arnett, D.K., Atwood, L.D., *et al.* (2001). Genome scan for quantitative trait loci linked to high-density lipoprotein cholesterol: The NHLBI Family Heart Study. *Arteriosclerosis Thrombosis and Vascular Biology*, 21, 1823–8.

Perola, M., Kainulainen, K., Pajukanta, P., *et al.* (2000). Genome-wide scan of predisposing loci for increased diastolic blood pressure in Finnish siblings. *Journal of Hypertension*, 18, 1579–85.

Perusse, L., Rice, T., Despres, J.P., *et al.* (1997). Familial resemblance of plasma lipids, lipoproteins and postheparin lipoprotein and hepatic lipases in the HERITAGE Family Study. *Arteriosclerosis Thrombosis and Vascular Biology*, 17, 3263–9.

Poulsen, P., Kyvik, K.O., Vaag, A., and Beck-Nielsen, H. (1999). Heritability of type II (non-insulin-dependent) diabetes mellitus and abnormal glucose tolerance—a population-based twin study. *Diabetologia*, 42, 139–45.

Rainwater, D.L., Almasy, L., Blangero, J., *et al.* (1999). A genome search identifies major quantitative trait loci on human chromosomes 3 and 4 that influence cholesterol concentrations in small LDL particles. *Arteriosclerosis Thrombosis and Vascular Biology*, 19, 777–83.

Rice, T., Rankinen, T., Province, M.A., *et al.* (2000). Genome-wide linkage analysis of systolic and diastolic blood pressure: the Quebec Family Study. *Circulation*, 102, 1956–63.

Rice, T., Rankinen, T., Chagnon, Y.C., *et al.* (2002). Genomewide linkage scan of resting blood pressure: HERITAGE Family Study. Health, Risk Factors, Exercise Training, and Genetics. *Hypertension*, 39, 1037–43.

Risch, N. (1990). Linkage strategies for genetically complex traits. 1. Linkage strategies for genetically complex traits. I. Multilocus models. *American Journal of Human Genetics*, 46, 222–8.

Risch, N. and Zhang, H. (1995). Extreme discordant sib pairs for mapping quantitative trait loci in humans. *Science*, 268, 1584–9.

Rosenson, R.S. and Tangney, C.C. (1998). Antiatherothrombotic properties of statins: implications for cardiovascular event reduction. *Journal of American Medical Association*, 279, 1643–50.

Ross, R. (1993). The pathogenesis of atherosclerosis: a perspective for the 1990s. *Nature*, 362, 801–9.

Rubins, H.B., Robins, S.J., Collins, D., *et al.* (1995). Distribution of lipids in 8,500 men with coronary artery disease. Department of Veterans Affairs HDL Intervention Trial Study Group. *American Journal of Cardiology*, 75, 1196–201.

Rust, S., Rosier, M., Funke, H., *et al.* (1999). Tangier disease is caused by mutations in the gene encoding ATP-binding cassette transporter 1. *Nature Genetics*, **22**, 352–5.

Sacco, R.L., Benson, R.T., Kargman, D.E., *et al.* (2001). High-density lipoprotein cholesterol and ischemic stroke in the elderly: the Northern Manhattan Stroke Study. *Journal of American Medical Association*, **285**, 2729–35.

Sagnella, G.A. (2001). Why is plasma renin activity lower in populations of African origin? *Journal of Human Hypertension*, **15**, 17–25.

Saltiel, A.R. and Kahn, C.R. (2001). Insulin signalling and the regulation of glucose and lipid metabolism. *Nature*, **414**, 799–806.

Siffert, W. (1998). G proteins and hypertension: an alternative candidate gene approach. *Kidney International*, **53**, 1466–70.

Shachter, N.S. (2001). Apolipoproteins C-I and C-III as important modulators of lipoprotein metabolism. *Current Opinion Lipidology*, **12**, 297–304.

Sharma, P., Fatibene, J., Ferraro, F., *et al.* (2000). A genome-wide search for susceptibility loci to human essential hypertension. *Hypertension*, **35**, 1291–6.

She, J.X. (1996). Susceptibility to type I diabetes: HLA-DQ and DR revisited. *Immunol Today*, **17**, 323–9.

She, J.X. and Marron, M.P. (1998). Genetic susceptibility factors in type 1 diabetes: linkage, disequilibrium and functional analyses. *Current Opinion Immunology*, **10**, 682–9.

Simon, D.B., Karet, F.E., Hamdan, J.M., DiPietro, A., Sanjad, S.A., and Lifton, R.P. (1996). Bartter's syndrome, hypokalaemic alkalosis with hypercalciuria, is caused by mutations in the Na-K-2Cl cotransporter NKCC2. *Nat Genet*, **13**, 183–8.

Simon, D.B. and Lifton, R.P. (1996). The molecular basis of inherited hypokalemic alkalosis: Bartter's and Gitelman's syndromes. *American Journal Physiology*, **271**, F961–6.

Stamler, J. (1997). The INTERSALT Study: background, methods, findings, and implications. *American Journal of Clinical Nutrition*, **65**, 626S–642S.

Stamler, J., Daviglus, M.L., Garside, D.B., Dyer, A.R., Greenland, P., and Neaton, J.D. (2000). Relationship of baseline serum cholesterol levels in 3 large cohorts of younger men to long-term coronary, cardiovascular, and all-cause mortality and to longevity. *Journal of American Medical Association*, **284**, 311–18.

Stengard, J.H., Zerba, K.E., Pekkanen, J., Ehnholm, C., Nissinen, A., and Sing, C.F. (1995). Apolipoprotein E polymorphism predicts death from coronary heart disease in a longitudinal study of elderly Finnish men. *Circulation*, **91**, 265–9.

Stoffers, D.A., Ferrer, J., Clarke, W.L., and Habener, J.F. (1997). Early-onset type-II diabetes mellitus (MODY4) linked to IPF1. *Nature Genetics*, **17**, 138–9.

Stumvoll, M. and Haring, H. (2002). The Peroxisome Proliferator-Activated Receptor-gamma2 Pro12Ala Polymorphism. *Diabetes*, **51**, 2341–7.

Tabor, H.K., Risch, N.J., and Myers, R.M. (2002). Opinion: Candidate-gene approaches for studying complex genetic traits: practical considerations. *Nature Reviews Genetics*, **3**, 391–7.

Talmud, P.J. and Humphries, S.E. (2001). Genetic polymorphisms, lipoproteins and coronary artery disease risk. *Current Opinion Lipidology*, **12**, 405–9.

Thomson, G. and Esposito, M.S. (1999). The genetics of complex diseases. *Trends Cell Biology*, **9**, M17–20.

Tsai, H.J., Sun, G., Weeks, D.E., *et al.* (2001). Type 2 diabetes and three calpain-10 gene polymorphisms in Samoans: no evidence of association. *American Journal of Human Genetics*, **69**, 1236–44.

Tsuang, D., Larson, E.B., Bowen, J., *et al.* (1999). The utility of apolipoprotein E genotyping in the diagnosis of Alzheimer disease in a community-based case series. *Archives Neurology,* **56,** 1489–95.

Ward, R. (1990). Familial aggregation and genetic epidemiology of blood pressure. In: *Hypertension: pathophysiology, diagnosis and management* (eds J.H. Laragh and B.M. Brenner), pp. 81–100. Raven Press Ltd, New York.

Weijnen, C.F., Rich, S.S., Meigs, J.B., Krolewski, A.S., and Warram, J.H. (2002). Risk of diabetes in siblings of index cases with Type 2 diabetes: implications for genetic studies. *Diabetic Medicine,* **19,** 41–50.

Weiss, K.M. and Clark, A.G. (2002). Linkage disequilibrium and the mapping of complex human traits. *Trends Genetics,* **18,** 19–24.

Whelton, P.K. (1994). Epidemiology of hypertension. *Lancet,* **344,** 101–6.

Wilson, P.W., Myers, R.H., Larson, M.G., Ordovas, J.M., Wolf, P.A., and Schaefer, E.J. (1994). Apolipoprotein E alleles, dyslipidemia, and coronary heart disease. The Framingham Offspring Study. *Journal of American Medical Association,* **272,** 1666–71.

Wiltshire, S., Hattersley, A.T., Hitman, G.A., *et al.* (2001). A genomewide scan for loci predisposing to type 2 diabetes in a U.K. population (the Diabetes UK Warren 2 Repository): analysis of 573 pedigrees provides independent replication of a susceptibility locus on chromosome 1q. *American Journal of Human Genetics,* **69,** 553–69.

Xu, X., Rogus, J.J., Terwedow, H.A., *et al.* (1999*a*). An extreme-sib-pair genome scan for genes regulating blood pressure. *American Journal of Human Genetics,* **64,** 1694–701.

Xu, X., Yang, J., Rogus, J., Chen, C., and Schork, N. (1999*b*). Mapping of a blood pressure quantitative trait locus to chromosome 15q in a Chinese population. *Human Molecular Genetics,* **8,** 2551–5.

Zhu, D.L., Wang, H.Y., Xiong, M.M., *et al.* (2001). Linkage of hypertension to chromosome 2q14–q23 in Chinese families. *Journal of Hypertension,* **19,** 55–61.

Chapter 5

Animal models of stroke: implications for genetic studies of human stroke

Speranza Rubattu, Bruna Gigante,
Rosita Stanzione, and Massimo Volpe

5.1 Introduction

Stroke represents a multifactorial and polygenic trait, resulting from a complex interaction between the genetic background and several environmental determinants (Rubattu *et al.* 2000). Evidence for heritability of stroke comes primarily from epidemiological surveys that show a pattern of familial aggregation (Gifford 1966, Marshall 1971, Ostfeld *et al.* 1974, Diaz *et al.* 1986, Welin *et al.* 1987, Kiely *et al.* 1993, Jousilati *et al.* 1997), from twin studies documenting excess disease concordance in monozygotic as compared to dizygotic twins (Brass *et al.* 1992), from studies in adoptive sibships and, finally, from the analysis of monogenic syndromes associated with stroke (Boers *et al.* 1985, Palsdottir *et al.* 1988, Levy *et al.* 1990, Joutel *et al.* 1996). The mode of inheritance of stroke appears to be rather complex, raising several major difficulties for the identification of the stroke-causing genes in humans. Thus, an important tool for investigating the genetic basis of stroke, as well as of other cardiovascular traits such as hypertension, has been provided by available experimental animal models.

In fact, animal models for human diseases, in general, provide a reductionist approach that circumvents the complexity of human disease. In particular, fully inbred animals avoid the problem of genetic heterogeneity. In addition, animal experimentation allows a much more precise control of environmental factors than is possible in clinical studies. Most importantly, the possibility to create a large cross-bred hybrid population with specific genetic constellation provides a powerful tool for carrying out genetic linkage analysis. Therefore, the availability of the appropriate animal model along with the recent developments in the methods and applications of molecular genetics has improved our capacity to dissect out the genetic determinants of cardiovascular traits.

5.2 The stroke-prone spontaneously hypertensive rat as a model for human stroke

In regard to the stroke phenotype, the most widely used animal model is the stroke-prone spontaneously hypertensive rat (SHRsp), that was originally obtained by selective inbreedings from the spontaneously hypertensive rat (SHR) (Okamoto *et al.* 1974). This procedure implies that, from the original colony of SHR, those rats displaying the stroke phenotype were used for selective breeding over several generations until the trait appeared to be fixed. Then, a repetitive brother/sister mating was performed, for at least 20 generations, to achieve full genetic homogeneity. The stroke-free SHR rats, on the other hand, underwent a parallel similar inbreeding procedure in order to become the most appropriate homogenous control of the SHRsp.

The stroke-prone spontaneously hypertensive strain is characterized by a very high frequency of cerebrovascular events as compared to its matched control. The occurrence of the stroke phenotype can be greatly enhanced and anticipated by feeding the rats with a high salt, low potassium, low protein dietary regimen (Japanese-style diet) (Yamori *et al.* 1984). Under this experimental condition stroke occurs in the presence of blood pressure levels substantially comparable to those observed in the stroke-resistant SHR (Rubattu *et al.* 1996). The relatively early onset of stroke in SHRsp fed with a Japanese-style diet provides a very profitable phenotype and a almost unique opportunity to investigate the genetic basis of a cardiovascular accident.

It is important to point out that the stroke-prone rat strain shares several similarities with the human disease. In fact, hypertension and dietary factors behave as predisposing risk factors for both rats and humans. In particular, a high salt dietary intake represents an exacerbating factor whereas potassium supplementation behaves as a protective factor towards stroke (Tobian *et al.* 1984, Khaw *et al.* 1987, Volpe *et al.* 1990, Slivka 1991, Hansson 1996, Ascherio *et al.* 1998, Klungel *et al.* 1999). As in humans, stroke is mostly ischaemic rather than haemorrhagic, further supporting the concept that high blood pressure is not the sole determinant of cerebrovascular accidents. In particular, the typical cerebrovascular lesions observed in the SHRsp are ischemia (44%), haemorrhage (36%), and haemorrhagic infarction (19%). These occur as a result of the fibrinoid angionecrosis of small cerebral vessels typically seen in this rat model (Rubattu *et al.* 1996). Finally, the objective manifestations of stroke in rats strikingly resemble those of humans (hemiplegia, hemiparesis, convulsions, akinesia, etc.). Thus, the animal model of the SHRsp represents a suitable model for investigating the etiopathogenetic mechanisms underlying human stroke.

On this basis, the SHRsp has been largely used in the past for the characterization of hormonal and functional abnormalities associated with occurrence of cerebrovascular accidents, and, most recently, to understand the mechanisms underlying genetic susceptibility to stroke. In particular, several pathophysiological aspects, potentially involved in the pathogenic process of stroke in SHRsp, have been thoroughly analysed over two decades or so and numerous peculiarities of the SHRsp strain have been highlighted as potential mechanisms. These include abnormalities of extracellular fluid volume, enhanced vascular reactivity to pressor agents, endothelial dysfunction, activation of central or autonomic nervous system, changes in renal haemodynamics, and abnormalities of the renin–angiotensin system (Volpe and Rubattu 1994).

Overall, the pathophysiological characterization of the stroke-prone rat strain has certainly improved our comprehension of the complex pathogenetic network underlying occurrence of stroke, and has identified mechanisms in common with the human condition such as endothelial dysfunction. In this regard, an important finding was the observation that the SHRsp strain showed, when compared to the stroke-resistant SHR, an impaired acetylcholine-induced vasorelaxation that associated and co-segregated with occurrence of cerebrovascular events (Volpe *et al.* 1996). Endothelial dysfunction is known to occur prior to the manifestation of overt cardiovascular diseases in humans as well (Luscher and Vanhoutte 1990), and based on current studies from our group, can be detected in hypertensive subjects with a family history of stroke but not in those without history of stroke (unpublished observations). Therefore intriguing parallels between the rat and the human disease were established by these pathophysiological studies. However, no final conclusion about the primary causes of stroke in this rat strain could be achieved through this approach.

5.3 Genetic dissection of the stroke in the SHRsp

Preliminary studies performed soon after the establishment of the stroke-prone strain indicated that the relative abundance of SHRsp gene dosage correlated with the time to develop stroke in crossbred animals, and suggested a recessive model of inheritance (Nagaoka *et al.* 1976). Furthermore, susceptibility to infarcts after middle cerebral artery occlusion in SHRsp rats appeared to be related to a single gene which affected the development of collateral flow, and was transmitted in an autosomal recessive manner (Coyle and Heistad 1991).

The genetic dissection of stroke predisposition in the SHRsp strain has been attempted only recently through the co-segregation and linkage analysis approach. This procedure relies on the genetic principles and independent assortment of alleles or genes (Struk *et al.* 1996). It is applied to intercross populations of F2-hybrids derived from the mating of the diseased and non-diseased strains. In an intercross population all loci segregate freely. Only those different among the parental strains and truly relevant for expression of the phenotype of interest, that is, stroke, will remain associated with the disease in the hybrid progeny (since they are, in fact, determining the phenotype). Therefore, these studies are able to test whether any part of the disease genome co-segregates with the occurrence of the phenotype of interest. In practice, one tests for the presence of co-segregation of the disease phenotype parameters and one or more polymorphic markers. A polymorphic marker represents a difference between the two parental strains that is based on DNA sequence variations.

For the genetic dissection of stroke in the SHRsp researchers have used the so-called 'reverse genetic approach'. This is a genome-wide screening with polymorphic markers, mostly anonymous, not gene-linked, that are evenly distributed across the chromosomes. Such a 'grid' of individual map points can be used to determine the approximate localization of a disease-relevant gene by linkage analysis. In fact, a positive finding establishes that a primary, disease-causing gene resides in a particular chromosomal region.

The two major linkage studies in the SHRsp performed the genotype/phenotype co-segregation analysis by using F2-hybrid populations derived either from the SHRsp/SHR or from the SHRsp/WKY cross (Rubattu *et al.* 1996, Jeffs *et al.* 1997). They used two different stroke phenotypes: the number of days necessary to develop stroke under the stroke permissive dietary regimen (stroke-proneness) (Rubattu *et al.* 1996), and the extent of ischemic damage after middle cerebral artery occlusion (stroke-sensitivity) (Jeffs *et al.* 1997). Both studies were able to demonstrate the existence of different genes involved in the two distinct phenotypes which exerted a direct pathogenetic role on stroke associated with hypertension, independently from the blood pressure levels. In fact, stroke-proneness appeared to be directly determined by at least three genetic components, exerting either a causative or a protective effect (Rubattu *et al.* 1996), whereas stroke-sensitivity was explained by a single genetic locus on rat chromosome 5 (Jeffs *et al.* 1997). Specifically stroke-proneness was linked to a major locus on rat chromosome 1 containing a stroke causing gene and to other loci on rat chromosomes 4 and 5 containing genes with a delaying effect towards the disease (Fig. 5.1).

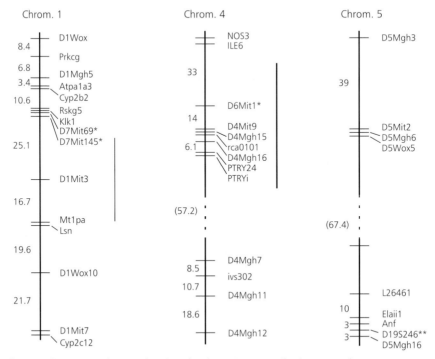

Fig. 5.1 Chromosomal maps showing the three QTLs contributing to stroke (stroke-proneness under a Japanese-style diet) in the SHRsp. The bars indicate the extension of the areas of linkage.

A significant epistatic interaction was observed between the chromosome 5 and the chromosome 1 quantitative tract loci (QTLs). Thus, evidence for a complex and poly-genic origin of stroke was obtained through these studies. An additional linkage analysis was performed in a different F2-hybrid cohort, obtained from SHR/WKY crossbreeding, by using the brain weight as a quantitative phenotype. As a result, a quantitative trait locus on chromosome 4 was identified (Ikeda *et al.* 1996).

Due to the large size of the chromosomal linkage areas which contain million of genes, the precise localization and identification of the specific stroke-causing genes can be achieved only after a laborious and time consuming approach, aimed at the progressive narrowing of the initial area (from about 15 up to 50 cM) down to the size required for the positional cloning (about 1 cM). Such an approach requires the genera-tion first of congenic strains, and then of congenic substrains, carrying smaller and smaller pieces of the original QTL and still showing the disease phenotype. The small-est area still linked to the disease phenotype can be physically reconstructed in order to obtain a map of the corresponding expressed sequences that can be ultimately analysed in search for significant disease-related abnormalities (Knoblauch *et al.* 1999). In fact, this work is currently in progress for some of the QTLs identified in the two linkage studies (Rubattu *et al.* 1999*a*).

Another feasible follow up of linkage studies is the search for obvious candidate genes contained within the QTL, followed by a careful comparative analysis in the attempt to identify structural, functional or regulatory differences between the disease and the con-trol strains. It is clear that 'candidates' are all those genes encoding proteins, hormones, or enzymes with known biological activities potentially related to the targeted pheno-type, that is, stroke. Remarkably, when such an approach was applied to the QTLs for stroke proneness, some interesting evidence was obtained. In fact, the adrenomedullin gene appeared to map in close proximity to the peak of linkage of the chromosome 1 QTL (Rubattu *et al.* 1998), and the genes for the atrial and brain natriuretic peptides mapped exactly at the peak of linkage of the QTL on chromosome 5. Interestingly, adrenomedullin, atrial and brain natriuretic peptides share natriuretic, diuretic and vasorelaxant properties, thus exerting important regulatory functions on the cardio-vascular system (Sakata *et al.* 1993, Rubattu and Volpe 2001). They also interact with each other. In fact, a modulatory role of adrenomedullin on atrial natriuretic peptide gene expression is known to take place in myocardiocytes (Sato *et al.* 1997).

Of note, a detailed analysis of the atrial natriuretic peptide gene revealed structural, functional, and regulatory alterations in the disease strain only (Rubattu *et al.* 1999*b*). In particular, two mutations were identified, one coding and one regulatory. The cod-ing mutation, responsible for a Gly to Ser transposition within the prosegment of proANP, was associated with differential processing and higher intracellular cGMP production. On the other hand, the regulatory mutation, involving an enhancer element, was associated with reduced gene transcription (Rubattu *et al.* 2002*a*). Moreover, an impaired endothelium-dependent vasorelaxation in response to ANP in

Table 5.1 Differences in the atrial naturetic gene (ANP) between the stroke-prone (SHRsp) and the stroke-resistant (SHRsr) rat strains

1. Coding mutation causing a Gly to Ser transposition within the prosegment of proANP peptide.
2. Regulatory mutation, affecting a PEA2 enhancer element, associated with a lower degree of ANP gene promoter activity both at baseline and after stimulation.
3. Differential intra- and extra-cellular processing of the SHRsp proANP peptide as compared to the SHRsr proANP peptide.
4. Differential brain, but not cardiac, expression of ANP between the two strains as well as among the F_2 rats carrying the –sp- allele versus the F_2 rats carrying the –sr- allele.

aortic rings from stroke-prone rats, as compared to stroke-resistant rats, was demonstrated (Russo *et al.* 1998). Therefore, the finding of altered structure, regulation, and function of the gene encoding ANP in the disease strain only strongly supported its candidacy as a stroke gene (Table 5.1). Of note, *in vitro* studies performed from other groups have recently documented an anti-proliferative effect of the ANP peptide in rat cultured vascular cells (Itoh *et al.* 1990, Morishita *et al.* 1994). Moreover, these investigations have shown that exposure of rat endothelial cells to the ANP peptide stimulates the process of apoptosis through the induction of p53 and the inhibition of BCl2 proteins (Suenobu *et al.* 1999).

In regard to the relationship between ANP gene and stroke occurrence, the major finding came from the structural analysis of the human ANP gene and, in particular, from the comparison of affected and non-affected individuals derived from a North American Caucasian population of male physicians (PHS). In fact, a twofold increase in the risk of stroke was discovered in carriers of a coding mutation within exon 1 of the gene (responsible for a Val to Met transposition in the prosegment of proANP) as compared to non-carriers (Rubattu *et al.* 1999c). A further study has associated an exon 3 mutation of the human ANP gene (responsible for the synthesis of a 30 instead of 28 amino acid peptide) with an increased risk of ischemic stroke in males from a case–control Italian cohort (Rubattu *et al.* 2002b). The two described coding mutations of the human atrial natriuretic peptide gene are shown in Fig. 5.2. Although these two studies support a role for the ANP gene in human stroke one study has failed to replicate the association with the exon 1 polymorphism in ischaemic stroke (Hassan *et al.* 2001).

Thus, the major lessons learned from these studies on the genetic basis of stroke is that there is an important parallelism between the stroke-prone animal model and human stroke. This parallelism goes behind the pathophysiological aspects and it rather involves, at least in part, its genetic origin. On the basis of this suggestive concordance between the genetic determinants of cerebrovascular disease in rats and in humans, the need to elucidate the functional relevance of the atrial natriuretic peptide gene mutations becomes an important goal. In this regard, *in vitro* studies represent

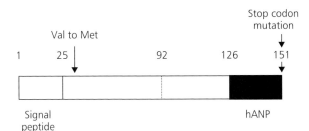

Fig. 5.2 Schematic representation of the human gene encoding the atrial natriuretic peptide. Two coding mutations are shown: one in exon 1 (responsible for a Val to Met transposition), and a second one located in the stop codon (responsible for the synthesis of a 30 rather than 28 amino acid mature peptide).

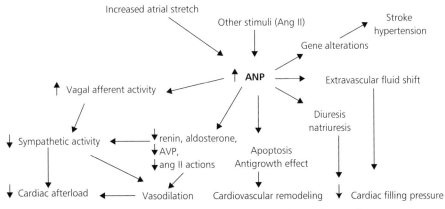

Fig. 5.3 Functional roles of the atrial natriuretic peptide on the cardiovascular system.

the most appropriate experimental approach to detect the possible contribution of both rat and human ANP gene mutations in the pathogenesis of vascular diseases. Of note, the *in vitro* approach, while providing us with important clues on the mutation-dependent disease mechanisms, may also open the way to new therapeutic strategies against stroke, which obviously represents the most important clinical end point. Finally, it has become clear that the evidence so far accumulated has changed our common view of ANP as a regulator of cardiovascular functions and has highlighted the potential role of the ANP gene as a possible determinant of stroke (Fig. 5.3).

5.4 **Genetic dissection of intermediate disease phenotypes**

In order to achieve a more complete understanding of the genetic basis of stroke in the SHRsp animal model, a complementary approach has been used. This involves the identification of so-called 'intermediate phenotypes' which can be used for linkage analysis. This approach, allowing the selective analysis of specific components of the disease process, may increase the power and sensitivity to detect underlying responsible genes (Stoll *et al.* 2001, Deschepper *et al.* 2002). The intermediate phenotype of endothelial dysfunction was characterized in an F2-intercross obtained from the SHRsp/SHR cross by measuring the maximal acetylcholine-induced vasorelaxation after maximal phenylephrine-induced vasoconstriction, and a phenotype/genotype co-segregation analysis was carried out to detect the genetic determinants. No evidence of linkage between endothelial dysfunction and a series of potential candidate genes was obtained (Rubattu *et al.* 2000*a,b*). The candidate gene analysis included genes of the renin–angiotensin system, of the natriuretic peptide system, the endothelial nitric oxide synthase and kallikrein. In contrast, a more recent wide genome screen covering the rat chromosomes with a 10 cM inter-marker distance has highlighted a few chromosomal areas showing a modest degree of linkage to endothelial dysfunction (Gigante *et al.* 2002).

5.5 Other experimental models of stroke

In the search for stroke-related genes, another experimental model was investigated, the SHR with middle cerebral artery occlusion induced ischaemic stroke. In particular, a differential display procedure was applied to the injured cerebral area and a likely candidate for stroke, the gene encoding adrenomedullin, was identified. In fact, this gene was overexpressed in brains of the SHR after MCAO-induced ischaemic stroke but not in the control SHR (Wang *et al.* 1995). Of note, the same gene was found to map within one of the stroke-QTLs identified in the SHRsp/SHR intercross, as mentioned above. However, although its candidacy as a stroke gene has become more relevant, no evidence of strain, stroke-related, specific peculiarities has ever been obtained for the adrenomedullin gene. In addition, its characterization in human populations, such as the Physicians Health study, did not reveal any positive association with stroke occurrence (unpublished observations).

Finally, mouse models were used to test the role of endothelial and neuronal nitric oxide synthase genes as putative candidates for stroke susceptibility. Whereas their direct contribution to stroke phenotypes had been previously excluded by linkage analysis in the rat model, the endothelial nitric oxide synthase (eNOS) gene knock-out mouse has demonstrated that eNOS is an important modulator of the degree of cerebral ischemia after stroke, by maintaining local cerebral blood flow (Samdani *et al.* 1997). Whether this finding relates to a primary or secondary involvement of the eNOS gene in stroke in this model remains to be determined.

5.6 Summary and outlook

There is always a certain expectation that genes identified as pathogenetically relevant in an animal model will have homologues involved in the pathogenesis of the disease in humans. Applying genetic experimental data to humans, however, is often not an easy task. In fact, very few genes discovered in animal models were subsequently confirmed in humans. Although this still remains a hope, nevertheless the use of animal models to investigate cardiovascular diseases may still provide useful advances in understanding genetics of human disease in a number of ways. They offer the opportunity to develop and apply novel molecular and statistical strategies useful for subsequent human investigation and, may allow identification of disease genes which improve our understanding of disease mechanisms. The experience gained with the studies on the animal model of the SHRsp is, from this point of view, very intriguing. In fact, it was only through the analysis of SHRsp that the ANP gene was identified as a candidate for stroke.

References

Ascherio, A., Rimm, E.B., Hernan, M.A., *et al.* (1998). Intake of potassium, magnesium, calcium, and fiber and the risk of stroke among US men. *Circulation*, **98**, 1198–204.

Boers, G.H., Smals, A.G., Trisbels, F.S., *et al.* (1985). Heterozigosity for homocistinuria in premature peripheral and cerebral occlusive arterial disease. *New England Journal of Medicine*, **313**, 709–15.

Brass, L.M., Isaacson, J.L., Merikangas, K.R., and Robinette, C.D. (1992). A study of twin and stroke. *Stroke*, **23**, 221–3.

Coyle, P. and Heistad, D.D. (1991). Development of collaterals in the cerebral circulation. *Blood Vessels*, **28**, 183–9.

Deschepper, C.F., Boutin-Ganache, I., Zahabi, A., and Jiang, Z. (2002). In search of cardiovascular candidate genes. Interactions between phenotypes and genotypes. *Hypertension*, **39** (Suppl. 2): 332–6.

Diaz, J.F., Hachinski, V.C., Pederson, L.L., and Donald, A. (1986). Aggregation of multiple risk factors for stroke in siblings of patients with brain infarction and transient ischemic attacks. *Stroke*, **17**, 1239–42.

Gifford, A.J. (1966). An epidemiological study of cerebrovascular disease. *American Journal of Public Health*, **56**, 452–61.

Gigante, B., Rubattu, S., Stanzione, R., *et al.* (2002). Three chromosomal regions modulate an impaired endothelial dependent vasorelaxation in the stroke-prone spontaneously hypertensive rat. *American Journal of Hypertension*, **15**(4), 149A.

Hansson, L. (1996). The benefits of lowering elevated blood pressure: a critical review of studies of cardiovascular morbidity and mortality in hypertension. *Journal of Hypertension*, **14**, 537–44.

Hassan, A., Ali, N., Dong, Y., Carter, N.D., and Markus, H.S. (2001). Atrial natriuretic peptide gene G664A polymorphism and the risk of ischemic cerebrovascular disease. *Neurology*, **577**, 1726–8.

Ikeda, K., Nra, Y., Matumoto, C., Massimo, T., Tamada, T., and Sawamura, M. (1996). The region responsible for stroke on chromosome 4 in the stroke-prone spontaneously hypertensive rat. *Biochemical Biophysic Research Communications*, **229**, 658–62.

Itoh, H., Pratt, R.E., and Dzau, V.J. (1990). Atrial natriuretic polypeptide inhibits hypertrophy of vascular smooth muscle cells. *Journal of Clinical Investigation*, **86**, 1690–7.

Jeffs, B., Clark, J.S., Anderson, N.H., *et al.* (1997). Sensitivity to cerebral ischemic insult in a rat model of stroke is determined by a single genetic locus. *Nature Genetics*, **16**, 364–7.

Jousilati, P., Rastenyte, D., Tuomilheto, J., *et al.* (1997). Parental history of cardiovascular disease and the risk of stroke. A prospective follow-up of 14371 middle-aged men and women in Finland. *Stroke*, **28**, 1361–6.

Joutel, A., Corpechot, C., Ducros, A., *et al.* (1996). Notch-3 mutations in CADASIL, a hereditary adult-onset condition causing stroke and dementia. *Nature*, **383**, 707–10.

Khaw, K.T. and Barrett-Connor, E. (1987). Dietary potassium and stroke-associated mortality: a 12-year prospective population study. *New England Journal of Medicine*, **316**, 235–40.

Kiely, D.K., Wolf, P.A., Cupples, L.A., Beiser, A.S., and Myers, R.H. (1993). Familial aggregation of stroke. The Framingham Study. *Stroke*, **24**, 1366–71.

Klungel, O.H., Stricker, B.H., Paes, A.H., *et al.* (1999). Excess stroke among hypertensive men and women attributable to undertreatment of hypertension. *Stroke*, **30**, 1312–18.

Knoblauch, M., Struk, B., Rubattu, S., and Lindpaintner, K. (1999). Genetic and congenic mapping of loci for blood pressure and blood pressure-related phenotypes in the rat. In *Molecular genetics of hypertension* (eds A.F. Dominiczak, J.M.C. Connell, and F. Soubrier), pp. 53–72. BIOS Scientific Publishers, Oxford.

Levy, E., Carman, M.D., Fernandez-Madrid, I.S., *et al.* (1990). Mutation of the Alzheimer's disease amyloid gene in hereditary cerebral hemorrhage, Dutch type. *Science*, **248**, 1124–6.

Luscher, T.F. and Vanhoutte, P.M. (1990). The endothelium: modulator of cardiovascular function. CRC Press, Boca Ranton.

Marshall, J. (1971). Familial incidence of cerebrovascular disease. *Journal of Medical Genetics*, **8**, 84–9.

Morishita, R., Gibbons, G.H., Pratt, R.E., *et al.* (1994). Autocrine and paracrine effects of atrial natriuretic peptide gene transfer on vascular smooth muscle and endothelial cell growth. *Journal of Clinical Investigation*, **94**, 824–9.

Nagaoka, A., Iwatsuka, H., Suzuoki, Z., and Okamoto, K. (1976). Genetic prediposition to stroke in spontaneously hypertensive rats. *American Journal of Physiology*, **230**, 1354–9.

Okamoto, K., Yamori, Y., and Nagaoka, A. (1974). Establishment of the stroke-prone spontaneously hypertensive rat (SHR). *Circulation Research*, **33/34** (Suppl. I), I43–I53.

Osfteld, A.M., Shekelle, R.B., Klawans, H., and Tufo, H.M. (1974). Epidemiology of stroke in an elderly welfare population. *American Journal of Public Health*, **64**, 450–8.

Palsdottir, A., Abrahamson, M., Thorsteinsson, L., *et al.* (1988). Mutation in cystatin C gene causes hereditary brain hemorrhage. *Lancet*, **2**, 603–4.

Rubattu, S., Volpe, M., Kreutz, R., Ganten, U., Ganten, D., and Lindpaintner, K. (1996). Chromosomal mapping of quantitative trait loci contributing to stroke in a rat model of complex human disease. *Nature Genetics*, **13**, 429–32.

Rubattu, S., Russo, R., Vecchione, C., *et al.* (1998). Identification of adrenomedullin as a candidate gene in the stroke-prone phenotype of spontaneously hypertensive rats (SHRsp). *American Journal of Hypertension*, **11**, 5A.

Rubattu, S., Ganten, U., Volpe, M., and Lindpaintner, K. (1999*a*). Increased incidence of stroke in congenic rats carrying the SHRSP-derived stroke-related locus, STR-1. *Circulation*, **100** (Suppl. I), I-275.

Rubattu, S., Lee, M.A., De Paolis, P., *et al.* (1999*b*). Altered structure, regulation and function of the gene encoding atrial natriuretic peptide in the stroke-prone spontaneously hypertensive rat. *Circulation Research*, **85**, 900–5.

Rubattu, S., Ridker, P.M., Stampfer, M., Hennekens, C.H., Volpe, M., and Lindpaintner, K. (1999*c*). The gene encoding atrial natriuretic peptide and the risk of human stroke. *Circulation*, **100**, 1722–5.

Rubattu, S., Giliberti, R., Russo, R., Ganten, U., Gigante, B., and Volpe, M. (2000*a*). Genetic analysis of the endothelium-dependent impaired vasorelaxation in the stroke-prone spontaneously hypertensive rat: a candidate gene approach. *Journal of Hypertension*, **13**, 161–5.

Rubattu, S., Giliberti, R., and Volpe, M. (2000*b*). Etiology and pathophysiology of stroke as a complex trait. *American Journal of Hypertension*, **13**, 1139–48.

Rubattu, S. and Volpe, M. (2001). The atrial natriuretic peptide: a changing view. *Journal of Hypertension*, **19**, 1923–31.

Rubattu, S., Giliberti, R., De Paolis, P., *et al.* (2002*a*). Effect of a regulatory mutation on the rat atrial natriuretic peptide gene transcription. *Peptides*, **23**, 555–60.

Rubattu, S., Stanzione, R., Spinsanti, P., *et al.* (2002*b*). The gene encoding atrial natriuretic peptide and the risk of ischemic stroke in males. *American Journal of Hypertension*, **15**(4), 12A.

Russo, R., Vecchione, C., Cosentino, F., *et al.* (1998). Impaired vasorelaxant responses to natriuretic peptides in the stroke-prone phenotype of spontaneously hypertensive rats. *Journal of Hypertension*, **16**, 151–6.

Sakata, J., Shimokubo, T., Kitamura, K., *et al.* (1993). Molecular cloning and biological activities of rat adrenomedullin, a hypotensive peptide. *Biochemical Biophysic Research Communications*, **195**, 921–7.

Samdani, A.F., Dawson, T.M., and Dawson, V.L. (1997). Nitric oxide synthase in models of focal ischemia. *Stroke*, **28**, 1283–8.

Sato, A., Canny, B.J., and Autelitano, D.J. (1997). Adrenomedullin stimulates cAMP accumulation and inhibits atrial natriuretic peptide gene expression in cardiomyocytes. *Biochemical Biophysic Research Communications*, **230**(92), 311–14.

Slivka, A. (1991). Effect of antihypertensive therapy on focal stroke in spontaneously hypertensive rats. *Stroke*, **22**, 884–8.

Stoll, M., Cowley, A.W., Jr., Tonellato, P.J., *et al.* (2001). A genomic-systems biology map for cardiovascular function. *Science*, **294**, 1723–6.

Struk, B., Cai, L., Niu, T., *et al.* (1996). Genetic linkage analysis: principles and practice. In *Molecular reviews in cardiovascular medicine* (eds K. Lindpaintner and D. Ganten), pp. 8–11. Chapman and Hall, London.

Suenobu, N., Shichiri, M., Iwashina, M., Marumo, F., and Hirata, Y. (1999). Natriuretic peptides and nitric oxide induce endothelial apoptosis via a cGMP-dependent mechanism. *Arteriosclerosis Thrombosis Vascular Biology*, **19**, 140–6.

Tobian, L., Lange, J.M., Ulm, K.M., Wold, L.J., and Iwai, J. (1984). Potassium prevents death from stroke in hypertensive rats without lowering blood pressure. *Journal of Hypertension*, **2** (Suppl.), 363–6.

Volpe, M., Camargo, M.J., Mueller, F.B., *et al.* (1990). Relation of plasma renin to end organ damage and to protection of K feeding in stroke-prone hypertensive rats. *Hypertension*, **15**, 318–26.

Volpe, M., Iaccarino, G., Vecchione, C., *et al.* (1996). Association and co-segregation of stroke with impaired endothelium-dependent vasorelaxation in stroke-prone, spontaneously hypertensive rats. *Journal of Clinical Investigation*, **98**, 256–61.

Volpe, M. and Rubattu, S. (1994). Pathophysiological aspects of genetically determined hypertension in rats, with special emphasis on stroke-prone spontaneously hypertensive rats. In *Handbook of hypertension, Vol. 16: Experimental and genetic models of hypertension* (eds D. Ganten and W. de Jong), pp. 365–94. Elsevier Science, Amsterdam.

Wang, X., Yue, T., Barone, F.C., *et al.* (1995). Discovery of adrenomedullin in rat ischemic cortex and evidence for its role in exacerbating focal brain ischemic damage. *Proceedings of National Academy of Science USA*, **92**, 11480–4.

Welin, L., Svardsudd, K., Wilhelmsen, L., Larsson, B., and Tibblin, G. (1987). Analysis of risk factors for stroke in a cohort of men born in 1913. *New England Journal of Medicine*, **317**, 521–6.

Yamori, Y., Horie, R., Tanase, H., Fujiwara, K., Nara, Y., and Lovenberg, W. (1984). Possibile role of nutritional factors in the incidence of cerebral lesions in stroke-prone spontaneously hypertensive rats. *Hypertension*, **6**, 49–53.

Chapter 6

Monogenic causes of ischaemic stroke

Martin Dichgans

6.1 **Introduction**

This chapter focuses on monogenic causes of ischaemic stroke. Within recent years most of the major gene loci have been mapped. Many of the genes have been cloned thus allowing a direct diagnosis in the index patient and its relatives. Moreover, cloning of the genes has provided new insights into the molecular mechanisms underlying these disorders. Thus, for example, the identification of the genes implicated in CADASIL and hereditary haemorrhagic telangiectasia revealed cell signalling pathways involved into angiogenesis.

In order to recognize Mendelian stroke syndromes it is essential to perform a systematic family inquiry and to search for neurological and non-neurological signs and symptoms in index cases and relatives. The diagnosis may have implications both for therapeutic decisions and genetic counselling. At present, there is no uniform classification for Mendelian stroke syndromes. Criteria that may be useful for clinical practice include underlying mechanisms (Table 6.1), mode of inheritance, and the presence or absence of associated symptoms. This chapter summarizes present data regarding clinical, genetic and pathophysiological aspects of monogenic conditions associated with ischaemic stroke. Diseases are considered in categories according to the classification in Table 6.1.

6.2 **Small vessel disease**

6.2.1 **Cerebral autosomal dominant arteriopathy with subcortical infarcts and leukoencephalopathy**

Cerebral autosomal dominant arteriopathy with subcortical infarcts and leuko-encephalopathy (CADASIL) is an autosomal dominantly inherited non-amyloid angiopathy caused by mutations in Notch3 (Joutel *et al.* 1996, Dichgans *et al.* 1998). Previous descriptions of families with 'hereditary multi-infarct dementia', 'chronic familial vascular encephalopathy', and 'familial subcortical dementia' represent early reports of the same condition. In 1993, Tournier-Lasserve mapped the gene to chromosome 19 and coined the acronym CADASIL (Tournier-Lasserve *et al.* 1993). Since then several hundreds of families have been reported from all over the world. In Germany there are more than

Table 6.1 Monogenic causes of ischaemic stroke

Small vessel disease
  CADASIL
  CARASIL
  Cerebroretinal vasculopathy and HERNS

Large artery disease
  Moya–Moya disease
  Ehlers–Danlos syndrome type IV
  Marfan syndrome
  Pseudoxanthoma elasticum
  Neurofibromatosis type I

Disorders affecting both small *and* large arteries
  Fabry disease
  Homocystinuria
  Sickle cell disease

Embolic causes of stroke
  Hereditary haemorrhagic telangiectasia
  Familial cardiomyopathies and dysrythmias

Prothrombotic disorders

Mitochondrial disorders

Familial hemiplegic migraine

180 families (Dichgans *et al.* unpublished data). Narrowing of the disease gene locus (Dichgans *et al.* 1996, Ducros *et al.* 1996) eventualy led to the identification of Notch3 as the responsible gene (Joutel *et al.* 1996). It was further shown that the expression of Notch3 is strongly restricted to vascular smooth muscle cells, a key element in small vessel pathology (Joutel *et al.* 2000*a*). This has opened an entire avenue for studying the mechanisms of vessel wall degeneration and microangiopathy-related ischaemic lesions.

Clinical phenotype

CADASIL patients usually present with one of the following four manifestations: ischaemic episodes, cognitive deficits, migraine with aura, and psychiatric disturbance. Ischaemic episodes (TIA or stroke) are the most frequent presentation found in about 85 per cent of symptomatic individuals (Chabriat *et al.* 1995*b*, Dichgans *et al.* 1998, Desmond *et al.* 1999). Mean age at onset for ischaemic episodes is around 46 years with a range of 30–70 years. In many cases ischaemic episodes present as a classic lacunar syndrome (pure motor stroke, ataxic hemiparesis/dysarthria-clumsy hand syndrome, pure sensory stroke, sensorimotor stroke) but other lacunar syndromes (brainstem or hemispheric) are also observed. They are often recurrent leading to severe disability with gait disturbance, urinary incontinence, and pseudobulbar palsy. Strokes involving the territory of a large artery have occasionally been reported (Rubio *et al.* 1997).

However, those observations may be coincidental. Without doubt, strokes related to small vessel pathology are the main manifestation of the disease.

Cognitive deficits are the second most frequent feature observed in about 60 per cent of symptomatic individuals. By the age of 65 two-thirds of the cases have become demented (Dichgans *et al.* 1998). Cognitive impairment includes deficits in episodic memory, attention, executive, and visuospatial functions, usually accompanied by psychomotor slowing and a narrowing of the field of interest. In most cases cognitive decline is slowly progressive with additional stepwise deterioration.

Migraine with aura is among the early manifestations of CADASIL and is found in about 30 per cent of the cases. Aura symptoms tend to involve the visual and sensory system. However, in a considerable number of cases symptoms are those of hemiplegic migraine, basilar migraine, or isolated aura which may be difficult to differentiate from ischaemic episodes. In fact, the relationship between 'migraine with aura' and 'TIA with headache' is an important pathophysiologic aspect of the disease. In an individual patient the type of aura may vary or be invariantly the same. In most patients who develop migraine, it is the first symptom (onset usually before age 40 years). Also, the frequency of migraine attacks seems to decrease after the first stroke (Dichgans *et al.* 1998). A reversible encephalopathy, often preceded by a migraine episode, has recently been reported. (Schon *et al*, 2003).

Mood disorders are the most frequent psychiatric manifestations and occur in about 30 per cent of the cases. Many patients develop adjustment disorder or moderate depression. Severe major depression is seen only in some cases. Other manifestations include manic depressive disorder, panic disorder, hallucinatory syndromes and delusional episodes. Rarely, CADASIL may present with a picture of schizophrenia. Up to 10 per cent of the CADASIL cases develop epileptic seizures which may require treatment. There have been single reports on spinal cord signs (Hutchinson *et al.* 1995) or infarcts (Sourander and Walinder 1977, Gutierrez-Molina *et al.* 1994), intracerebral haemorrhages (Sourander and Walinder 1977), and episodes of raised intracranial pressure (Baudrimont *et al.* 1993, Feuerhake *et al.* 2002).

The overall course of CADASIL is highly variable even within single families. Some patients remain asymptomatic until their seventies whereas others are severely disabled by the age of 50. Early onset does not necessarily predict rapid progression. In a large population of patients the duration from onset to death varied between 3 and 43 years with a mean of 23 years (Dichgans *et al.* 1998). Advanced stages correspond to the clinical syndrome of severe Binswanger's encephalopathy (Caplan 1995). Mean age at death is about 60 years (Chabriat *et al.* 1995*b*, Dichgans *et al.* 1998, Desmond *et al.* 1999).

Neuroimaging

Magnetic resonance imaging reveals two major types of abnormalities (Fig. 6.1) (Chabriat *et al.* 1998, Auer *et al.* 2001*a*): First, small circumscribed regions that are isointense to free cerebrospinal fluid (CSF) on T1- and T2-weighted images. Many of

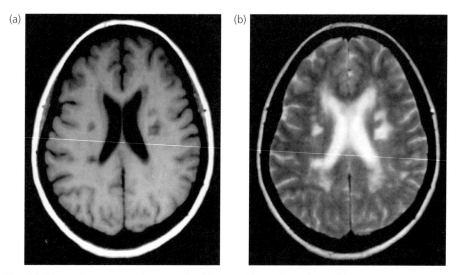

Fig. 6.1 Magnetic resonance images of a 45-year-old female patient with CADASIL.
(a) T1-weighted image showing multiple small deep infarcts as well as periventricular signal
hypointensities; (b) T2-weighted image showing diffuse signal-hyperintensities in the
periventricular and deep white matter (*see also* fig. 13.2 for example of characteristic anterior
temporal pole involvement).

these lesions are suggestive of lacunar infarcts regarding size, shape, and location.
Second, less well-demarcated T2-hyperintensities of variable size that may show different degrees of hypointensity on T1-weighted images but are clearly distinct from free
CSF. The majority of these lesions are located in the subcortical white matter but similar lesions may be seen in other brain regions including the subcortical grey matter
(Chabriat *et al.* 1998, Auer *et al.* 2001*a*). Small irregular T2-hyperintensities of the
periventricular and deep white matter are usually the first sign seen in younger individuals. As individuals get older, lesions tend to become confluent eventually affecting
a large proportion of the white matter. In addition, patchy areas of variable T1-signal
hypointensity become apparent within confluent lesions indicating progressive tissue
damage within T2-visible lesions. Apparently, the onset of MRI visible lesions and the
rate of progression show considerable variation (Chabriat *et al.* 1995*b*, Dichgans *et al.*
1999*a*), even though by about age 35 years all gene carriers have developed lesions on
MRI (Chabriat *et al.* 1995*b*). The pattern of MRI lesions (Chabriat *et al.* 1998, Yousry
et al. 1999) shares many similarities with sporadic small vessel disease (sSVD).
However, there are two important signs that have turned out to be particularly helpful
in the identification of disease gene carriers. First, T2-signal hyperintensities within the
temporopolar white matter (O'Sullivan *et al.* 2001, Auer *et al.* 2001*a*), and second,
involvement of the subcortical U-fibers within temporopolar and superior frontal
regions (Auer *et al.* 2001*a*). Conventional angiography is not contributory. In fact,
CADASIL patients are at an increased risk of developing angiographic complications
(Dichgans and Petersen 1997).

Cerebral blood supply in CADASIL is reduced below demand, as demonstrated by an increased oxygen extraction rate both in asymptomatic and demented CADASIL individuals (Chabriat *et al.* 1995*a*). Studies on brain perfusion and brain metabolism found significant reductions of cerebral blood flow, cerebral blood volume, and cerebral glucose utilization (Chabriat *et al.* 1995*a*, Mellies *et al.* 1998, Chabriat *et al.* 2000, Brüning *et al.* 2001, Pfefferkorn *et al.* 2001). Altogether these data suggest an early and important role of impaired cerebral perfusion in CADASIL. The arterio-venous transit time is markedly prolonged in CADASIL patients compared to controls (Liebetrau *et al.* 2002). This finding agrees with the underlying angiopathy which mainly affects small arteries, arterioles, and capillaries.

Using different methodological approaches two recent studies found a marked impairment of cerebral vasoreactivity (Chabriat *et al.* 2000, Pfefferkorn *et al.* 2001) which is in accordance with the observed degeneration of vascular smooth muscle cells (VSMC) in small arteries and arterioles (Ruchoux *et al.* 1995). Interestingly, a reduced cerebral vasoreactivity has similarly been documented in sporadic small vessel disease (Molina *et al.* 1999, Terborg *et al.* 2000) which is likewise associated with a degeneration of vascular smooth muscle cells. Altogether these findings underline the critical role of VSMC pathology in cerebral small vessel disease. Obviously, the observed functional alterations might be relevant to the occurrence of ischaemic lesions. Thus they could be a promising target for therapeutic efforts (Forteza *et al.* 2001). An increased fragility of cerebral microvessels in CADASIL is suggested by a high frequency of cerebral microbleeds in autopsy material (Dichgans *et al.* 2002). Microbleeds may be detected *in vivo* by gradient-echo MRI. They are also found in cerebral amyloid angiopathy, hypertensive small vessel disease and age related white matter changes suggesting that microbleeds are a common property of cerebral small vessel disease.

Using different approaches such as MR spectroscopy (Auer *et al.* 2001*b*), diffusion tensor imaging (Chabriat *et al.* 1999), and magnetization transfer imaging (Iannucci *et al.* 2001), recent studies have provided evidence for subtle tissue alterations (demyelination, axonal loss, gliosis, enlargement of the extracellular spaces) outside T2-visible lesions in the white and grey matter. Both the total volume of lesions (Dichgans *et al.* 1999*a*, Iannucci *et al.* 2001) and the extent of signal alterations within lesions (Chabriat *et al.* 1999, Iannucci *et al.* 2001, Auer *et al.* 2001*b*) correlate with clinical parameters, indicating that these measures might be used as outcome measures in future therapeutic trials.

Pathology

Most autopsy studies have been carried out on patients with advanced disease. Macroscopic examination of the brain reveals a pronounced rarefication of the subcortical white matter with periventricular preference (Ruchoux and Maurage 1997). Other consistent findings are lacunar infarcts located predominantly within the basal ganglia, thalamus, and brain stem (in particular the pons). Histopathological examination shows various degress of demyelination, axonal loss, enlargement of the extracellular space, and mild astrocytic gliosis compatible with chronic ischaemia. The underlying vascular lesion is a unique non-arteriosclerotic, amyloid-negative angiopathy involving small arteries (100–400 μm) and capillaries primarily in the brain but also in other organs. The diagnosis may therefore be established by a simple skin biopsy (Ruchoux *et al.* 1994, Mayer *et al.* 1999, Joutel *et al.* 2001). Ultrastructural examination reveals characteristic granular osmiophilic deposits within the vascular basal lamina which are considered diagnostic (Fig. 6.2). These deposits are often seen in direct contact with vascular smooth muscle cells which degenerate and eventually disappear. They have not been characterized biochemically and their origin remains unresolved. Even though CADASIL is a generalized angiopathy, vascular complications appear to be limited to the brain. This discrepancy might in part be related to the predominant involvement of leptomeningeal and long penetrating arteries of the brain. However, additional factors such as properties of the blood brain barrier may be suspected (Ruchoux and Maurage 1997, Dichgans *et al.* 1999*b*).

Genetics and molecular mechanisms

CADASIL patients carry mutations in the Notch3 gene (Fig. 6.3) (Joutel *et al.* 1996). Notch3 is one of four mammalian homologues of Drosophila Notch (Weinmaster 1997).

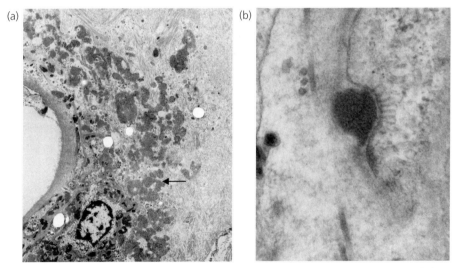

Fig. 6.2 Granular osmiophilic material (GOM) in two patients with CADASIL. This can only be detected on electron microscopy as in the following images. (a) A post mortem brain specimen of a small artery showing large amounts of GOM, seen as grey material (one example is arrowed). (b) A skin biopsy specimen showing a single GOM deposit (sample kindly processed by Dr Safa Al Sarraj (a) and Ray Moss (b), London, UK). (Copyright with Hugh Markus).

Notch genes code for large transmembrane receptors involved into cell fate decisions during embryonic development (Artavanis-Tsakonas *et al*. 1999). The Notch3 receptor is proteolytically processed in the *trans*-Golgi network as it trafficks from the endoplasmatic reticulum to the plasma membrane (Fig. 6.4). Proteolytic cleavage results in a large extracellular fragment and a small intracellular fragment that contains the transmembrane region.

Like all Notch receptors, Notch3 contains a large number of tandemly arranged epidermal growth factor-like (EGF-like) repeat domains which account for most of the extracellular part of the protein. All CADASIL mutations are located in EGF-like repeat domains with a strong cluster at the N-terminus (Fig. 6.3) (Joutel *et al*. 1997, Dichgans *et al*. 2000). The mutational spectrum includes missense mutations (Joutel *et al*. 1997, Oberstein *et al*. 1999, Dichgans *et al*. 2000), splice site mutations (Joutel *et al*. 2000*b*) and small in-frame deletions (Dichgans *et al*. 2000, 2001) (Fig. 6.5). Most patients (about 95%) have missense mutations with some being particularly common. However, there are many private mutations (Joutel *et al*. 1997, Dichgans *et al*. 2000). Mutations show a highly stereotyped nature: they all involve highly conserved cysteine residues (Figs 6.3 and 6.5) (Joutel *et al*. 1997, Dichgans *et al*. 2000, 2001). As a consequence, the usual number of six cysteine residues within wild type EGF-like repeat domains is changed to an odd number. It has been suggested that the unpaired cysteine residue generated by the mutations could cause aberrant interactions of Notch3 with other Notch3 molecules or other proteins. In fact, recent data have provided evidence for multimerization of mutant Notch3 (Joutel *et al*. 2000*a*).

Expression of the human Notch3 receptor is restricted to VSMC and pericytes. In CADASIL there is an excessive accumulation of the ectodomain of the Notch3 receptor within blood vessels (Joutel *et al*. 2000*a*). Accumulation takes place at the cytoplasmic membrane of VSMC and pericytes in close vicinity to, but not within, the deposits that characterize the disease. Notch3 immunostaining of dermal blood vessels derived from skin biopsies has been shown to be diagnostic (Joutel *et al*. 2001).

Recent data suggest that the Notch3 receptor may have a role in promoting vascular smooth muscle cell survival. Rat embryonic aorta cells transfected with the constitutively active intracellular form of the Notch3 receptor show enhanced resistance to Fas-ligand induced apoptosis (Wang *et al*. 2002). Moreover, in an *in vivo* model of arterial injury expression of Notch3 was shown to be upregulated in neointimal tissue (Wang *et al*. 2002). Taken together these data suggest a critical role for Notch3 in vascular remodelling.

Genotype–phenotype correlations

So far more than 50 different mutations have been reported from all over the world. A founder effect has been documented for the Finnish population but not for others. Recent data have raised the possibility that specific Notch3 mutations may be associated with particular phenotypes (Joutel *et al*. 2000*b*, Lesnik Oberstein *et al*. 2001,

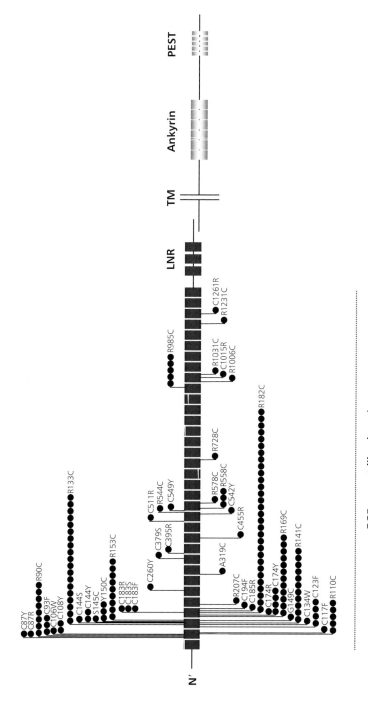

EGF-repeat-like domains

Fig. 6.3 Graphical illustration of the human Notch3 receptor and spectrum of mutations; pooled data from (Joutel *et al.* 1997, Oberstein *et al.* 1999, Dichgans *et al.* 2000, Arboleda-Velasquez *et al.* 2002, Dichgans *et al.* unpublished data): CADASIL mutations are located in epidermal growth factor (EGF)-like repeat domains of the Notch3 receptor with a strong cluster at the N-terminus.

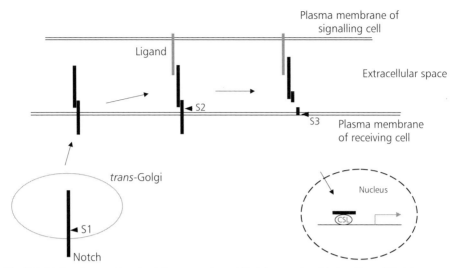

Fig. 6.4 Maturation and proteolytic processing of Notch receptor: Maturation of Notch receptors involves a constitutive cleavage in the trans-Golgi network as the receptor traffics toward the plasma membrane. Cleavage at the S1 site results in a larger extracellular fragment containing all the EGF-repeat like domains and a smaller intracellular fragment which contains the transmembrane region. Only the heterodimeric proteins are present at the cell surface. The next step is binding of the ligand. Ligands of Notch are presented by neighbouring cells. Binding of the ligand facilitates cleavage within the extracellular juxtamembrane region (S2 site). S2 cleavage induces a third intracellular cleavage within the transmembrane region (S3 site). S3 cleavage results in the release of the intracellular portion of Notch. Upon release, the intracellular domain translocates to the nucleus where it modifies transcription of target genes.

Arboleda-Velasquez *et al.* 2002). However, evidence from various sources suggests that genotype–phenotype correlations in CADASIL are weak at best (Dichgans *et al.* 1998, 1999*a*, 2001). These observations are in line with the stereotyped nature of the mutations. There is a single report on a homozygous CADASIL patient from Finland (Tuominen *et al.* 2001). The phenotype in this patient was at the severe end of the disease but still within the normal spectrum. Thus CADASIL seems to follow the classic definition of dominance according to which homozygotes and heterozygotes are phenotypically indistinguishable. Another important observation is the identification of a de novo Notch3 mutation in a sporadic patient (Joutel *et al.* 2000*c*). This finding has implications for diagnostic considerations.

Treatment

So far there is no specific treatment for the disease. Managment focuses on the control of symptoms such as headache, mood disturbances, urinary incontinence, and sleep disturbances. Motor disabilities require formal rehabilitation. Forced crying and

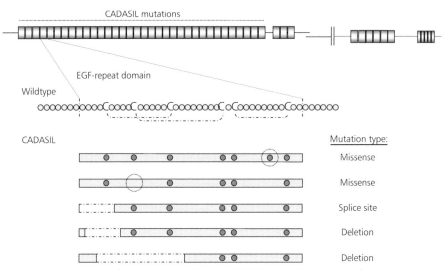

Fig. 6.5 Consequences of CADASIL mutations on EGF-like repeat domains of Notch3: Each domain contains a stretch of about 40 amino acids including an invariant number of six cysteine residues. The six cysteine residues form three disulfide bridges within the respective domain (Dichgans *et al.* 2000). The mutational spectrum includes missense mutations (>90%), small in-frame deletions, and splice site mutations. All CADASIL mutations result in an odd number of cysteine residues within a given EGF-like repeat domain, which leaves an unpaired cysteine residue within the respective domain.

laughing may respond to selective serotonin reuptake inhibitors. When oral hydration and feeding become insufficient, the patient should receive additional tube feeding.

6.2.2 Cerebral autosomal recessive arteriopathy with subcortical infarcts and leukoencephalopathy (CARASIL)

A syndrome of cerebral small vessel disease in combination with orthopedic problems and alopecia has repeatedly been described in families of Japanese origin (Fukutake and Hirayama 1995, Yanagawa *et al.* 2002). To date, a total of about 20 patients have been reported. Consanguinity has been demonstrated for most families suggesting an autosomal recessive mode of inheritance. The male to female ratio is about 3 : 1 (Yanagawa *et al.* 2002).

Age at onset for cerebral manifestations is between 20 and 40 years. Some patients present with a typical stroke; about 50 per cent in the series reported by Fukutake and Hirayama (1995). In others the course is slowly progressive with additional stepwise deterioration. Over the time most patients become demented. Neurologic symptoms include pyramidal tract signs, gait disturbance, pseudobulbar palsy, urinary incontinence, and extrapyramidal signs like in classical Binswanger's disease (Caplan 1995). Orthopedic complications include intervertebral disc disease and miscellaneous manifestations of osseous structures in particular, kyphosis, degenerative arthropathy, ossification of intraspinal canal ligaments, and deformity of elbows. The course is relentlessly progressive. Most patients die within 10–20 years following onset (Fukutake and Hirayama 1995, Yanagawa *et al.* 2002).

MR imaging reveals extensive, largely symmetrical white matter signal abnormalities (hyperintense on T2-weighted images) and small lacunar lesions. Postmortem pathology of the brain shows diffuse demyelination and small cystic infarcts in the white matter and the basal ganglia. Vascular alterations are most pronounced in small penetrating arteries of the brain with a caliber of about 100–400 μm. Changes include concentric narrowing of the lumen by severe fibrous intimal proliferation, hyaline degeneration of the media and fragmentation of the internal elastica. Similar changes may be found in vessels from other organs. However, the sensitivity of biopsies (e.g. from the skin) is unknown. In contrast with CADASIL, vessels do not stain for PAS and there is no granular osmiophilic basal lamina material on ultrastructural examination. Identification of the gene will help to understand the mechanisms of this complex disorder. There is no specific treatment so far.

6.2.3 Cerebroretinal vasculopathy and hereditary endotheliopathy with retinopathy, nephropathy, and stroke

Microangiopathy of the brain in combination with a vascular retinopathy are the leading features of cerebroretinal vasculopathy (CRV) and hereditary endotheliopathy with retinopathy, nephropathy, and stroke (HERNS) (Grand *et al.* 1988, Jen *et al.* 1997). Inheritance is autosomal dominant with a high penetrance. Both conditions are exceptionally rare. A distinctive feature of CRV and HERNS is the presence of progressive subcortical contrast-enhancing lesions with surrounding oedema (pseudotumours) typically located within the fronto-parietal white matter (Fig. 6.6).

Clinical symptoms include progressive visual loss, headache, seizures, focal neurologic deficits and progressive cognitive worsening. Onset is usually in the third or fourth decades of life. Visual disturbances (blind spots) are the initial symptom in most cases. Within a few years patients develop focal neurologic deficits. They are usually of sudden onset (stroke-like). Brain magnetic resonance images reveals contrast enhancing lesions with surrounding vasogenic edema most commonly in the frontoparietal region (Fig. 6.6). Upon biopsy, small intracerebral vessels exhibit amorphous thickening of their walls with adventitial fibrosis. Retinal abnormalities include telangiectatic capillaries and microaneurysms, preferentially around the posterior pole, which may be seen even in asymptomatic individuals on fluorescein angiography (Ophoff *et al.* 2001). Advanced stages are characterized by occlusion of branches of large retinal arteries and avascular areas in the retinal periphery. Renal insufficiency and proteinuria has been reported in some members from a family of Chinese origin reported by Jen *et al.* (1997). Another prominent feature in that family was migraine

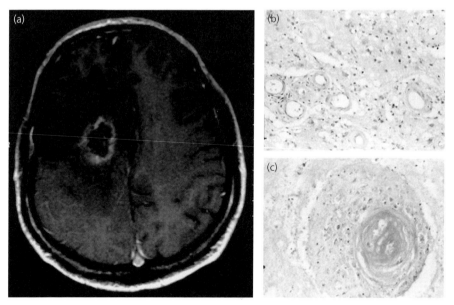

Fig. 6.6 A distinctive feature of CRV and HERNS is the presence of progressive subcortical contrast-enhancing lesions with surrounding oedema (pseudotumours) typically located within the fronto-parietal white matter. Gadolinium-DTPA enhanced T1-weighted image from a 35 year old male patient showing a typical mass lesion in the right frontal lobe. There is marked perifocal oedema and irregular enhancement following administration of the contrast agent; (b) and (c) histopathologic specimens taken from a left frontal mass lesion of the patients mother: (b) white matter with pathologic microvessels, oedema, and reactive gliosis; (c) necrotic vessel with thrombosis in an area of coagulative white matter necrosis (kindly provided by S. Weil, Neurologische Klinik, Klinikum Großhadern, München) (see Plate 1).

(see below). Ultrastructural examination of microvessels from different organs including the brain, kidney, and skin revealed multilayered capillary basal membranes. Based on these findings the authors suspected a primary endothelial injury and coined the acronym HERNS.

CRV and HERNS represent allelic disorders. Both conditions have recently been mapped to a single locus chromosome 3p21.1–p21.3 (Ophoff *et al.* 2001). A third condition, hereditary vascular retinopathy (HVR) has been mapped to the same genetic interval. White matter T2-hypersignals where observed in some patients. Yet, stroke does not appear to be part of the syndrome. The single family with HVR reported so far is remarkable for a high frequency of migraine and Raynaud syndrome (Terwindt *et al.* 1998). However, upon genetic analysis the relationship between the HVR haplotype and the occurrence of migraine and Raynaud phenomenon turned out to complex (Ophoff *et al.* 2001).

The differential diagnosis of CRV/HERNS/HVR includes diabetic retinopathy, hypertensive small vessel disease, and Susac syndrome (Papo *et al.* 1998). Corticosteroids have been advocated for the treatment of oedema in the acute stage of CRV/HERNS. Surgical resection of the pseudotumour has not helped those who underwent this procedure.

6.3 Large artery disease

6.3.1 Moya–Moya disease

Spontaneous occlusion of the circle of Willis (Moya–Moya disease) is a chronic progressive condition of unknown cause that is characterized primarily by the angiographic finding of bilateral stenosis or occlusion at the terminal carotid artery associated with telangiectatic vessels at the base of the brain (Ikezaki *et al.* 1997). Suzuki and Takaku observed that these collateral vessels give the appearance of a puff of smoke on arteriography and coined the name Moya–Moya (Suzuki *et al.* 1969). The disease is uncommon in non-Asian populations whereas its estimated prevalence in Japan is ≥3 to 100,000 persons. Moya–Moya occurs more frequently in females (male-to-female ratio 2:3).

Hemiplegia of sudden onset and epileptic seizures constitute the prevailing presentation in childhood. Other manifestations include sensory impairment, involuntary movements, and headache. They are caused by cerebral ischaemia due to the narrowing or occlusion of the circle of Willis. Progressive narrowing of the carotid fork results in gradual development of collateral circulation with formation of fragile new vessels. Eventual rupture of these abnormal vessels causes haemorrhage (subarachnoid, intraventricular, or intracerebral)—the predominant manifestation of Moya–Moya disease in patients older than 30 years (Ikezaki *et al.* 1997).

Most cases appear to be sporadic, but about 10 per cent occur as familial cases (Fukuyama *et al.* 1991, Fukui 1997). Non-invasive diagnostic methods such as magnetic resonance imaging (MRI) and magnetic resonance angiography (MRA) have assisted in identifying asymptomatic family members thus increasing the number of familial cases. About 70 per cent of cases of Moya–Moya disease among family members occur in siblings, whereas 24 per cent occur in a parent and offspring. Linkage has been reported to loci on chromosomes 3p24.2–26 and 17q25 reaching maximum LOD scores of 3.46 and 4.58, respectively (Ikeda *et al.* 1999, Yamauchi *et al.* 2000).

Hypotheses concerning additional aetiologies of Moya–Moya disease include infection with subsequent autoimmune response and environmental agents. So far, none of these hypotheses have been definitely confirmed. Instead, there is accumulating evidence that the condition is largely caused by genetic factors with multiple genes involved (Graham *et al.* 1997). The concordance rate in monozygotic twins is high.

Moya–Moya-like vascular changes have been described in association with a variety of conditions such as neurofibromatosis type 1 (NF 1; von Recklinghausen disease), sickle cell disease, tuberous sclerosis, Marfan syndrome, and pseudoxanthoma elasticum.

Histologically there is a cellular fibrous thickening, or eccentric fibrosis, of the intima. The internal elastic lamina shows duplication and tortuosity, whereas the media shows atrophy and thinning (Oka *et al.* 1981). The adventitia is without major changes. The most severely affected site is confined to the carotid fork. However, similar vascular changes have been found in other organs (Aoyagi *et al.* 1996). Recent studies on vascular smooth muscle cells derived from patients with Moya–Moya disease suggest an increase in elastin synthesis within arterial smooth muscle cells and elastin accumulation (Yamamoto *et al.* 1997).

Patients have been treated with antiplatelet agents, rheologic therapy, cortico-steroids, and calcium-channel blockers, although the efficacy of these treatments has not been proven. Anticoagulants should be avoided because of the risk of bleeding. Good results have been reported with surgical revascularization such as superficial temporal artery to MCA anastomosis (reviewed in Han *et al.* 2000).

6.3.2 Ehlers–Danlos syndrome type IV

Ehlers–Danlos syndrome (EDS) type IV, the vascular or ecchymotic type, is an auto-somally dominantly inherited disorder that results from mutations in the COL3A1, the gene for collagen type III. The clinical diagnosis is made on the basis of at least two of the following clinical criteria: easy bruising, translucent skin with visible veins, characteristic facial features, and rupture of arteries, uterus, or intestines (Pepin *et al.* 2000). Patients often have unexplained ecchymoses in well-protected areas. Hyperextensibility of the skin is unusual in the vascular type of EDS. Also, large-joint mobility is generally normal, with hypermobility limited to small joints of the hand. The diagnosis is confirmed by mutational screening or biochemical studies (cultured fibroblasts synthesize abnormal type III procollagen). The mutational spectrum is broad with more than 200 different mutations reported thus far (Pepin *et al.* 2000) and http://www.le.ac.uk/genetics/collagen/col3a1.html. All of them lead to synthesis of an abnormal type III procollagen protein. New mutations are common and about one-half of the index cases have no apparent family history for the disorder.

Neurovascular complications include intracranial aneurysms (IA), arterial dissection and spontaneous rupture of large-and medium-sized arteries (Schievink *et al.* 1994, North *et al.* 1995). IAs may be saccular or fusiform, and they are commonly located in the cavernous sinus (Schievink 1997). Rupture of these aneurysms results in spontaneous carotid-cavernous sinus fistula. In a large series including 220 index cases and 199 of their affected relatives 10.5 per cent of the individuals were found to have arterial complications of the central nervous system with a mean age of onset of 32.8 years (Pepin *et al.* 2000). Fistulae involving the carotid artery and cavernous sinus were the most common complication (2.4%) followed by aneurysm (1.2%) and rupture (0.5%).

The main cause of death in EDS type IV is arterial dissection or rupture mostly of the thoracic or abdominal artery. Other causes include organ rupture (uterus, liver, spleen, heart) and gastrointestinal rupture. The median survival time is around 48 years (Pepin *et al.* 2000). Rupture of any artery into a free space, such as the pleural cavity, requires immediate intervention, even thought the tissues are friable and repair may be difficult. In contrary rupture into a confined space may be sealed by tamponade, and in such cases, surgery may be deleterious. Arteriography carries special risks and should be avoided if possible. Whether incidental aneurysms should be treated is still unclear. Prompt surgical intervention is crucial in the treatment of bowel rupture. Women with EDS type IV who become pregnant have to be considered at high risk for uterine and vessel rupture and should therefore be followed at specialized centers.

6.3.3 Marfan syndrome

Marfan syndrome (MFS) is an autosomal dominant disorder characterised by abnormalities of the musculoskeletal system, cardiovascular system and eye (Pyeritz 2000). The condition is caused by mutations in the gene encoding fibrillin-1 (FBN1) on chromosome 15. Major diagnostic criteria include pectus carinatum or excavatum, reduced upper to lower segment ratio or arm span to height ratio >0.5 (Fig. 6.7), scoliosis >20°, ectopia lentis, and dilation of the ascending aorta with or without regurgitation. Clinical expression of the genetic defect may vary both within and between families (Pereira *et al.* 1994). Molecular diagnosis is feasible but labourious since the majority of patients with MFS have private mutations in a very large gene.

Neurovascular complications of MFS are less frequent than previously assumed. In a recent hospital based study including 513 patients with MFS the frequency of neurovascular complications was found to be 3.5 per cent (Wityk *et al.* 2002). Transient ischaemic attacks were the most frequent manifestation (2%) followed by cerebral infarction (0.4%), spinal cord infarction (0.4%), subdural hematoma (0.4%), and spinal subarachnoid hemorrhage (0.2%). Neurovascular manifestations were found to be associated with cardiac sources of embolism, in particular prosthetic heart valves and atrial fibrillation. However, there was no association with aortic disease. The same study failed to confirm an association between cerebral artery dissection and TIA or stroke (Wityk *et al.* 2002). Chronic anticoagulant therapy was the likely cause in 2 of 3 patients with hemorrhagic events. Gott *et al.* (1999) reported postoperative cerebral embolic events in 25 of 675 patients (3.7%) undergoing aortic root replacement. An association between MFS and IA has been repeatedly proposed but also challenged (van den Berg *et al.* 1996, Schievink 1997, Conway *et al.* 1999). Conway reviewed 25 patients with MFS who came to autopsy and found a prevalence of IA not statistically different from the general population (Conway *et al.* 1999). Moreover, a review of

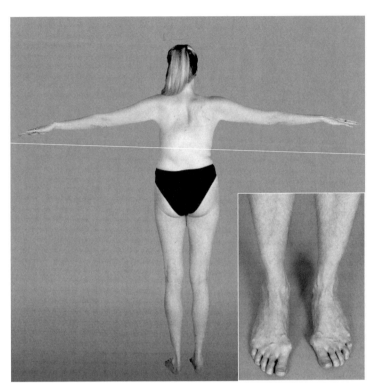

Fig. 6.7 Back view of a 33-year-old female patient with Marfan syndrome and cerebrovascular complications. Note the characteristic skeletal abnormalities (scoliosis, reduced upper to lower segment ratio, arm span to height ratio >0.5, pes planus) (see Plate 2).

750 neurosurgical patients treated for IA revealed no patients with MFS. Many of the vascular complications of MFS are due to the changes in elastic arteries, which are age-dependent and localized primarily in the media. They include fragmentation and disarray of elastic fibers, degeneration of smooth muscle cells, and separation of muscle fibers by collagen and pools of mucopolysaccharide. As a result the ascending aorta becomes less distensible and stiffer than usual.

Individuals with MFS should avoid intense physical or emotional stress. Patients should be considered for β-adrenergic blockade. Close follow-up of aortic root diamter by serial ultrasound measurements is recommended. In some cases surgery may become necessary. Individuals with MFS should use routine antibiotic prophylaxis before dental and other procedures that carry a high risk of introducing bacteria into the blood stream.

6.3.4 Pseudoxanthoma elasticum

Pseudoxanthoma elasticum (PXE) is a connective tissue disorder characterized by calcification of elastic fibers in the skin, eye, and cardiovascular system. The prevalence is estimated to be about 1 in 100,000. Typical skin changes consist in yellowish grouped papules beginning on the lateral aspect of the neck. Opthalmoscopic examination reveals mottled appearance of the retina as well as angioid streaks which are due to the breakdown of the elastic lamina of Bruch's membrane. The diagnosis may be confirmed by histologic examination of a skin biopsy. Mutations in ABCC6, a member of the ATP-binding cassette (ABC) gene subfamily C have been shown to cause autosomal recessive and autosomal dominant variants of the disease (Ringpfeil *et al.* 2000). However, the mechanisms by which these mutations become pathogenic are still unknown.

Cardiovascular complications are common due to calcification of the internal elastic lamina of mostly medium-sized arteries. Patients with PXE are at an increased risk of developing ischaemic infarction (Schievink *et al.* 1994, van den Berg *et al.* 2000). Focal cerebral ischaemia in PXE may be caused by large artery disease, or less frequently small vessel disease. Hypertension, also common in PXE, acts as an accelerating factor (van den Berg *et al.* 2000). A network of abnormal vessels between the external carotid and internal carotid system (rete mirabile) associated with carotid hypoplasia has repeatedly been reported in patients with PXE (Schievink *et al.* 1994). There are several case reports on a co-occurrence of PXE with IA or spontaneous dissection of cervical arteries. However, these observations are likely to be fortuitous (van den Berg *et al.* 2000). Platelet inhibitors, high systemic blood pressure, and contact sports should be avoided because of an increased risk of bleeding. Patients should be followed by an ophthalmologist. Nutritional restrictions (calcium) are controversial.

6.3.5 Neurofibromatosis type I

Neurofibromatosis type 1 (NF1) is one of the most common autosomal dominant disorders with a prevalence of about 1 in 3500 live births and virtually complete penetrance by adulthood. NF1 is a progressive systemic disease involving tissues of meso- and ectodermal origin. There is a high rate of neomutations (Riccardi 1991) with about 50 per cent of all NF1 patients having no family history. The NF1 gene codes for neurofibromin, a large (12 kB transcript) tumor supressor protein (Gutmann *et al.* 1993, Seizinger 1993). As of January 2002, the Human Gene Mutation Database listed more than 438 different NF1 mutations (http://archive.uwcm.ac.uk/uwcm/mg/ hgmd0.html). The majority of them leads to a truncated protein and can be detected at the protein level. Diagnosis is based on clinical criteria (Gutmann and Collins 1997).

Clinical features of NF1 include neurofibromas, café-au-lait spots, Lisch nodules, malignancies (central nervous system tumours and pheochromocytoma), skeletal deformities (thinning of the cortex of long bones, pseudoarthrosis, scoliosis), and vascular occlusive disease. Cerebrovascular symptoms are a rare though accepted complication of the disease (Rizzo and Lessell 1994). Stenosis, and eventually occlusion of the supraclinoid internal carotid artery is the most commonly reported abnormality. Intracranial arterial occlusions are often associated with a Moya–Moya-like pattern of collateral vessels (see above), which indicates that stenosis develops early in life. There have been a number of case reports on IA in NF1 (Schievink 1997). However, there is no evidence for an association between IAs and NF1 (Conway *et al.* 2001). The vascular pathology in NF1 includes concentric growth of the intima, disruption of the elastica, and nodular aggregates of proliferating smooth muscle cells. These findings are in agreement with studies that have demonstrated a vascular expression of NF1 within smooth muscle cells and vascular endothelium (Norton and Gutmann 1995). The impact of NF1 mutations on the vascular pathology is further corroborated by a mouse model of mutations in p120-rasGAP and NF1 genes (Henkemeyer *et al.* 1995). Like p120-rasGAP, Neurofibromin has been shown to act as a GTPase activating protein (GAP) on Ras. Disruption of p120-rasGAP in mice affects the ability of endothelial cells to organize into vascularised networks, and mutations in GAP and NF1 genes have a synergistic effect on the observed phenotype which includes thinning and rupture of large and medium sized arteries during embryonic development. There is no specific therapy for cerebrovascular complications in NF1.

6.4 Disorders affecting both small and large arteries

6.4.1 Fabry disease

Fabry disease is an X-linked disorder resulting from mutations of the α-galactosidase A gene at Xq22. The mutational spectrum is broad with more than 150 different mutations identified so far. Mutations result in a very low specific activity of the lysosomal hydrolase α-galactosidase A (Desnick 1995). The deficiency of this enzyme results in progressive accumulation of glycosphingolipids, particularly globotriaosylceramide (GB3) in various organs, predominantly in the vascular endothelial and smooth muscle cells, myocardium, renal epithelium, and the central nervous system. Dermal vessels undergo dilation and proliferation to form angiokeratoma. The incidence has been estimated to be $1:117,000$ births (Meikle *et al.* 1999).

Onset usually occurs in childhood or adolescence with severe debilitating neuropathic pain in the extremities and acroparesthesia, anhidrosis, skin, and mucosal angiokeratoma. Ophtalmologic examination often reveals corneal opacities, retrolenticular cataracts and tortuous retinal blood vessels. Severe morbidity follows cardiac, renal, and cerebrovascular involvement and tends to occur in the fourth decade (Desnick 1995, Brady and Schiffmann 2000). Prior to the introduction of enzyme replacement therapy the median age at death was 55 years in males.

Cerebrovascular symptoms seem to be mediated both by large- and small-artery involvement with a preference for the posterior circulation (Grewal 1994, Mitsias and Levine 1996, Crutchfield *et al.* 1998, Moore *et al.* 2001). Small artery involvement is characterized by progressive occlusion of blood vessels, secondary to deposition of Gb3 within the vascular wall (Fig. 6.5). The most frequent sign of large artery disease is dolichoectasia of the basilar and vertebral arteries. Large infarcts involving the cortex have been explained by artery-to-artery embolism from ectatic vessels. There is accumulating evidence for a prothrombotic state in Fabry disease (DeGraba *et al.* 2000). However, the pathophysiology of strokes in Fabry disease is far from being understood. For example, recent studies have shown that cerebral blood flow (CBF) is *increased* in patients with Fabry disease, particularly in the posterior and vertebrobasilar circulation (Moore *et al.* 2001, 2002). Following enzyme replacement therapy there was a significant reduction in regional CBF (Moore *et al.* 2001) and CBF velocity (Moore *et al.* 2002). Based on enhanced nitrotyrosine staining in dermal and cerebral blood vessels, Moore *et al.* (2001) suggested a chronic alteration of the nitric oxide pathway. Plethysmographic measurements have revealed an exaggerated blood flow response to intra-arterial acetylcholine in gene carriers compared to controls (Altarescu *et al.* 2001). However, evidence exists that enhanced blood flow response in Fabry disesae is mediated by non-NO endothelium-dependent vasodilatory pathways (e.g. involving endothelium-derived hyperpolarizing factor). Some patients may develop intracranial haemorrhage which may be caused by vessel degeneration as well as uncontrolled hypertension from renal failure. In hemizygous patients the penetrance for cerebrovascular involvement on MRI is complete by about 54 years (Crutchfield *et al.* 1998). In female heterozygotes the penetrance and expressivity of the phenotype is much lower. The diagnosis of Fabry disease may be suspected based on the typical skin changes that characterize the disease (angiokeratoma corporis diffusum): clustered non-blanching angiectases primarily over the lower part of the trunk, buttocks, and scrotum. Another frequent finding are painful paresthesias due to small fiber neuropathy (involvement of the vasa nervorum). The diagnosis is confirmed by skin biopsy (lipid inclusions in the vascular endothelium, Fig. 6.8) and biochemical studies.

So far there is no completely effective treatment. Carbamazepine or phenytoin may offer relief from the painful paraesthesias. Enzyme replacement therapy (ERT) has been shown to be effective in ameliorating some of the symptoms (Schiffmann *et al.* 2001). In a recent double blind placebo-controlled trial 26 hemizygous male patients were randomized to receive α-galactosidase A (α-gal A) or placebo. α-gal A was administered intravenously at a dosage of 0.2 mg/kg given every other week (12 doses total). Compared with placebo treatment with α-gal A reduced the level of neuropathic pain (the primary outcome measure), improved glomerular histology, reduced the QRS interval on electrocardiography, and partially corrected the underlying metabolic defect as reflected by significant Gb3 reductions and weight gain. After completing the initial trial, all patients were enrolled in a 1-year open-label continuation trial of ERT. After 12 or 18 months of therapy some haemodynamic abnormalities of the brain had largely resolved. Intravenous administration of α-gal A appears to be safe particularly when given over 40 minutes. ERT offers promise as an effective management strategy for patients with Fabry disease.

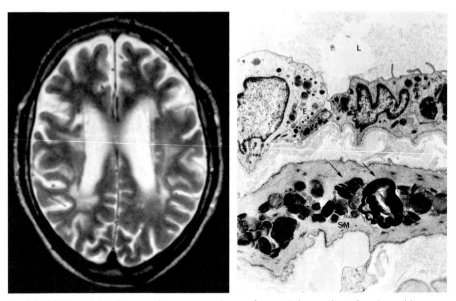

Fig. 6.8 (a) T2-weighted magnetic resonance image from a Fabry patient showing white periventricular and deep white matter high signal, and (b) electron microscopy image of a dermal vessel from the same individual showing multi-lamellated zebra bodies (arrows) within vascular smooth muscle cells (L = vessel lumen; E = endothelial cell; SM = smooth muscle cell) (x16500; kindly provided by J Müller-Höcker, Munich).

6.4.2 **Homocystinuria**

Of the several autosomal recessive enzyme deficiencies that cause homocystinuria, cystathionine beta-synthase (CBS) deficiency, in which the conversion of homocysteine to cytstathionine is impaired, is the most common form (Mudd *et al.* 1995). The estimated incidence of CBS deficiency varies from 1 in 50,000 to 1 in 400,000. Over 90 different mutations have been described, with most being quite rare (Kraus *et al.* 1999 and http://www.uchsc.edu/sm/cbs). Homocystinuria may also result from disturbances in the conversion of homocysteine to methionine by a pathway that requires the formation of methylated derivatives of both folate and vitamin B12.

The disease should be considered in any child with stroke, mental retardation, or atraumatic (mostly downward) dislocation of lenses. Other features include skeletal abnormalities (marfanoid habitus) and premature atherosclerosis and thrombosis. The separation of homocystinuria from Marfan syndrome represents one of the earliest and best examples of the concept of phenocopies. The propensity toward vascular thrombosis is the major life-threatening manifestation of the disease. Twenty-five per cent of untreated patients with CBS deficiency will have had a thromboembolic event by the age of 20 years.

Cerebrovascular accidents account for about one third of thromboembolic complications. Damage to the endothelium is suspected to be a critical step of the atherosclerotic process (Doshi *et al.* 1999). Homocysteine has been shown to directly damage endothelial cells and increase smooth muscle cell proliferation *in vitro*. Putative factors whereby homocysteine may induce vascular injury further include extracellular matrix modification, lipoprotein oxidation, and effects on platelet survival time and coagulation (Bellamy *et al.* 1997). Arteries show marked fibrous intimal thickening and abnormalities of the vascular media. Patients with concurrent homocystinuria and factor V Leiden have an increased risk of thrombosis (Mandel *et al.* 1996).

Homocysteine in the urine is easily detected by an amino acid analysis. CBS deficiency must be differentiated from other defects that can cause homocystinuria. In CBS deficiency, plasma levels of methionine are elevated (usually in the range of 500–2000 µM). Based on observations that some patients with CBS deficiency may respond to pyridoxine (vitamin B6) therapy, two major subgroups have traditionally been defined: pyridoxine responsive homocystinuria and pyridoxine non-responsive homocystinuria. Those that are responsive tend to have a later onset, a milder phenotype and a better prognosis. Mild to moderate elevations of plasma homocysteine have been established as an independent risk factor for extracranial carotid-artery stenosis and cardiovascular complications including stroke (Selhub *et al.* 1995, Welch and Loscalzo 1998) and see Chapter 7.

Early diagnosis of homocystinuria is critical, as the frequency of clinical complications can be minimized by instituting an appropriate (methionine-restricted) diet and, in some forms of the disease, large daily doses of pyridoxine (50–500 mg/day) (Mudd *et al.* 1985). Betaine, a methyl donor that recycles homocysteine to methionine, is recommended for those who do not tolerate a methionine-restricted diet and do not respond to pyridoxine. Folate is recommended because of a secondary deficiency. Antiplatelet agents are given to prevent thromboembolic complications. Patients with homocystinuria are at increased risk for surgery and need special perioperative care (Weksler 1995).

6.4.3 Sickle cell disease

Sickle cell disease (SCD) comprises a group of inherited haemoglobinopathies. Haemoglobin S (HbS) results from an amino acid substitution in the β-chain. SCD disease may be caused by the homozygous state for HbS or by the compound heterozygous state with other haemoglobinopathies (e.g. HbC or mild β-thalassaemia) (Old 2002).

Neurological complications are common and include transient ischaemic attacks (TIA), stroke, cognitive decline, myelopathy, and seizures (Prengler *et al.* 2002). Based on data from more than 4000 patients it has been estimated that 25 per cent of patients with HbSS and 10 per cent of those with HbSC disease will have had a stroke by the age of 45 years (Ohene-Frempong *et al.* 1998). Patients with SCD may develop both ischaemic and haemorrhagic stroke. The risk for haemorrhagic stroke is highest between age 20 and 29 years. In contrast the incidence of ischaemic stroke shows two peaks (between 2 and 5 years and >50 years) and decreases between 20 and 29 years (Ohene-Frempong *et al.* 1998). The recurrence rate for stroke is high (up to 67%).

At least three mechanisms account for ischaemic stroke in SCD: (1) small vessel disease (intravascular sickling or sludging phenomenon), (2) large artery disease (intimal hyperplasia and thrombus formation), and (3) hemodynamic insufficiency. Large vessel disease is usually confined to the distal supraclinoid internal carotid artery (ICA) and the proximal portions of the middle cerebral artery (MCA) and anterior cerebral artery (ACA). Such lesions have been demonstrated in about 80 per cent of SCD patients who presented with a stroke (Adams 2001). In advanced stages angiography may show Moya–Moya-like vascular changes. In fact, Moya–Moya disease and SCD share the risk of early infarction coupled with a later risk of haemorrhage possibly due to rupture of dilated weakened colateral vessels. The cause of intimal hyperplasia, and why it occurs at specific sites in the anterior circulation is unknown. Ischaemic infarcts are often located in borderzone regions, in particular the anterior and deep borderzone region (Pavlakis *et al.* 1988). In a series of 320 patients 22 per cent showed typical infarcts and 13 per cent showed silent infarcts (Moser *et al.* 1996). Silent infarcts are associated with stroke (Miller *et al.* 2001) and cognitive decline (Armstrong *et al.* 1996).

Strokes may be precipitated by pain crisis, infection, and other systemic illnesses. Hypoxia and acute worsening of anaemia are associated with a higher risk for stroke (Prengler *et al.* 2002). Risk factors for ischaemic stroke in SCD include prior TIA, recent episodes of chest pain, and increased blood pressure. Haemorrhagic strokes are associated with a high mortality rate (26% within 2 weeks following the event)(Ohene-Frempong *et al.* 1998).

There are three main approaches to therapy: (1) transfusion, (2) hydroxyurea, and (3) bone marrow transplantation (Adams 2001, Prengler *et al.* 2002). The aim of transfusion therapy is to normalize cerebral perfusion acutely and to prevent stroke recurrence. Transcranial doppler sonography (TCD) has been shown to be valuable in selecting patients at high risk for stroke (Adams *et al.* 1992). Patients with flow velocities in the middle cerebral artery or distal internal carotid artery of 200 cm/s or higher had a 40 per cent risk for stroke over 3 years. The Stroke Prevention Trial in SCD (STOP study) tested whether long-term transfusion therapy can reduce the risk of first stroke in high-risk children selected by screening with TCD (Adams *et al.* 1998). As a result of this trial it was recommended to place all patients with middle cerebral artery blood flow velocities >200 cm/s on transfusion (National Heart, Lung, and Blood Institute Clinical Alert). Perfusion MRI has recently been shown to be sensitive in detecting CBF changes in SCD (Kirkham *et al.* 2001). Whether perfusion MRI is valuable for guiding the management in individual patients needs to be determined. Bone marrow transplantation may be curative. In 10 patients with a history of stroke, there was stabilization on neuroimaging within 1 year (Walters *et al.* 2000, Adams 2001, Prengler *et al.* 2002). However, there is a considerable risk of peritransplant complications. Hydroxyurea elevates the percentage of fetal haemoglobin and is associated with improvements in rheology and red blood cell survival. Hydroxyurea has been shown to successfully reduce the frequency of pain, acute chest syndrome, and need for transfusions (Charache *et al.* 1995). However, its effects on stroke are unknown.

6.5 Embolic causes of stroke

6.5.1 Hereditary haemorrhagic telangiectasia

Hereditary haemorrhagic telangiectasia (HHT; Osler–Weber–Rendu disease) is an autosomal dominant vascular dysplasia that is inherited with high penetrance and variable expressivity. The estimated prevalence is up to 1 in 50,000. A family history of HHT is present in most patients. Vascular malformations may occur in various organs, including the lung, liver, kidney, and brain.

Clinically, the condition is characterized by mucocutaneous telangiectasias, severe recurrent epistaxis, gastrointestinal haemorrhage, and a high incidence of vascular malformations in the lung and brain (Guttmacher *et al.* 1995). Telangiectasias tend to enlarge and multiply over time. Pulmonary arteriovenous malformations (AVMs) are frequently accompanied by dyspnea or haemoptysis. Neurologic complications may arise from pulmonary AVMs or cerebrovascular malformations (CVMs) which include classic AVM, cavernous malformations, venous malformations, and indeterminate CVMs (Fulbright *et al.* 1998). In a large systematic study the frequency of classic AVMs was found to be 11 per cent (Willemse *et al.* 2000). AVMs are mostly low grade (Spetzler-Martin grade I or II), are frequently multiple, and occur both supratentorially and infratentorially. Intracranial AVMs may cause intraparenchymal or subarachnoid haemorrhage but the risk of bleeding is relatively low (Willemse *et al.* 2000, Maher *et al.* 2001). In a large series of 321 cases with HHT the frequency of intracranial haemorrhage (ICH) was found to be 2.1 per cent with a mean age of onset for ICH of 25.4 years (Maher *et al.* 2001). All patients with ICH had a favourable outcome at a mean follow up interval of six years. Other manifestations of CVMs include seizures as well as headache. The most frequent cause of neurologic complications is embolism from pulmonary AVM. About 20 per cent of patients with HHT develop pulmonary AVM, and about one third of those with pulmonary AVM will develop cerebrovascular complications (Maher *et al.* 2001). Paradoxial embolism is the most common mechanism. However, rarely a thrombus may form within the fistula itself. Transient ischaemic attacks during haemoptysis may be caused by air embolism from a bleeding pulmonary arteriovenous fistula. Moreover, brain abscess from septic emboli occur in 5–9 per cent of HHT patients with pulmonary AVM.

Most HHT families have mutations in one of two known genes. HHT1 is the endoglin gene on chromosome 9q33. Endoglin is a homodimeric transmembrane receptor which is highly expressed on endothelial cells. Endoglin binds transforming growth factor-beta (TGFβ) isoforms 1 and 3 in combination with the signalling complex of TGFβ receptors types I and II. Its expression increases during angiogenesis, wound healing, and inflammation, all of which are associated with TGFβ signalling and alterations in vascular structure. Mouse embryos lacking both copies of the endoglin gene die due to defects in vessel and heart development (Bourdeau *et al.* 1999, Arthur *et al.* 2000). HHT2 is the activin receptor-like kinase 1 gene (ALK1) on chromosome 12q13 (Johnson *et al.* 1996). Like endoglin, ALK1 is a cell-surface receptor for the TGFβ superfamily of ligands that is heavily expressed in endothelial and vascular smooth muscle cells. Mice deficient in ALK1 show severe vascular abnormalities characterized by fusion of capillary plexes into cavernous vessels (Urness *et al.* 2000). Thus both HHT1 and HHT2 highlight the role of receptors for TGFβ family members in the regulation of vascular differentiation.

The treatment of HHT is usually limited to the management of complications. In some cases resection or occlusion of pulmonary arteriovenous fistulas may be recommended. In patients with recurrent bleeding chronic iron administration and periodic transfusion may be necessary.

6.5.2 Familial cardiomyopathies and familial dysrythmias

Cardiomyopathies are classified as hypertrophic (HCM), dilated (DCM), arrythmogenic right ventricular (ARVC), and restrictive cardiomyopathy (RCM). A genetic cause has been demonstrated in 50 per cent of patients with HCM, 35 per cent with DCM, and about 30 per cent with ARVC. Multiple genetic loci and genes have been identified for each of these conditions (Franz *et al.* 2001). Inheritance is usually autosomal dominant. HCM is common (~1 in 500 young adults) and has been identified as an important cause of sudden unexpected death. DCM (~1 in 20,000) and ARVC are less frequent.

Embolic stroke or TIA may occur as a complication of all types of cardiomyopathy, with atrial fibrillation (AF) being the major determinant. Other potential mechanisms include mural thrombi. Of 900 patients followed over a mean of 7 ± 7 years, 44 (4.9%) developed an ischaemic stroke (Maron *et al.* 2002). Of these 89 per cent (39) had AF. Twenty per cent (10) died as a direct consequence of their event. Apart from AF, stroke was independtly associated with congestive symptoms and advanced age. Prophylactic warfarin treatment was associated with a marked reduction of cerebrovascular events. There is little data regarding the frequency and determinants of stroke in patients with DCM and ARVC. The frequency of white matter lesions and cerebral infarcts was found to be significantly higher in patients with DCM aged <50 years than in matched controls (Dusleag *et al.* 1992). Because of its clinical heterogeneity there is no uniform treatment strategy for cardiomyopathy. Apart from treatment, prophylaxis of sudden death is important even in symptom-free patients.

There are several forms of primary cardiac arrythmia which may be classified depending on whether they involve superventricular structures (e.g. familial atrial fibrillation), the conduction system, or the ventricular system (e.g. long QT syndrome, reviewed in Roberts and Brugada 2000). Most frequently inheritance is autosomal dominant. Many of the genes have been mapped to specific chromosomal regions. Some of them have been shown to encode ion channels (Keating and Sanguinetti 2001). Stroke has repeatedly been reported in families with primary cardiac arrhythmia (Natowicz and Kelley 1987, Brugada et al. 1997) albeit there are no systematic studies addressing the frequency of cerebrovascular events in this group of disorders.

6.6 Prothrombotic disorders

Several genetic defects of proteins that regulate blood coagulation have been identified including deficiencies of the natural anticoagulants (antithrombin III, protein C, protein S), and point mutations in coagulation molecules such as factor V Leiden (1691G/A) or the prothrombin gene (20210G/A).

An association between inherited thrombophilias and venous thrombosis is firmly established (Rosendaal 1999). However, an association with ischaemic stroke has been questioned. In fact, most association studies have been negative (Hassan and Markus 2000, Hankey et al. 2001). Their role in multifactorial stroke is reviewed in Chapter 7. There is some evidence that coagulation disorders are relevant to the pathogenesis of stroke in young people (Martinez et al. 1993, Barinagarrementeria et al. 1994, Munts et al. 1998, Gunther et al. 2000 and Section 12.8.4). However, further studies are warranted to settle this issue. Theoretically, thrombophilia may exacerbate stroke whether it is embolic or atherothrombotic, while venous thrombosis could cause stroke in patients with a cardiac right to left shunt. It has been suggetsed that the co-occurrence of multiple coagulation defects potentiates the risk for ischaemic stroke (Koller et al. 1994, Chaturvedi and Dzieczkowski 1999, Chaturvedi et al. 1999).

Routine laboratory testing for inherited thrombophilias is unwarranted in all patients with ischaemic stroke. However, testing may be useful in selected patients. Factors that increase the pre-test probability include: (i) venous or arterial thrombosis in patients aged ≤45 years, (ii) recurrent thrombosis without precipitating factors, (iii) a family history of thrombosis, (iv) thrombosis during pregnancy, (v) resistance to heparin (ATIII deficiency), and (vi) warfarin induced skin-necrosis (protein C or protein S deficiencies) (Bushnell et al. 2000). A number of aspects need to be considered before ordering these tests, since test results are influenced by physiological, pharmacological, and hematological factors: First, testing should be avoided in the acute phase (i.e. until 2 months post-stroke). Second, patients should not be on warfarin for at least 2 weeks. Third, tests shoud be repeated after several weeks for confirmation and, fourth, testing family members should be considered if there is a family history of thrombosis (Bushnell et al. 2000).

Patients with ischaemic stroke who are found to have an inherited thrombophilia are often treated empirically with anticoagulants based on the assumptions that the association is causal and that anticoagulants are the most effective treatment. Neither of these assumptions are evidence-based.

6.7 **Mitochondrial disorders**

Mitochondrial disease (MD) is an important cause of stroke particularly in young individuals. Data regarding the prevalence of MD among stroke patients vary considerably depending on the age of the population under investigation, the type of stroke, and the methods used to diagnose MD (Martinez-Fernandez et al. 2001). Mitochondrial myopathy, encephalopathy, lactic acidosis, and stroke-like episodes (MELAS) is associated with several mutations in mitochondrial DNA (mtDNA). Most cases (approximatley 80%) result from a point mutation (A3243G) in the tRNA[leucine (UUR)] gene which is associated with respiratory chain complex I deficiency. Muscle biopsy reveals abnormal mitochondria and ragged-red fibers.

The phenotype of MELAS is highly variable ranging from asymptomatic cases to severe childhood multisystem disease with lactic acidosis. Stroke-like episodes usually occur before age 40. The mechanisms underlying these episodes are incompletely understood. In many cases 'stroke' regions are not limited to vascular territories and cerebral angiography does not reveal embolic or stenotic lesions. These observations indicate that mechanisms other than cerebral infarction may be involved. Some authors have suggested a disturbance of the blood–brain barrier, presumably due to mitochondrial respiratory failure in the vascular endothelium (Yoneda et al. 1999). Others suspected an impaired autoregulation of cerebral blood supply secondary to metabolic abnormalities within precapillary sphincters (Sakuta and Nonaka 1989, Ohama et al. 1987). Both hypotheses are supported by studies that have indicated increased numbers of enlarged and structurally abnormal mitochondria in endothelial cells, pericytes, and vascular smooth muscle cells of capillaries and small arteries (Ohama et al. 1987, Sakuta and Nonaka 1989, Mizukami et al. 1992, Tsuchiya et al. 1999). In addition, primary defects in neuronal oxidative metabolism may be involved in the pathogenesis of stroke-like episodes in MELAS. Cerebral lesions often involve the occipital–parietal regions (Fig. 6.9 and Fig. 13.3). MR spectroscopy is useful to demonstrate elevated levels of lactate within 'stroke' lesions (see Fig. 13.4), although a simlar peak is often seen acutely with other causes of ischaemic infarction. These lesions may markedly regress on subsequent scans.

Several anecdotal reports have advocated the use of coenzyme Q, dichloroacetate, creatine, or vitamins in MELAS. However, in one of very few controlled trials there was no significant effect of coenzyme Q and multiple vitamins in mitochondrial diseases. Intravenous administration of L-Arginine, the precursor of nitric oxide, given within 1 h of onset of stroke-like episodes has been reported to result in dramatic improvement of ischaemic symptoms (Koga 2002).

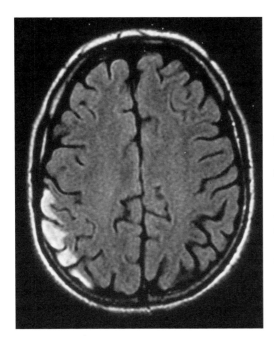

Fig. 6.9 Magnetic resonance image (FLAIR sequence) showing a cortical 'infarction' in an 18-year-old male patient with MELAS and a typical A3243G mutation in the tRNA$^{leucine (UUR)}$ gene. The patient presented with hemianopia and status epilepticus. Further neuroimaging appearances of MEALS are shown in Figs 13.3. and 13.4.

A rigorous epidemiological study was carried out for the A3243G mutation for mitochondrial encephalopathy, lactic acidosis, and stroke-like episodes (MELAS syndrome) in the adult population of Northern Ostrobothnia, a province in northern Finland (Majamaa *et al*. 1998). This mutation was found in 11 pedigrees, and its frequency was calculated to be no less than 16.3 per 100,000 in the adult population of the region (95% CI, 11.3–21.4 per 100,000). Mitochondrial DNA haplotyping indicated that the mutation had arisen in the population at least nine separate times. The most common symptoms associated with the point mutation were hearing impairment, cognitive decline, and short stature. The authors point out that Finland is known to harbour at least 30 heritable disorders at a greater prevalence than other countries. This may be due in part to a founder effect and to the isolation of the population. Until epidemiological studies of MELAS have been conducted in other populations, it is not possible to know whether the prevalence of the mutation is higher in Finland than elsewhere.

6.8 Familial hemiplegic migraine

Familial hemiplegic migraine (FHM) is a rare autosomal dominantly inherited disorder characterized by attacks of transient hemiparesis followed by a migraine headache (International Headache Classification Committee of the International Headache Society 1988). It may be divided into pure FHM (80% of families), and FHM with permanent cerebellar signs. FHM is genetically heterogenous. Mutations in CACNA1A are present in 50 per cent of families with hemiplegic migraine, including all those with cerebellar signs (Ophoff *et al.* 1996, Ducros *et al.* 2001). CACNA1A encodes the α1A subunit of voltage-gated P/Q-type calcium channels in neurons. A minority of families with pure FHM map to a second locus on Chromosome 1 (Gardner *et al.* 1997, Joutel *et al.* 2001) and there is evidence for at least one additional locus.

Onset of symptoms is usually in childhood or adolescence (mean 17 years, range 1–51 years) (Ducros *et al.* 2001, Thomsen *et al.* 2002). In addition to hemiplegic attacks, patients with FHM most often have other typical aura symptoms (sensory, visual, aphasic, and motor). A significant proportion of patients have attacks fullfilling the criteria for basilar migraine (Thomsen *et al.* 2002), and about one third have attacks with decreased consciousness or coma (Ducros *et al.* 2001, Thomsen *et al.* 2002). Attacks may be precipitated by minor head trauma or conventional angiography (Joutel *et al.* 1993, Ducros *et al.* 2001, Kors *et al.* 2001, Thomsen *et al.* 2002). In FHM the duration of both the aura and headache is often prolonged. Aura symptoms may last up to several weeks (Vahedi *et al.* 2000). Some patients develop permanent cerebellar signs, in particular nystagmus, ataxia, and dysarthria. These symptoms develop gradually and may be accompanied by progressive cerebellar atrophy. Epileptic seizures (mostly generalized) are found in up to 7 per cent of the patients (Thomsen *et al.* 2002). They may occur in the context of severe migraine attacks and independently.

Stroke has repeatedly been mentioned in patients with FHM. However, so far there is no conclusive evidence for an association between FHM and stroke. In the series by Thomsen 5 out of 147 patients (3.4%) were reported to have had a stroke. However, details regarding age at onset or the type of infarcts were not provided. In the series by Ducros, which included 117 patients with a documented CACNA1A mutation, stroke was not reported. There are some remarkable phenotypic similarities between FHM and CADASIL, including attacks of hemiplegic migraine and an increased risk for angiographic complications (Joutel *et al.* 1993, Hutchinson *et al.* 1995, Dichgans *et al.* 1997). However, in contrast to CADASIL there is no evidence for an increased frequency of infarcts or subcortical white matter abnormalities on MRI in FHM.

Ketamine (a glutamate NMDA receptor antagonist) has been used with success to treat aura symptoms in FHM. In a small open label study ketamine given intranasally in the early aura phase reproducibly reduced the severity and duration of neurologic deficits in 5/11 patients with FHM (Kaube *et al.* 2000). There have been anecdotal reports on a therapeutic response to verapamil and acetazolamide. However, these reports await further confirmation.

References

Adams, R., McKie, V., Nichols, F., *et al.* (1992). The use of transcranial ultrasonography to predict stroke in sickle cell disease. *New England Journal of Medicine*, **326**, 605–10.

Adams, R.J. (2001). Stroke prevention and treatment in sickle cell disease. *Archives of Neurology*, **58**, 565–8.

Adams, R.J., McKie, V.C., Hsu, L., *et al.* (1998). Prevention of a first stroke by transfusions in children with sickle cell anemia and abnormal results on transcranial Doppler ultrasonography. *New England Journal of Medicine*, **339**, 5–11.

Altarescu, G., Moore, D.F., Pursley, R., *et al.* (2001). Enhanced endothelium-dependent vasodilation in Fabry disease. *Stroke*, **32**, 1559–62.

Aoyagi, M., Fukai, N., Yamamoto, M., Nakagawa, K., Matsushima, Y., and Yamamoto, K. (1996). Early development of intimal thickening in superficial temporal arteries in patients with moyamoya disease. *Stroke*, **27**, 1750–4.

Arboleda-Velasquez, J.F., Lopera, F., Lopez, E., *et al.* (2002). C455R notch3 mutation in a Colombian CADASIL kindred with early onset of stroke. *Neurology*, **59**, 277–9.

Armstrong, F.D., Thompson, R.J., Jr., Wang, W., *et al.* (1996). Cognitive functioning and brain magnetic resonance imaging in children with sickle cell disease. Neuropsychology Committee of the Cooperative Study of Sickle Cell Disease. *Pediatrics*, **97**, 864–70.

Artavanis-Tsakonas, S., Rand, M.D., and Lake, R.J. (1999). Notch signaling: cell fate control and signal integration in development. *Science*, **284**, 770–6.

Arthur, H.M., Ure, J., Smith, A.J., *et al.* (2000). Endoglin, an ancillary TGFbeta receptor, is required for extraembryonic angiogenesis and plays a key role in heart development. *Developmental Biology*, **217**, 42–53.

Auer, D.P., Putz, B., Gossl, C., Elbel, G.K., Gasser, T., and Dichgans, M. (2001*a*). Differential lesion patterns in CADASIL and sporadic subcortical arteriosclerotic encephalopathy: MR imaging study with statistical parametric group comparison. *Radiology*, **218**, 443–51.

Auer, D., Schirmer, T., Heidenreich, J.O., Herzog, J., Pütz, B., and Dichgans, M. (2001*b*). Altered white and gray matter metabolism in CADASIL as detected by chemical shift imaging and single voxel ^{1}H-MRS. *Neurology*, **56**, 635–42.

Barinagarrementeria, F., Cantu-Brito, C., De La, P.A., and Izaguirre, R. (1994). Prothrombotic states in young people with idiopathic stroke. A prospective study. *Stroke*, **25**, 287–90.

Baudrimont, M., Dubas, F., Joutel, A., Tournier-Lasserve, E., and Bousser, M.G. (1993). Autosomal dominant leukoencephalopathy and subcortical ischemic stroke. A clinicopathological study. *Stroke*, **24**, 122–5.

Bellamy, M.F. and McDowell, I.F. (1997). Putative mechanisms for vascular damage by homocysteine. *Journal of Inherited Metabolic Diseases*, **20**, 307–15.

Bourdeau, A., Dumont, D.J., and Letarte, M. (1999). A murine model of hereditary hemorrhagic telangiectasia. *Journal of Clinical Investigation*, **104**, 1343–51.

Brady, R.O. and Schiffmann, R. (2000). Clinical features of and recent advances in therapy for Fabry disease. *Journal of the American Medical Association*, **284**, 2771–5.

Brugada, R., Tapscott, T., Czernuszewicz, G.Z., *et al.* (1997). Identification of a genetic locus for familial atrial fibrillation. *New England Journal of Medicine*, **336**, 905–11.

Brüning, R., Dichgans, M., Berchtenbreiter, C., *et al.* (2001). CADASIL: decrease in regional cerebral blood volume in hyperintense subcortical lesions inversely correlates with disability and cognitive performance. *AJNR American Journal of Neuroradiology*, **22**, 1268–74.

Bushnell, C.D. and Goldstein, L.B. (2000). Diagnostic testing for coagulopathies in patients with ischemic stroke. *Stroke*, **31**, 3067–78.

Caplan, L.R. (1995). Binswanger's disease—revisited. *Neurology*, **45**, 626–33.

Chabriat, H., Bousser, M.G., and Pappata, S. (1995*a*). Cerebral autosomal dominant arteriopathy with subcortical infarcts and leukoencephalopathy: a positron emission tomography study in two affected family members. *Stroke*, **26**, 1729–30.

Chabriat, H., Vahedi, K., Iba-Zizen, M.T., *et al.* (1995*b*). Clinical spectrum of CADASIL: a study of 7 families. Cerebral autosomal dominant arteriopathy with subcortical infarcts and leukoencephalopathy. *Lancet*, **346**, 934–9.

Chabriat, H., Levy, C., Taillia, H., *et al.* (1998). Patterns of MRI lesions in CADASIL. *Neurology*, **51**, 452–7.

Chabriat, H., Pappata, S., Poupon, C., *et al.* (1999). Clinical severity in CADASIL related to ultrastructural damage in white matter: in vivo study with diffusion tensor MRI. *Stroke*, **30**, 2637–43.

Chabriat, H., Pappata, S., Ostergaard, L., *et al.* (2000). Cerebral hemodynamics in CADASIL before and after acetazolamide challenge assessed with MRI bolus tracking. *Stroke*, **31**, 1904–12.

Charache, S., Terrin, M.L., Moore, R.D., *et al.* (1995). Effect of hydroxyurea on the frequency of painful crises in sickle cell anemia. Investigators of the Multicenter Study of Hydroxyurea in Sickle Cell Anemia. *New England Journal of Medicine*, **332**, 1317–22.

Chaturvedi, S. and Dzieczkowski, J.S. (1999). Protein S deficiency, activated protein C resistance and sticky platelet syndrome in a young woman with bilateral strokes. *Cerebrovascular Diseases*, **9**, 127–30.

Chaturvedi, S., Joshi, N., and Dzieczkowski, J. (1999). Activated protein C resistance in young African American patients with ischemic stroke. *Journal of Neurological Sciences*, **163**, 137–9.

Conway, J.E., Hutchins, G.M., Tamargo, R.J. (1999). Marfan syndrome is not associated with intracranial aneurysms. *Stroke*, **30**, 1632–6.

Conway, J.E., Hutchins, G.M., and Tamargo, R.J. (2001). Lack of evidence for an association between neurofibromatosis type I and intracranial aneurysms: autopsy study and review of the literature. *Stroke*, **32**, 2481–5.

Crutchfield, K.E., Patronas, N.J., Dambrosia, J.M., *et al.* (1998). Quantitative analysis of cerebral vasculopathy in patients with Fabry disease. *Neurology*, **50**, 1746–9.

DeGraba, T., Azhar, S., Dignat-George, F., *et al.* (2000). Profile of endothelial and leukocyte activation in Fabry patients. *Annals of Neurology*, **47**, 229–33.

Desmond, D.W., Moroney, J.T., Lynch, T., Chan, S., Chin, S.S., and Mohr, J.P. (1999). The natural history of CADASIL: a pooled analysis of previously published cases. *Stroke*, **30**, 1230–3.

Desnick, R.J. (1995). α-Galactosidase A deficiency: Fabry disease. In *The metabolic bases of inherited disease* (eds C.R. Scriver, A.L. Beaudet, W.S. Sly, and D. Valle), pp. 2741–84. McGraw Hill, New York.

Dichgans, M., Mayer, M., Muller-Myhsok, B., Straube, A., and Gasser, T. (1996). Identification of a key recombinant narrows the CADASIL gene region to 8 cM and argues against allelism of CADASIL and familial hemiplegic migraine. *Genomics*, **32**, 151–4.

Dichgans, M. and Petersen, D. (1997). Angiographic complications in CADASIL. *Lancet*, **349**, 776–7.

Dichgans, M., Mayer, M., Uttner, I., *et al.* (1998). The phenotypic spectrum of CADASIL: clinical findings in 102 cases. *Annals of Neurology*, **44**, 731–9.

Dichgans, M., Filippi, M., Bruning, R., *et al.* (1999*a*). Quantitative MRI in CADASIL: correlation with disability and cognitive performance. *Neurology*, **52**, 1361–7.

Dichgans, M., Wick, M., and Gasser, T. (1999*b*). Cerebrospinal fluid findings in CADASIL. *Neurology*, **53**, 233.

Dichgans, M., Herzog, J., and Gasser, T. (2001). *Notch3* in-frame deletion involving three cysteine residues causes typical CADASIL. *Neurology*, **57**, 1714–7.

Dichgans, M., Ludwig, H., Müller-Höcker, J., Messerschmidt, A., and Gasser, T. (2000). Small in-frame deletions and missense mutations in CADASIL: 3D models predict misfolding of Notch3 EGF-like repeat domains. *European Journal of Human Genetics*, **8**, 280–5.

Dichgans, M., Holtmannspötter, K., Herzog, J., Peters, N., Bergmann, M., and Yousry, T.A. (2002). Cerebral microbleeds in CADASIL: a gradient-echo MRI and autopsy study. *Stroke*, **33**, 67–71.

Doshi, S.N., Goodfellow, J., Lewis, M.J., and McDowell, I.F. (1999). Homocysteine and endothelial function. *Cardiovascular Research*, **42**, 578–82.

Ducros, A., Denier, C., Joutel, A., *et al.* (2001). The clinical spectrum of familial hemiplegic migraine associated with mutations in a neuronal calcium channel. *New England Journal of Medicine*, **345**, 17–24.

Ducros, A., Nagy, T., Alamowitch, S., *et al.* (1996). Cerebral autosomal dominant arteriopathy with subcortical infarcts and leukoencephalopathy, genetic homogeneity, and mapping of the locus within a 2-cM interval. *American Journal of Human Genetics*, **58**, 171–81.

Dusleag, J., Klein, W., Eber, B., *et al.* (1992). Frequency of magnetic resonance signal abnormalities of the brain in patients aged less than 50 years with idiopathic dilated cardiomyopathy. *American Journal of Cardiology*, **69**, 1446–50.

Feuerhake, F., Volk, B., Ostertag, B., *et al.* (2002). Reversible coma with raised intracranial pressure: an unusual clinical manifestation of CADASIL. *Acta Neuropathologica (Berlin)*, **103**, 188–92.

Forteza, A.M., Brozman, B., Rabinstein, A.A., Romano, J.G., and Bradley, W.G. (2001). Acetazolamide for the treatment of migraine with aura in CADASIL. *Neurology*, **57**, 2144–5.

Franz, W.M., Muller, O.J., and Katus, H.A. (2001). Cardiomyopathies: from genetics to the prospect of treatment. *Lancet*, **358**, 1627–37.

Fukui, M. (1997). Current state of study on moyamoya disease in Japan. *Surgical Neurology*, **47**, 138–43.

Fukutake, T. and Hirayama, K. (1995). Familial young-adult-onset arteriosclerotic leukoencephalopathy with alopecia and lumbago without arterial hypertension. *European Neurology*, **35**, 69–79.

Fukuyama, S., Kanai, M., and Osawa, M. (1991). Clinical genetic analysis on the moyamoya disease. In *Annual report 1990* (ed. M. Fukui), pp. 53–9. The research committee on sponataneous occlusion of the circle of willis (moyamoya disease) of the ministry of health and welfare, Fukuoka.

Fulbright, R.K., Chaloupka, J.C., Putman, C.M., *et al.* (1998). MR of hereditary hemorrhagic telangiectasia: prevalence and spectrum of cerebrovascular malformations. *Ameriacn Journal of Neuroradiology*, **19**, 477–84.

Gardner, K., Barmada, M.M., Ptacek, L.J., and Hoffman, E.P. (1997). A new locus for hemiplegic migraine maps to chromosome 1q31. *Neurology*, **49**, 1231–8.

Gott, V.L., Greene, P.S., Alejo, D.E., *et al.* (1999). Replacement of the aortic root in patients with Marfan's syndrome. *New England Journal of Medicine*, **340**, 1307–13.

Graham, J.F. and Matoba, A. (1997). A survey of moyamoya disease in Hawaii. *Clinics in Neurology and Neurosurgery*, **99**, (Suppl 2), S31–S35.

Grand, M.G., Kaine, J., Fulling, K., *et al.* (1988). Cerebroretinal vasculopathy. A new hereditary syndrome. *Ophthalmology*, **95**, 649–59.

Grewal, R.P. (1994). Stroke in Fabry's disease. *Journal of Neurology*, **241**, 153–6.

Gunther, G., Junker, R., Strater, R., *et al.* (2000). Symptomatic ischemic stroke in full-term neonates: role of acquired and genetic prothrombotic risk factors. *Stroke*, **31**, 2437–41.

Gutierrez-Molina, M., Caminero, R.A., Martinez, G.C., Arpa, G.J., Morales, B.C., and Amer, G. (1994). Small arterial granular degeneration in familial Binswanger's syndrome. *Acta Neuropathologica (Berlin)*, **87**, 98–105.

Gutmann, D.H., Aylsworth, A., Carey, J.C., *et al.* (1997). The diagnostic evaluation and multidisciplinary management of neurofibromatosis 1 and neurofibromatosis 2. *Journal of the American Medical Association*, **278**, 51–7.

Gutmann, D.H. and Collins, F.S. (1993). The neurofibromatosis type 1 gene and its protein product, neurofibromin. *Neuron*, **10**, 335–43.

Guttmacher, A.E., Marchuk, D.A., and White, R.I. (1995). Hereditary hemorrhagic telangiectasia. *New England Journal of Medicine*, **333**, 918–24.

Han, D.H., Kwon, O.K., Byun, B.J., *et al.* (2000). A co-operative study: clinical characteristics of 334 Korean patients with moyamoya disease treated at neurosurgical institutes (1976–1994). The Korean Society for Cerebrovascular Disease. *Acta neurochirurgica (Wien)*, **142**, 1263–73.

Hankey, G.J., Eikelboom, J.W., Van Bockxmeer, F.M., Lofthouse, E., Staples, N., and Baker, R.I. (2001). Inherited thrombophilia in ischemic stroke and its pathogenic subtypes. *Stroke*, **32**, 1793–9.

Hassan, A. and Markus, H.S. (2000). Genetics and ischaemic stroke. *Brain*, **123**, 1784–812.

Henkemeyer, M., Rossi, D.J., Holmyard, D.P., *et al.* (1995). Vascular system defects and neuronal apoptosis in mice lacking ras GTPase-activating protein. *Nature*, **377**, 695–701.

Hutchinson, M., O'Riordan, J., Javed, M., *et al.* (1995). Familial hemiplegic migraine and autosomal dominant arteriopathy with leukoencephalopathy (CADASIL). *Annals of Neurology*, **38**, 817–24.

Iannucci, G., Dichgans, M., Rovaris, M., *et al.* (2001). Correlations between clinical findings and magnetization transfer imaging metrics of tissue damage in individuals with cerebral autosomal dominant arteriopathy with subcortical infarcts and leukoencephalopathy. *Stroke*, **32**, 643–8.

Ikeda, H., Sasaki, T., Yoshimoto, T., Fukui, M., and Arinami, T. (1999). Mapping of a familial moyamoya disease gene to chromosome 3p24.2–p26. *American Journal of Human Genetics*, **64**, 533–7.

Ikezaki, K., Han, D.H., Kawano, T., Kinukawa, N., and Fukui, M. (1997). A clinical comparison of definite moyamoya disease between South Korea and Japan. *Stroke*, **28**, 2513–17.

Jen, J., Cohen, A.H., Yue, Q., *et al.* (1997). Hereditary endotheliopathy with retinopathy, nephropathy, and stroke (HERNS). *Neurology*, **49**, 1322–30.

Johnson, D.W., Berg, J.N., Baldwin, M.A., *et al.* (1996). Mutations in the activin receptor-like kinase 1 gene in hereditary haemorrhagic telangiectasia type 2. *Nature Genetics*, **13**, 189–95.

Joutel, A., Bousser, M.G., Biousse, V., *et al.* (1993). A gene for familial hemiplegic migraine maps to chromosome 19. *Nature Genetics*, **5**, 40–5.

Joutel, A., Corpechot, C., Ducros, A., *et al.* (1996). Notch3 mutations in CADASIL, a hereditary adult-onset condition causing stroke and dementia. *Nature*, **383**, 707–10.

Joutel, A., Vahedi, K., Corpechot, C., *et al.* (1997). Strong clustering and stereotyped nature of Notch3 mutations in CADASIL patients. *Lancet*, **350**, 1511–15.

Joutel, A., Andreux, F., Gaulis, S., *et al.* (2000*a*). The ectodomain of Notch3 receptor accumulates within the cerebrovasculature of CADASIL patients. *Journal of Clinical Investigation*, **105**, 597–605.

Joutel, A., Chabriat, H., Vahedi, K., *et al.* (2000*b*). Splice site mutation causing a 7 amino-acids Notch3 in frame deletion in CADASIL. *Neurology*, **54**, 1874–5.

Joutel, A., Dodick, D.D., Parisi, J.E., Cecillon, M., Tournier-Lasserve, E., and Bousser, M.G. (2000*c*). De novo mutation in the Notch3 gene causing CADASIL. *Annals of Neurology*, **47**, 388–91.

Joutel, A., Favrole, P., Labauge, P., *et al.* (2001). Skin biopsy immunostaining with a Notch3 monoclonal antibody for CADASIL diagnosis. *Lancet*, **358**, 2049–51.

Kaube, H., Herzog, J., Kaufer, T., Dichgans, M., and Diener, H.C. (2000). Aura in some patients with familial hemiplegic migraine can be stopped by intranasal ketamine. *Neurology*, **55**, 139–41.

Keating, M.T. and Sanguinetti, M.C. (2001). Molecular and cellular mechanisms of cardiac arrhythmias. *Cell*, 104, 569–80.

Kirkham, F.J., Calamante, F., Bynevelt, M., *et al.* (2001). Perfusion magnetic resonance abnormalities in patients with sickle cell disease. *Annals of Neurology*, 49, 477–85.

Koga, Y., Ishibashi, M., Ueki, I., *et al.* (2002). Effects of L-arginine on the acute phase of strokes in three patients with MELAS. *Neurology*, 58, 827–8.

Koller, H., Stoll, G., Sitzer, M., Burk, M., Schottler, B., and Freund, H.J. (1994). Deficiency of both protein C and protein S in a family with ischemic strokes in young adults. *Neurology*, 44, 1238–40.

Kors, E.E., Terwindt, G.M., Vermeulen, F.L., *et al.* (2001). Delayed cerebral edema and fatal coma after minor head trauma: role of the CACNA1A calcium channel subunit gene and relationship with familial hemiplegic migraine. *Annals of Neurology*, 49, 753–60.

Kraus, J.P., Janosik, M., Kozich, V., *et al.* (1999). Cystathionine beta-synthase mutations in homocystinuria. *Human Mutation*, 13, 362–75.

Lesnik Oberstein, S.A., van den, B.R., Van Buchem, M.A., *et al.* (2001). Cerebral microbleeds in CADASIL. *Neurology*, 57, 1066–70.

Liebetrau, M., Herzog, J., Hamann, G., and Dichgans, M. (2002). Prolonged cerebral transit time in CADASIL: a transcranial ultrasound study. *Stroke*, 33, 509–12.

Maher, C.O., Piepgras, D.G., Brown, R.D., Jr., Friedman, J.A., and Pollock, B.E. (2001). Cerebrovascular manifestations in 321 cases of hereditary hemorrhagic telangiectasia. *Stroke*, 32, 877–82.

Majamaa, K., Moilanen, J.S., Uimonen, S., *et al.* (1998). Epidemiology of A3243G, the mutation for mitochondrial encephalomyopathy, lactic acidosis, and strokelike episodes: prevalence of the mutation in an adult population. *American Journal of Human Genetics*, 63, 447–54.

Mandel, H., Brenner, B., Berant, M., *et al.* (1996). Coexistence of hereditary homocystinuria and factor V Leiden—effect on thrombosis. *New England Journal of Medicine*, 334, 763–8.

Maron, B.J., Olivotto, I., Bellone, P., *et al.* (2002). Clinical profile of stroke in 900 patients with hypertrophic cardiomyopathy. *Journal of the American College of Cardiology*, 39, 301–7.

Martinez-Fernandez, E., Gil-Peralta, A., Garcia-Lozano, R., *et al.* (2001). Mitochondrial disease and stroke. *Stroke*, 32, 2507–10.

Martinez, H.R., Rangel-Guerra, R.A., and Marfil, L.J. (1993). Ischemic stroke due to deficiency of coagulation inhibitors. Report of 10 young adults. *Stroke*, 24, 19–25.

Mayer, M., Straube, A., Bruening, R., *et al.* (1999). Muscle and skin biopsies are a sensitive diagnostic tool in the diagnosis of CADASIL. *Journal of Neurology*, 246, 526–32.

Meikle, P.J., Hopwood, J.J., Clague, A.E., Carey, W.F. (1999). Prevalence of lysosomal storage disorders. *Journal of the American Medical Association*, 281, 249–54.

Mellies, J.K., Baumer, T., Muller, J.A., *et al.* (1998). SPECT study of a German CADASIL family: a phenotype with migraine and progressive dementia only. *Neurology*, 50, 1715–21.

Miller, S.T., Macklin, E.A., Pegelow, C.H., *et al.* (2001). Silent infarction as a risk factor for overt stroke in children with sickle cell anemia: a report from the Cooperative Study of Sickle Cell Disease. *Journal of Pediatrics*, 139, 385–90.

Mitsias, P. and Levine, S.R. (1996). Cerebrovascular complications of Fabry's disease. *Annals of Neurology*, 40, 8–17.

Mizukami, K., Sasaki, M., Suzuki, T., *et al.* (1992). Central nervous system changes in mitochondrial encephalomyopathy: light and electron microscopic study. *Acta Neuropathologica (Berlin)*, 83, 449–52.

Molina, C., Sabin, J.A., Montaner, J., Rovira, A., Abilleira, S., and Codina, A. (1999). Impaired cerebrovascular reactivity as a risk marker for first-ever lacunar infarction: a case-control study. *Stroke*, **30**, 2296–301.

Moore, D.F., Altarescu, G., Ling, G.S., *et al.* (2002). Elevated cerebral blood flow velocities in Fabry disease with reversal after enzyme replacement. *Stroke*, **33**, 525–31.

Moore, D.F., Scott, L.T., Gladwin, M.T., *et al.* (2001). Regional cerebral hyperperfusion and nitric oxide pathway dysregulation in Fabry disease: reversal by enzyme replacement therapy. *Circulation*, **104**, 1506–12.

Moser, F.G., Miller, S.T., Bello, J.A., *et al.* (1996). The spectrum of brain MR abnormalities in sickle-cell disease: a report from the Cooperative Study of Sickle Cell Disease. *AJNR American Journal of Neuroradiology*, **17**, 965–72.

Mudd, S.H., Levy, H.L., and Skovby, F. (1995). Disorders of transsulfuration. In *The metabolic basis of inherited disease* (eds C.R. Scriver, A.L. Beaudet, W.S. Sly, and D. Valle), pp. 1279–327. McGraw Hill, New York.

Mudd, S.H., Skovby, F., Levy, H.L., *et al.* (1985). The natural history of homocystinuria due to cystathionine beta-synthase deficiency. *American Journal of Human Genetics* **37**, 1–31.

Munts, A.G., van Genderen, P.J., Dippel, D.W., van Kooten, F., and Koudstaal, P.J. (1998). Coagulation disorders in young adults with acute cerebral ischaemia. *Journal of Neurology*, **245**, 21–5.

Natowicz, M. and Kelley, R.I. (1987). Mendelian etiologies of stroke. *Annals of Neurology*, **22**, 175–92.

North, K.N., Whiteman, D.A., Pepin, M.G., and Byers, P.H. (1995). Cerebrovascular complications in Ehlers-Danlos syndrome type IV. *Annals of Neurology*, **38**, 960–4.

Norton, K.K., Xu, J., and Gutmann, D.H. (1995). Expression of the neurofibromatosis I gene product, neurofibromin, in blood vessel endothelial cells and smooth muscle. *Neurobiology of disease*, **2**, 13–21.

O'Sullivan, M., Jarosz, J.M., Martin, R.J., Deasy, N., Powell, J.F., and Markus, H.S. (2001). MRI hyperintensities of the temporal lobe and external capsule in patients with CADASIL. *Neurology*, **56**, 628–34.

Oberstein, S.A., Ferrari, M.D., Bakker, E., *et al.* (1999). Diagnostic Notch3 sequence analysis in CADASIL: three new mutations in Dutch patients. Dutch CADASIL Research Group. *Neurology*, **52**, 1913–15.

Ohama, E., Ohara, S., Ikuta, F., Tanaka, K., Nishizawa, M., and Miyatake, T. (1987). Mitochondrial angiopathy in cerebral blood vessels of mitochondrial encephalomyopathy. *Acta Neuropathologica (Berlin)*, **74**, 226–33.

Ohene-Frempong, K., Weiner, S.J., Sleeper, L.A., *et al.* (1998). Cerebrovascular accidents in sickle cell disease: rates and risk factors. *Blood*, **91**, 288–94.

Oka, K., Yamashita, M., Sadoshima, S., and Tanaka, K. (1981). Cerebral haemorrhage in Moyamoya disease at autopsy. *Virchows Archives*, **392**, 247–61.

Old, J. (2002). Hemoglobinopathies and thalassemias. In *Emery's and Rimoin's principles and practice of medical genetics* (eds D.I. Rimoin, J.M. Connor, R.E. Pyeritz, and B. Korf), pp. 1861–98. Churchill Livingstone, London.

Ophoff, R.A., DeYoung, J., Service, S.K., *et al.* (2001). Hereditary vascular retinopathy, cerebroretinal vasculopathy, and hereditary endotheliopathy with retinopathy, nephropathy, and stroke map to a single locus on chromosome 3p21.1–p21.3. *American Journal of Human Genetics*, **69**, 447–53.

Ophoff, R.A., Terwindt, G.M., Vergouwe, M.N., *et al.* (1996). Familial hemiplegic migraine and episodic ataxia type-2 are caused by mutations in the Ca2+ channel gene CACNL1A4. *Cell*, **87**, 543–52.

Papo, T., Biousse, V., Lehoang, P., *et al.* (1998). Susac syndrome. *Medicine (Baltimore)*, 77, 3–11.

Pavlakis, S.G., Bello, J., Prohovnik, I., *et al.* (1988). Brain infarction in sickle cell anemia: magnetic resonance imaging correlates. *Annals of Neurology*, 23, 125–30.

Pepin, M., Schwarze, U., Superti-Furga, A., and Byers, P.H. (2000). Clinical and genetic features of Ehlers-Danlos syndrome type IV, the vascular type (see comments). *New England Journal of Medicine*, 342, 673–80.

Pereira, L., Levran, O., Ramirez, F., *et al.* (1994). A molecular approach to the stratification of cardiovascular risk in families with Marfan's syndrome. *New England Journal of Medicine*, 331, 148–53.

Pfefferkorn, T., von Stuckrat-Barre, S., Herzog, J., Gasser, T., Hamann, G., and Dichgans, M. (2001). Reduced cerebrovascular C02 reactivity in CADASIL: a transcranial doppler sonography study. *Stroke*, 32, 17–21.

Prengler, M., Pavlakis, S.G., Prohovnik, I., and Adams, R.J. (2002). Sickle cell disease: the neurological complications. *Annals of Neurology*, 51, 543–52.

Pyeritz, R.E. (2000). The Marfan syndrome. *Annual Review of Medicine*, 51, 481–510.

Riccardi, V.M. (1991). Neurofibromatosis: past, present, and future. *New England Journal of Medicine*, 324, 1283–5.

Ringpfeil, F., Lebwohl, M.G., Christiano, A.M., and Uitto, J. (2000). Pseudoxanthoma elasticum: mutations in the MRP6 gene encoding a transmembrane ATP-binding cassette (ABC). transporter. *Proceedings of the National Academy Science USA*, 97, 6001–6.

Rizzo, J.F.III. and Lessell, S. (1994). Cerebrovascular abnormalities in neurofibromatosis type 1. *Neurology*, 44, 1000–2.

Roberts, R. and Brugada, R. (2000). Genetic aspects of arrhythmias. *American Journal of Medical Genetics*, 97, 310–18.

Rosendaal, F.R. (1999). Risk factors for venous thrombotic disease. *Thrombosis and Haemostasis*, 82, 610–19.

Rubio, A., Rifkin, D., Powers, J.M., *et al.* (1997). Phenotypic variability of CADASIL and novel morphologic findings. *Acta Neuropathologica (Berlin)*, 94, 247–54.

Ruchoux, M.M., Chabriat, H., Bousser, M.G., Baudrimont, M., and Tournier-Lasserve, E. (1994). Presence of ultrastructural arterial lesions in muscle and skin vessels of patients with CADASIL. *Stroke*, 25, 2291–2.

Ruchoux, M.M., Guerouaou, D., Vandenhaute, B., Pruvo, J.P., Vermersch, P., and Leys, D. (1995). Systemic vascular smooth muscle cell impairment in cerebral autosomal dominant arteriopathy with subcortical infarcts and leukoencephalopathy. *Acta Neuropathologica (Berlin)*, 89, 500–12.

Ruchoux, M.M. and Maurage, C.A. (1997). CADASIL: Cerebral autosomal dominant arteriopathy with subcortical infarcts and leukoencephalopathy. *Journal of Neuropathology and Experimental Neurology*, 56, 947–64.

Sakuta, R. and Nonaka, I. (1989). Vascular involvement in mitochondrial myopathy. *Annals of Neurology*, 25, 594–601.

Schievink, W.I. (1997). Genetics of intracranial aneurysms. *Neurosurgery*, 40, 651–62.

Schievink, W.I., Michels, V.V., and Piepgras, D.G. (1994). Neurovascular manifestations of heritable connective tissue disorders. A review. *Stroke*, 25, 889–903.

Schiffmann, R., Kopp, J.B., Austin, H.A., III *et al.* (2001). Enzyme replacement therapy in Fabry disease: a randomized controlled trial. *Journal of the American Medical Association*, 285, 2743–9.

Schon, F., Martin, R.J., Prevett, M., Clough, C., Enevoldson, T.P., and Markus H.S. (2003). 'CADASIL coma': an underdiagnosed acute encephalopathy. *Journal of Neurology, Neurosurgery and Psychiatry*, 74, 249–52.

Seizinger, B.R. (1993). NF1: a prevalent cause of tumorigenesis in human cancers? *Nature Genetics*, **3**, 97–9.

Selhub, J., Jacques, P.F., Bostom, A.G., *et al.* (1995). Association between plasma homocysteine concentrations and extracranial carotid-artery stenosis. *New England Journal of Medicine*, **332**, 286–91.

Sourander, P. and Walinder, J. (1977). Hereditary multi-infarct dementia. Morphological and clinical studies of a new disease. *Acta Neuropathologica (Berlin)*, **39**, 247–54.

Suzuki, J. and Takaku, A. (1969). Cerebrovascular 'moyamoya' disease. Disease showing abnormal net-like vessels in base of brain. *Archives of Neurology*, **20**, 288–99.

Terborg, C., Gora, F., Weiller, C., and Rother, J. (2000). Reduced vasomotor reactivity in cerebral microangiopathy: a study with near-infrared spectroscopy and transcranial Doppler sonography. *Stroke*, **31**, 924–9.

Terwindt, G.M., Haan, J., Ophoff, R.A., *et al.* (1998). Clinical and genetic analysis of a large Dutch family with autosomal dominant vascular retinopathy, migraine and Raynaud's phenomenon. *Brain*, **121**, 303–16.

Thomsen, L.L., Eriksen, M.K., Roemer, S.F., Andersen, I., Olesen, J., and Russell, M.B. (2002). A population-based study of familial hemiplegic migraine suggests revised diagnostic criteria. *Brain*, **125**, 1379–91.

Tournier-Lasserve, E., Joutel, A., Melki, J., *et al.* (1993). Cerebral autosomal dominant arteriopathy with subcortical infarcts and leukoencephalopathy maps to chromosome 19q12. *Nature Genetics*, **3**, 256–9.

Tsuchiya, K., Miyazaki, H., Akabane, H., *et al.* (1999). MELAS with prominent white matter gliosis and atrophy of the cerebellar granular layer: a clinical, genetic, and pathological study. *Acta Neuropathologica (Berlin)*, **97**, 520–4.

Tuominen, S., Juvonen, V., Amberla, K., *et al.* (2001). Phenotype of a homozygous CADASIL patient in comparison to 9 age-matched heterozygous patients with the same R133C Notch3 mutation. *Stroke*, **32**, 1767–74.

Urness, L.D., Sorensen, L.K., and Li, D.Y. (2000). Arteriovenous malformations in mice lacking activin receptor-like kinase-1. *Nature Genetics*, **26**, 328–31.

Vahedi, K., Denier, C., Ducros, A., *et al.* (2000). CACNA1A gene de novo mutation causing hemiplegic migraine, coma, and cerebellar atrophy. *Neurology*, **55**, 1040–2.

van den Berg, J.S., Hennekam, R.C., Cruysberg, J.R., *et al.* (2000). Prevalence of symptomatic intracranial aneurysm and ischaemic stroke in pseudoxanthoma elasticum (In Process Citation). *Cerebrovascular Diseases*, **10**, 315–19.

van den Berg, J.S., Limburg, M., and Hennekam, R.C. (1996). Is Marfan syndrome associated with symptomatic intracranial aneurysms? *Stroke*, **27**, 10–12.

Walters, M.C., Storb, R., Patience, M., *et al.* (2000). Impact of bone marrow transplantation for symptomatic sickle cell disease: an interim report. Multicenter investigation of bone marrow transplantation for sickle cell disease. *Blood*, **95**, 1918–24.

Wang, W., Prince, C., Mou, Y., and Pollman, M.J. (2002). Notch3 signaling in vascular smooth muscle cells induces c-FLIP expression via ERK/MAPK activation: resistance to FasL-induced apoptosis. *Journal of Biological Chemistry*, **277**, 231665–71.

Weinmaster, G. (1997). The ins and outs of notch signaling. *Molecular and Cellular Neuroscience*, **9**, 91–102.

Weksler, B.B. (1995). Hematologic disorders and ischemic stroke. *Current Opinion in Neurology*, **8**, 38–44.

Welch, G.N. and Loscalzo, J. (1998). Homocysteine and atherothrombosis. *New England Journal of Medicine*, 338, 1042–50.

Willemse, R.B., Mager, J.J., Westermann, C.J., Overtoom, T.T., Mauser, H., and Wolbers, J.G. (2000). Bleeding risk of cerebrovascular malformations in hereditary hemorrhagic telangiectasia. *Journal of Neurosurgery*, 92, 779–84.

Wityk, R.J., Zanferrari, C., and Oppenheimer, S. (2002). Neurovascular complications of Marfan syndrome: a retrospective, hospital-based study. *Stroke*, 33, 680–4.

Yamamoto, M., Aoyagi, M., Tajima, S., *et al.* (1997). Increase in elastin gene expression and protein synthesis in arterial smooth muscle cells derived from patients with Moyamoya disease. *Stroke*, 28, 1733–8.

Yamauchi, T., Tada, M., Houkin, K., *et al.* (2000). Linkage of familial moyamoya disease (spontaneous occlusion of the circle of Willis) to chromosome 17q25. *Stroke*, 31, 930–5.

Yanagawa, S., Ito, N., Arima, K., and Ikeda, S. (2002). Cerebral autosomal recessive arteriopathy with subcortical infarcts and leukoencephalopathy. *Neurology*, 58, 817–20.

Yoneda, M., Maeda, M., Kimura, H., Fujii, A., Katayama, K., and Kuriyama, M. (1999). Vasogenic edema on MELAS: a serial study with diffusion-weighted MR imaging. *Neurology*, 53, 2182–4.

Yousry, T.A., Seelos, K., Mayer, M., *et al.* (1999). Characteristic MR lesion pattern and correlation of T1 and T2 lesion volume with neurologic and neuropsychological findings in cerebral autosomal dominant arteriopathy with subcortical infarcts and leukoencephalopathy (CADASIL). *American Journal of Neuroradiology*, 20, 91–100.

Chapter 7

Polygenic ischaemic stroke including new genetic and statistical approaches

Ahamad Hassan and Hugh S. Markus

7.1 Introduction

Although the monogenic disorders are an important recognized cause of stroke, they comprise less than 1 per cent of all cases. In the vast majority of individuals, stroke is sporadic. In these cases, classical Mendelian patterns of inheritance cannot be demonstrated, although evidence from twin (Brass *et al.* 1992, Bak *et al.* 2002), family history (Jousilahti *et al.* 1997, Liao *et al.* 1997), and animal studies (Rubattu *et al.* 1996, Jeffs *et al.* 1997) still suggests that genetic factors are important. The identification and characterization of the responsible stroke genes has recently been highlighted as a 'field of need' (Boerwinkle *et al.* 1999), as it is envisaged that research will eventually lead to improved assessment of individual disease risk and may reveal new therapeutic pathways. In this chapter we review progress that has been made towards identifying the individual genetic factors in multifactorial ischaemic stroke, limitations of current techniques, and approaches which may be used in the future to overcome these limitations.

7.2 Genetic disease models of ischaemic stroke

Although genetic influences are recognized to be important in ischaemic stroke, before planning studies to identify specific genes it is useful to have a picture of how genetic factors could be operating in the disease. Most stroke geneticists consider a disease model similar to that adopted in other complex traits such as hypertension and diabetes, as being useful.

The principle features of this model are:

(1) That stroke is a polygenic disorder reflecting the influence of several genetic loci modulating different pathophysiological processes. The traditional view is that there may be many hundreds of genetic variants, each conferring equally small amounts of disease risk. However, studies in animal models (Rubattu *et al.* 1996, Jeffs *et al.* 1997), and more recently in man (Gretarsdottir *et al.* 2002), have supported the alternative notion there may be a few major stroke genes which confer the bulk of genetic risk.

(2) That genetic factors may express their influence only under certain conditions. This is a phenomenon which is referred to as variable penetrance and is responsible for complex patterns of inheritance seen in polygenic disorders such as stroke. Variable penetrance can arise for several reasons. For example, the presence of several genes may be required to increase the risk of disease in an additive manner (a gene dose effect), or a gene may have to first interact with another risk factor such as an environmental trigger, for example, smoking or another gene (epistatic interaction). Gene–environment or gene–gene interactions of this kind are usually synergistic with the net result being a multiplicative increase in disease risk.

(3) That genetic factors may be comparatively more important in early onset disease. It is hypothesized that early onset disease has a more homogenous substrate with genetic factors having comparatively more influence than environmental factors (Lander and Schork 1994). There is anecdotal evidence for this theory from other polygenic diseases, and direct evidence for stroke more recently from twin (Brass *et al*. 1998) and family history studies (Jousilahti *et al*. 1997).

Cerebral infarction is the end result of a number of complex pathophysiological processes. If one accepts that stroke is a polygenic condition, it is also helpful to consider at what level in the stroke pathway, genetic influences might be operating to increase disease risk (Fig. 7.1). Genes could be acting at the level of conventional risk factors such as hypertension, either by predisposing to the risk factors themselves or by modulating their effects on end organs. Alternatively genetic factors could be operating independent of these known risk factors by directly participating in the processes that lead to atherosclerosis, plaque rupture, and thromboembolism. Finally genetic factors

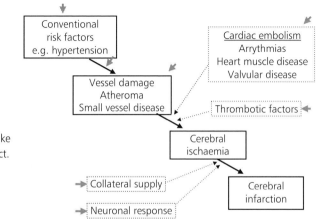

Fig. 7.1 There are multiple potential sites at which stroke susceptibility genes could act. These are illustrated on the flow diagram of stroke pathogenesis by the grey arrows.

could influence the response of brain tissue to ischaemia, for example, by determining collateral blood flow, or neuronal susceptibility to ischaemia.

7.3 Difficulties in identifying stroke genes

Although disease models facilitate our understanding of stroke genes, identifying individual molecular factors is still difficult, for several reasons. First, stroke is usually a late onset disease. This means that techniques which rely on available family members for genetic comparison are difficult to perform, as often the relevant individuals, such as parents or siblings will have died. Second, stroke may exhibit the phenomenon of locus heterogeneity, that is, many different disease alleles may predispose to the same phenotype. Third, stroke is a phenotypically heterogenous disorder, and different stroke subtypes have different underlying disease mechanisms. Recent advances in neuroimaging have made it easier to identify the underlying disease mechanisms and appropriately classify stroke in many cases, although in up to 30 per cent the mechanism may be undetermined. It is likely that the genetic risk profile at the molecular level may differ according to ischaemic stroke subtype. This is illustrated by the autosomal dominant disease CADASIL, described in detail in Section 6.2.1, which results in recurrent lacunar stroke secondary to cerebral small vessel disease, but does not predispose to other stroke subtypes such as large vessel disease or cardioembolism. In addition, it is possible that the overall importance of genetic factors varies between the individual stroke subtypes. For example, it has been hypothesized that genetic influences may be more important in lacunar and large vessel stroke, as opposed to cardioembolic strokes or stroke of undetermined aetiology (Polychronopoulos et al. 2002). In extreme circumstances genetic factors may have no role to play what so ever in an individual stroke because of random or environmental reasons. This is known as phenocopy and an example would be an ischaemic stroke as a result of traumatic arterial dissection. The main message from the above is that definition of stroke phenotype according to underlying mechanism is essential if genetic influences are not to be diluted and genetic risk factors are to be successfully identified. Stroke subtype classification systems which are frequently used include the TOAST (trial of org 10172 in acute stroke treatment) classification (for more detail see Section 1.3) (Adams, Jr. et al. 1993) or the Oxford Community Stroke Project Classification, (Bamford et al. 1991), although the latter system is primarily a clinical classification rather than a pathological system and therefore less precise and not so well suited to genetic association studies.

Other factors which make molecular genetic studies of stroke difficult are variable gene penetrance and the confounding effects of co-existent risk factors such as hypertension and diabetes. These risk factors may share some susceptibility genes with ischaemic stroke and therefore it may be difficult to dissect out the role of an individual gene in the disease.

7.4 Human studies of polygenic ischaemic stroke: the candidate gene approach

The current mainstay of genetic studies of stroke in human has been through the use of association studies. This involves first identifying a molecular variant or polymorphism within a functionally relevant gene (candidate gene), and then determining its role in conferring stroke risk by comparing its frequency amongst affected and unaffected individuals. Traditionally a case control or cohort method is employed, and the individuals tested are unrelated. It should be noted that a positive association does not necessarily imply causation, but may merely represent linkage disequilibrium due to the close proximity between a polymorphism and actual disease causing locus. Association studies are a powerful method to detect disease alleles as exemplified by the association of APOE alleles with Alzheimer's disease (Poirier *et al*. 1993). However, to date no single gene has been consistently implicated in human ischaemic stroke with most associations not replicated and at best remaining controversial. Both false associations (type I error) and missed associations (type II error) are common problems with this type of study. Potential causes of type II error include, small sample sizes, poor selection of phenotype including lack of subtyping, and study of older individuals where genetic factors may carry less influence than environmental factors. One of the most important causes of type I error is population stratification, which arises because of marked differences in the frequency of genetic polymorphisms within different ethnic populations. Other important causes are multiple hypothesis testing, which can lead to association through chance, and publication bias in favour of studies with positive findings. Some journal editors have recently set out standards for acceptance of association studies for publication (Editorial 1999, Bird *et al*. 2001). We would generally agree with these recommendations which are likely to produce the most successful and valuable studies. Some of these guidelines as applied to ischaemic stroke are listed in Table 7.1. Bias due to population stratification can be reduced by studying prospective populations. Most often a nested case–control design is performed where cases developing stroke during the follow up period are matched with individuals who do not develop stroke. This approach has a number of advantages but two main disadvantages. First, characterization of strokes with accurate phenotyping can be difficult. Individuals present with stroke at an unpredictable time and location. Second, the total number of strokes is usually small. For example, in the Physicians Health Study 14,916 men were followed up for 12 years (Zee *et al*. 2002). Three hundred and thirty-eight cases of stroke occurred. Even differentiating ischaemic stroke from haemorrhagic stroke was difficult. Furthermore assuming 20 per cent are due to primary haemorrhage, the number due to specific ischaemic stroke subtypes such as small vessel disease and large vessel disease is likely to only be about 50–70 subjects. This provides little statistical power to determine whether associations exist in these subgroups. Even with follow up of a population of 500,000 for 10 years in the

Table 7.1 Some recommendations for association studies in polygenic human stroke

Problem	Recommendations
Type II error	Adequate sample size, e.g. >300 cases and controls
	Well-phenotyped cases with ischaemic stroke subtyping
	Use intermediate phenotypes (see chapter 8)
	Studies of young subjects, e.g. <65 years
Type I error	
Population stratification	Match controls for ethnic group
	Replicate findings in 2nd independent population
	Use internal family controls (family-based association studies)
Plausibility	Plausible biological hypotheses
Multiple hypothesis testing	Bonferroni correction or other multiple comparisons adjustment
	More stringent p values, e.g. <0.01 or high odds ratio, e.g. >2
Publication bias	Editors should be more willing to publish well designed negative studies.

The role of studies using intermediate phenotypes and family-based association studies is discussed further in the text.

United Kingdom as is planned in the UK BioBank study only 4500 strokes would be expected to occur, resulting, for example, in only 800 cases of small vessel disease stroke or lacunar stroke. Therefore while prospective cohorts may be useful in identifying associations with genes which are risk factors for all types of stroke, they are less efficient at identifying associations with specific stroke phenotypes.

Candidate gene studies require an *a priori* understanding of stroke pathophysiology and therefore lack the ability to identify novel genes. However, a large number of potential candidate genes have been described with potentially functional polymorphisms, which has made this a practical and popular approach.

Ischaemic stroke genes can be considered as belonging to two broad categories: (i) those which influence stroke risk and (ii) those which influence infarct size after vessel occlusion by influencing vascular reactivity, collateral supply, and neuronal responses to injury. It should be remembered that these two categories are not mutually exclusive, because certain genes may predispose to both stroke and stroke outcome. An example of this would be the endothelial nitric oxide synthase gene (eNOS) which by modulating levels of nitric oxide (NO) could influence both development of atherosclerotic plaque and cerebral autoregulation of blood flow. Whilst genes in the second category may be equally relevant to all subtypes of stroke, those falling into the first category may be relevant only in certain stroke subtypes.

A large number of candidate genes has been investigated in stroke, in many cases following the demonstration of an association with ischaemic heart disease. However, it is likely that there are also stroke specific genes which are yet to be characterized. It is convenient to describe the important candidate genes according to their metabolic or biochemical roles. The groups include genes affecting (i) haemostasis, (ii) the renin angiotensin system, (iii) nitric oxide and endothelial dysfunction, (iv) homocysteine metabolism, (v) lipid metabolism, and (vi) proinflammatory genes. Over the last few years there has been a proliferation of association studies examining candidate genes from these systems and it would not be practical to list them all here. For the purposes of this review, and bearing in mind the guidelines which we have discussed above, we will focus primarily on large case–control or cohort studies of at least 600 individuals, smaller studies if stroke subtyping was performed and studies which focused on young stroke cases.

7.4.1 Haemostasis

Whilst inherited prothrombotic states are believed to be causal in many cases of venous thrombosis including cerebral vein thrombosis (Martinelli *et al.* 1998), a relationship with arterial thrombosis has been more difficult to prove. Most large case control studies have failed to find an association between inherited prothrombotic states such as activated protein C resistance, or the underlying factor V mutation, and ischaemic stroke in unselected individuals (Table 7.2). These gene defects may be responsible for stroke in some younger individuals (De Stefano *et al.* 1998, Margaglione *et al.* 1999) especially where there is a family history of premature stroke (De Lucia *et al.* 1997), and they may also be an important cause of childhood stroke (Nowak-Gottl *et al.* 1999). Because these variants are associated with venous thrombosis, in a case of young stroke it is important to exclude right to left shunting through an atrial septal defect or patent foramen ovale as a possible stroke mechanism. A recent meta-analysis of 3399 individuals indicated that the factor V Leiden variant might be a weak risk factor for ischaemic stroke (Wu and Tsongalis 2001). However, this meta-analysis was strongly influenced by a single study which indicated that the Leiden mutation was a strong risk factor for early onset disease (Margaglione *et al.* 1999). The same meta-analysis demonstrated no association between stroke and a factor II prothrombin variant. Therefore on balance, these variants are unlikely to be an important cause of stroke in middle aged and elderly individuals. They may be more important in paediatric and young adult onset stroke (see Section 12.8.3).

Genetic variants of other components of the coagulation cascade such as factor VII and fibrinogen have also been examined following prospective studies which demonstrated a role of these proteins in arterial disease (Meade *et al.* 1986, Heinrich *et al.* 1994, Smith *et al.* 1997). A factor VII gene polymorphism has been associated with lower levels of factor VIIc (Green *et al.* 1991), and was found to be protective in myocardial infarction (Iacoviello *et al*. 1998), but in a subsequent study no association was found between factor VII:C levels or the R353Q variant and ischaemic cerebrovascular disease (Heywood *et al*. 1997).

Raised fibrinogen levels may predispose to stroke both by accelerated atherosclerosis and also prothrombotic mechanisms. Homozygosity for a G→A substitution at position 455 of the β fibrinogen gene, which is associated with higher fibrinogen levels, was found to be increased in large vessel stroke (Kessler *et al*. 1997). A separate group examined the role of a different fibrinogen β chain variant (β448) and found an association with stroke in women but not men (Carter *et al*. 1997). The basis of this sex specific interaction remains unclear.

Studies in myocardial infarction suggest the formation of abnormal fibrin structures may be important in arterial thrombosis (Fatah *et al*. 1996). In normal physiology, this is dependent on both the function of factor XIII, which is involved in fibrin cross-linking and the activity of the fibrinolytic system. Raised levels of plasminogen activator inhibitor have been demonstrated in the acute and convalescent phase of stroke. However, no link could be demonstrated between an insertion deletion polymorphism (4G/5G), which is itself associated with levels of plasminogen activator inhibitor (Catto *et al*. 1997 and Stroke). A separate study examined the influence of this variant on post-stroke mortality and found that the 4G genotype, associated with higher PAI-1 levels, had a protective effect (Roest *et al*. 2000). The authors of this study speculate that the effect could be occurring independently of fibrinolysis. Higher PAI-1 levels might have a beneficial role by inhibiting tissue plasminogen activator which has proteolytic effects at both level of the atherosclerotic plaque and also the blood brain barrier through plasmin generation. A polymorphism in the factor XIII gene has also been examined in ischaemic stroke after reports that this variant was protective in myocardial infarction. It has been suggested that this polymorphism (Val34Leu) may be associated with weaker fibrin structures. However, there is controversy surrounding its role in ischaemic stroke (Catto *et al*. 1998, Elbaz *et al*. 2000*a*). It is possible that variants in the factor XIII gene may have a more important role in haemorrhagic stroke, through effects on vascular remodelling and increased bleeding tendency (Catto *et al*. 1998, Reiner *et al*. 2001).

The role of platelet glycoprotein (Gp) receptor polymorphisms has also been studied extensively in patients with ischaemic stroke. These molecules are members of the integrin family and when activated bind to fibrinogen, von Willebrand factor or collagen, and therefore promote platelet aggregation and thrombosis. The P1A2 variant of the platelet fibrinogen receptor has been reported as a risk factor for acute coronary syndromes, specifically in young patients (Carter *et al*. 1996, Weiss *et al*. 1996). A subgroup analysis in a case–control study suggested that that the P1A2 allele may also be an important risk factor in stroke patients <50 years of age (Carter *et al*. 1998). However studies in young women with stroke failed to demonstrate an association with this polymorphism (Wagner *et al*. 1998, Reiner *et al*. 2000), which would be consistent with

Table 7.2 Association studies in ischaemic stroke: haemostatic system

Gene	Reference	Polymorphism	Methodology	Phenotype	Result	Comments
Factor V	Catto *et al.* (1995, 1996a)	Q506 Leiden	Case control 348 cases 247 controls	Ischaemic stroke / stroke mortality	Negative	
	Longstreth *et al.* (1998)	Q506 Leiden	Case control 106 cases 391 controls	Ischaemic stroke young women 18–44	Negative	
	Margaglione *et al.* (1999)	Q506 Leiden	Case control 202 cases 1036 controls	Ischaemic stroke age 3–50 and subtype	Positive	OR 2.56 (1.28–5.14), risk greater in women
	Hankey *et al.* (2001)	Q506 Leiden	Case control 219 cases 205 controls	Ischaemic stroke and subtype	Negative	
	Zunker *et al.* (2001)	Q506 Leiden	Case control 489 cases 112 controls	Ischaemic stroke and subtype	Negative	
	Madonna *et al.* (2002)	Q506 Leiden	Case control 132 cases 262 controls	Ischaemic stroke 6–50 years	Negative	
	Szolnoki *et al.* (2001)	Q506 Leiden	Case control 664 cases 199 controls	Ischaemic stroke and subtype	Positive	Large vessel infarcts OR 2.25 (1.16–4.34)
	Wu *et al.* (2001)	Q506 Leiden	Meta-analysis 983 cases 2416 controls	Ischaemic stroke	Positive	OR 1.43 (1.03–1.97)
Prothrombin	Longstreth *et al.* (1998)	G20210A	Case control 106 cases 391 controls	Ischaemic stroke young women 18–44	Negative	
	De Stefano *et al.* (1998)	G20210A	Case control 72 cases 198 controls	Ischaemic stroke <50 years	Positive	OR 5.1 (1.6–6.3)
	Margaglione *et al.* (1999)	G20210A	Case control 202 cases 1036 controls	Ischaemic stroke 2–50 and subtype	Negative	
	Ridker *et al.* (1999)	G20210A	Nested case control 259 cases 1744 controls	Ischaemic stroke/ PICH	Negative	Weak association with DVT
	Wu *et al.* (2001)	G20210A	Meta-analysis 696 cases 2755 controls	Ischaemic stroke	Negative	

	Reference	Polymorphism	Study design	Outcome	Result	Comments
	Hankey et al. (2001)	G20210A	Case control 219 cases 205 controls	Ischaemic stroke and subtype	Negative	
	Madonna et al. (2002)	G20210A	Case control 132 cases 262 controls	Ischaemic stroke 6–50 years	Negative	
Factor VII	Heywood et al. (1997)	R353Q	Case control 286 cases 198 controls	Ischaemic stroke, subtype and stroke mortality	Negative	No association with stroke subtype or mortality
Fibrinogen	Kessler et al. (1997)	G455A	Case control 227 cases 225 controls	Ischaemic stroke and subtype	Positive	Homozygotes only in large vessel stroke
	Carter et al. (1997)	β448(1/2)	Case control 305 cases 197 controls	Ischaemic stroke and subtype	Positive	Genotype distribution different amongst females only
PAI 1	Catto et al. (1997)	4G/5G	Case control 421 cases 172 controls	Ischaemic stroke, subtype and mortality	Negative	No association with stroke subtype or mortality
	Roest et al. (2000)	4G/5G	Nested case control 114 cases 512 controls	Stroke mortality in women 52–67	Positive	4G allele associated with reduced risk of mortality
	Hindroff et al. (2002)	4G/5G	Case control 106 cases 385 controls	Stroke in women <45	Negative	
Factor XIII	Catto et al. (1998)	Val34Leu	Case control 529 cases 437 controls	Ischaemic stroke and subtype	Negative	Leu allele weak association with PICH. No association with ischaemic stroke subtype
	Elbaz et al. (2000a)	Val34Leu	Case control 456 cases 456 control	Ischaemic stroke and subtype	Positive	Leu allele protective OR 0.58 (0.44–0.75),

(continued)

Table 7.2 (continued)

Gene	Reference	Polymorphism	Methodology	Phenotype	Result	Comments
GpIIb/IIIa	Carter et al. (1998)	P1A2	Case control 505 cases 402 controls	Ischaemic stroke, subtype and mortality	Positive	Association with atherothrombotic stroke in non smokers and patients <50
	Wagner et al. (1998)	P1A2	Case control 63 cases 122 controls	Ischaemic stroke young women 15–44	Negative	
	Reiner et al. (2000)	P1A2	Case control 36 cases 346 controls	Ischaemic stroke women age 18–44	Negative	
	Wu et al. (2001)	P1A2	Meta-analysis 479 cases 1376 controls	Ischaemic stroke	Negative	
	Carter et al. (1999)	HPA3	Case control 515 cases 423 controls	Ischaemic stroke, subtype and mortality	Negative	AA and AB alleles were over-represented in post stroke survivors
	Reiner et al. (2000)	HPA3	Case control 36 cases 346 controls	Ischaemic stroke women 18–44	Negative	Positive association restricted to individuals with diabetes, hypertension or hyperhomocysteinaemia
GpIb/IX	Baker et al. (2001)	Kozak (T/C)	Case control 219 cases 205 controls	Ischaemic stroke and subtype	Positive	OR 1.6 (1.03–2.54)
	Frank et al. (2001)	Kozak (T/C)	Case control 106 cases 384 controls	Ischaemic stroke young women 18–44	Negative	
	Reiner et al. (2000)	HPA2	Case control 36 cases 346 controls	Ischaemic stroke women 18–44	Negative	

	Reference		Study design	Phenotype	Result	Comments
	Baker et al. (2001)	HPA2	Case control 219 cases and 205 controls	Ischaemic stroke and subtype	Negative	
	Carter et al. (1998)	VNTR	Case control 588 cases 422 controls	Ischaemic stroke, subtype and mortality	Negative	
	Baker et al. (2001)	VNTR	Case control 219 cases 205 controls	Ischaemic stroke and subtype	Negative	
Gpla/lla	Carlsson et al. (1999)	C807T	Case control 45 cases 41 controls	Ischaemic stroke ≤50 years	Positive	
	Reiner et al. (2000)	C807T	Case control 36 cases 346 controls	Ischaemic stroke 18–44	Positive	T_{807} allele associated with stroke in patients ≤50 years OR = 2.24 (0.99–5.06)

PAI = plasminogen activator inhibitor, Gp = glycoprotein, OR = odds ratio, DVT = deep vein thrombosis.

the results of a recent meta-analysis (Wu and Tsongalis 2001). The results of most large studies, with one exception, suggest that variants of the von Willebrand factor receptor GpIa/IIa are not risk factors for stroke (Baker *et al.* 2001). However, two small studies have suggested that a silent point mutation (GpIa C807T) in the gene encoding the glycoprotein Ia subunit of the platelet collagen receptor is a risk factor for young stroke (Carlsson *et al.* 1999, Reiner *et al.* 2000). This finding warrants further larger studies, especially as this polymorphism appears to have functional significance, correlating with increased expression of the collagen receptor *in vitro*.

7.4.2 Renin angiotensin pathway

The production of angiotensin II and the catabolism of bradykinin are important effects of angiotensin converting enzyme (ACE), and these peptides have important functions at the local vascular level, including regulation of vascular tone and endothelial function and smooth muscle cell proliferation. The ACE gene is probably the most extensively investigated candidate gene in ischaemic stroke (Table 7.3), following a report by Cambien and co-workers which suggested that an insertion/deletion (I/D) polymorphism was associated with myocardial infarction (Cambien *et al.* 1992). A number of studies have reported an association with stroke, usually with a relative risk of the order of 1.5–4, but other studies have failed to find a significant association. A meta-analysis has evaluated the risk of stroke in 1918 subjects versus 722 controls from seven studies and it was concluded that the ACE D allele conferred a modest effect with an odds ratio of 1.31 (95% CI 1.06–1.62), according to a recessive model of inheritance (Sharma 1998). A weaker association was seen under a dominant model. This meta-analysis may well have over-estimated the association because of confounding due to publication bias. Furthermore subtype analysis could not be performed because of methodological differences between studies.

The conflicting results of studies of the ACE gene insertion/deletion polymorphism, highlight some of the difficulties with using the candidate gene approach in stroke. Frequently studies have been small and under powered to detect effects, and a variety of control groups have been used ranging from randomly selected population controls to non-randomly selected hospital patients with other diseases. In some instances there may have also been mismatching of cases and controls according to ethnic origin leading to confounding results as a consequence of population stratification. One method of overcoming selection bias is to study population cohorts prospectively. Recently the role of the ACE genotype was investigated in the Physicians Heart Study cohort with a negative conclusion (Zee *et al.* 1999). However, prospective cohort studies tend to suffer from poor phenotyping and in this study both cases of haemorrhagic stroke and ischaemic stroke were not distinguished and no ischaemic stroke phenotyping was performed. This may be a serious shortcoming as several studies have specifically reported an association of ACE genotype with the lacunar stroke

Table 7.3 Major case control association studies in ischaemic stroke

Gene	Reference	Polymorphism	Methodology	Phenotype	Result	Comments
ACE	Markus et al. (1995)	I/D	Case control 100 cases and 137 controls	Ischaemic stroke and subtype	Positive	Association mainly with lacunar stroke
	Catto et al. (1996b)	I/D	Case control 418 cases 231 controls	Ischaemic stroke, subtype and mortality	Negative	No association with stroke or subtype. D allele associated with early mortality
	Ueda et al. (1995)	I/D	Case control 488 cases 188 controls	Ischaemic stroke and subtype	Negative	
	Doi et al. (1997)	I/D	Case control 181 cases 271 controls	Ischaemic stroke (atheroembolic/lacunar)	Positive	Association with young strokes <60 (possibly post stroke mortality)
	Zee et al. (1999)	I/D	Nested case control 348 cases 348 controls	Ischaemic stroke/PICH	Negative	No association following stratification for low risk
	Elbaz et al. (1998)	CT 2/3	Case control 510 cases 510 controls	Ischaemic stroke and subtype	Positive	2/2 genotype associated with lacunar stroke
	Sharma et al. (1998)	I/D	Meta-analysis 1918 cases and 722 controls	Ischaemic stroke	Positive	Moderate increase in risk associated with D allele under a recessive model of inheritance
eNOS	Yahashi et al. (1998)	ecNOS 4a/b	Case control 127 cases 91 controls	Atherothrombotic/lacunar/silent stroke	Negative	
	Hou et al. (2001)	ecNos 4a/b	Case control 364 cases 516 controls	Ischaemic stroke and subtype	Positive	OR 2.44 (1.6–3.7), all ischaemic stroke
	Elbaz et al. (2000b)	Glu298Asp	Case control 460 cases and 460 controls	Ischaemic stroke and subtype	Positive	Association highest for lacunar stroke GG genotype OR 2.0 (1.05–3.80)
	Markus et al. (1998)	Glu298Asp	Case Control 361 cases 236 controls	Ischaemic stroke and subtype	Negative	No association with carotid atheroma

(continued)

Table 7.3 (continued)

Gene	Reference	Polymorphism	Methodology	Phenotype	Result	Comments
p22PHOX	Ito et al. (2000a)	C242T	Case control 226 cases 301 controls	Iscahemic stroke and subtype	Positive	TC/TT OR 1.81 (1.15–2.86) Association highest for atheroembolic
MTHFR	Markus et al. (1997)	C677T	Case control 345 cases 161 controls	Ischaemic stroke and subtype	Negative	No association in folate deficient patients, young individuals or carotid atheroma
	Kristensen et al. (1999)	C677T	Case control 80 cases 41 controls	Ischaemic stroke 18–44	Negative	
	Soriente et al. (1998)	C677T	Case control 60 cases 182 controls	Early onset ischaemic stroke (4–49 years)	Positive	TT genotype OR 2.1 (C.I. 1.1–4.0)
	De Stefano et al. (1998)	C677T	Case control 72 cases 198 controls	Ischaemic stroke <50 yrs	Negative	
	Madonna et al. (2002)	C677T	Case control 132 cases 262 controls	Ischaemic stroke <51 yrs	Negative	
	Eikelboom et al. (2000)	C677T	Case control 219 cases 205 controls	Ischaemic stroke and subtype	Negative	
	Wu et al. (2002)	C677T	Meta-analysis 1337 cases, 1738 controls	Ischaemic stroke	Negative	
Apo E	Kessler et al. (1997)	Apoε2/ε3/ε4	Case control 227 cases 225 controls	Ischaemic stroke and subtype	Positive	ε4 association with large vessel disease
	Ferruci et al. (1997)	Apoε2/ε3/ε4	Cohort study 1664 subjects	Ischaemic stroke >71	Positive	ε2 protective in patients 70–79
	Basun et al. (1996)	Apoε2/ε3/ε4	Cohort study 1077 subjects	Ischaemic stroke in those >75 at baseline	Negative	

Reference	Polymorphism	Study design	Phenotype	Result	Comments
Kuusisto et al. (1995)	Apoe2/e3/e	Cohort study 1067 subjects	Ischaemic/ PICH 65–74 years at baseline	Negative	No association with stroke mortality
Catto et al. (2000)	Apoe2/e3/e4	Case control 532 cases 289 controls	Iscahemic stroke and subtype	Negative	
Kokubo et al. (2000)	Apoe2/e3/e4	Case control 201 cases 1126 controls	Ischaemic stroke and subtype	Positive	e2/e2 and e3/e4 genotypes associated with predominantly atherothrombotic stroke
Zhu et al. (2000)	Apoe2/e3/e4	Cohort study 1301 subjects	Ischaemic and haemorrhagic stroke	Negative	
McCarron et al. (1999)	Apoe2/e3/e4	Meta-analysis 926 cases 890 controls	Ischaemic stroke	Positive	e4 carriers OR 1.73 (1.34–2.23)
CD14					
Ito et al. (2000b)	C-260T	Case control 235 cases 309 controls	Ischaemic stroke and subtype	Negative	
Zee et al. (2002)	C-260T	Case controls 338 cases 338 controls	Ischaemic stroke	Negative	

PICH = primary intracerebral haemorrhage, OR = odds ratio.

(small vessel disease) phenotype (Markus *et al.* 1995, Elbaz *et al.* 1998, Szolnoki *et al.* 2001). In addition to the ACE gene, variants of the angiotensinogen gene have also been investigated, but the studies have been too small to draw any definite conclusions. Both ACE and angiotensinogen gene variants have also been studied in relation to intermediate phenotypes which are considered in more detail in Chapter 8.

7.4.3 Nitric oxide and endothelial dysfunction

The activity of the L-arginine/nitric oxide system is an important mediator of endothelial function. It has diverse effects, including regulation of the tone, integrity, growth, and thrombogenic properties of the vessel wall. Strong evidence from animal and human studies has indicated that the activity of this system is under genetic control. Studies using the stroke prone spontaneously hypertensive rat (Chapter 5), have suggested that impaired endothelial dysfunction is an important predisposing factor leading to stroke (Russo *et al.* 1998). In addition, knockout mice deficient in endothelial nitric oxide are highly sensitive to focal cerebral ischaemia (Samdani *et al.* 1997) and have marked vessel wall abnormalities (Rudic and Sessa 1999). An earlier study demonstrated that a functional variant of endothelial nitric oxide synthase (ecNOS 4a) was associated with an increased risk of coronary artery disease and myocardial infarction in smokers (Wang *et al.* 1996), and more recently an association with stroke was reported in a large Chinese stroke population (Hou *et al.* 2001). There was no difference in genotype distribution across stroke subtypes. One possible mechanism could be via effects on collateral blood flow, since in a recent study, a promoter variant in complete linkage disequilibrium (T786C) was found to be associated with increased cerebrovascular resistance and decreased cerebral blood flow (Nasreen *et al.* 2002), although the effect was again confined to smokers. Another polymorphism (Glu298Asp) encodes an amino acid change, and may possibly have some effect on enzyme activity. It has been suggested that this variant is a risk factor for lacunar stroke (Elbaz *et al.* 2000*b*). However, this finding was not confirmed in another study (Markus *et al.* 1998).

Endothelial dysfunction can also be influenced by oxidative stress and the generation of superoxide, which reduces the bioavailability of NO and favours the production of harmful NO free radicals. NADPH oxidase is an important source of superoxide in blood vessels and a polymorphism in a key component (p22phox) has been shown to influence the activity of this enzyme. Recently an association between this variant was found for both large vessel and lacunar strokes, although the association appeared to be stronger for those with stroke due to large vessel disease (Ito *et al.* 2000*a*). This would be consistent with the earlier reports that the polymorphism might be a risk factor for myocardial infarction (Inoue *et al.* 1998).

7.4.4 Homocysteine metabolism

Several inborn errors of metabolism can lead to very high levels of homocysteine in plasma and urine. Homocysteinuria is frequently associated with stroke and

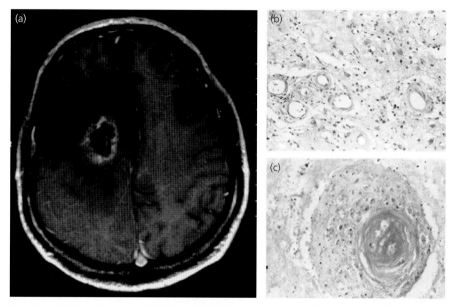

Plate 1 A distinctive feature of CRV and HERNS is the presence of progressive subcortical contrast-enhancing lesions with surrounding oedema (pseudotumours) typically located within the fronto-parietal white matter. Gadolinium-DTPA enhanced T1-weighted image from a 35 year old male patient showing a typical mass lesion in the right frontal lobe. There is marked perifocal oedema and irregular enhancement following administration of the contrast agent; (b) and (c) histopathologic specimens taken from a left frontal mass lesion of the patient's mother: (b) white matter with pathologic microvessels, oedema, and reactive gliosis; (c) necrotic vessel with thrombosis in an area of coagulative white matter necrosis (kindly provided by S. Weil, Neurologische Klinik, Klinikum Großhadern, München).

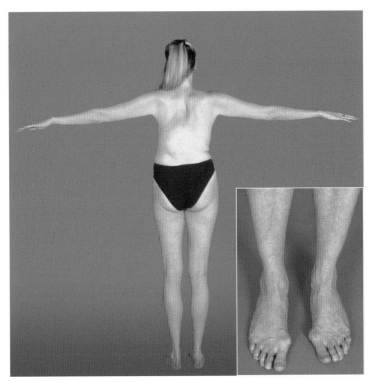

Plate 2 Back view of a 33-year-old female patient with Marfan syndrome and cerebrovascular complications. Note the characteristic skeletal abnormalities (scoliosis, reduced upper to lower segment ratio, arm span to height ratio >0.5, pes planus).

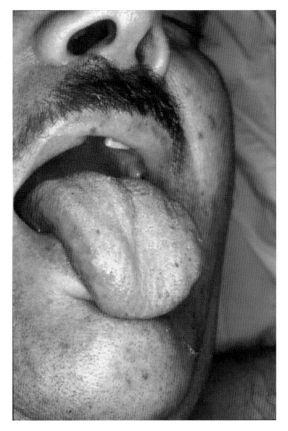

Plate 3 Telangectasia on the tongue of a patient with hereditary haemorrhagic telangectasia.

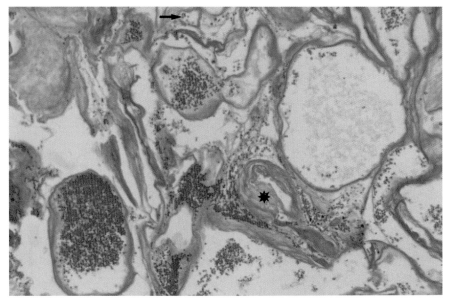

Plate 4 Histological section of a cerebral cavernous angioma. This shows juxtaposition of vascular cavities surrounded by a thin (arrow) or thick (star) endothelial wall. Note the absence of intervening brain parenchyma. (Modified Gomori trichrome stain, magnification ×200.) Courtesy of Professor Françoise Chapon.

atherosclerosis (Mudd *et al.* 1985), and this has generated significant interest in mild homocysteinaemia as a risk factor for vascular disease. Subsequent cross-sectional, case–control and prospective studies have established that mild to moderate elevations of serum homocysteine (>15 mmol/l), at levels below those associated with homocysteinuria, are also associated with increased risk (Brattstrom *et al.* 1998). The aetiology of hyperhomocysteinaemia within this range is likely to be multifactorial. Environmental factors, particularly folate intake, are believed to be important in addition to genetic factors. The most common mutation associated with homocysteinuria is a defect in the cystathione β–synthase gene. Heterozygotes possess approximately 30 per cent of normal enzyme activity and two small studies have indicated an excess of heterozygosity for cystathione β-synthase deficiency amongst individuals with vascular diseases including stroke (Boers *et al.* 1985, Clarke *et al.* 1991). However, as the background prevalence of heterozygotes is only around 1 per cent, these mutations are unlikely to be an important cause of sporadic stroke at a population level.

Very rarely patients with homocysteinuria have a complete deficiency of methylene tetrahydrofolate reductase (MTHFR), a folate dependent enzyme catalysing the rate limiting step in the methylation of homocysteine to methionine. In 1988, a common thermolabile variant of MTHFR associated with decreased enzyme activity and mildly elevated plasma homocysteine was identified (Kang *et al.* 1988). The underlying genetic basis for this is a common mutation (C→T at position 677), and the role of this polymorphism has been studied in the context of ischaemic stroke. Several studies, with one exception involving young stroke patients (Soriente *et al.* 1998), indicate that although the MTHFR genotype is a predictor of mild homocysteinaemia, it is not associated with increased stroke risk (Table 7.3). This would be consistent with findings from meta-analyses (Brattstrom *et al.* 1998, Wu and Tsongalis 2001). This apparent paradox is probably explained by other factors being more important in determining homocysteine levels. One of these is dietary intake of B vitamins and folic acid. A number of studies have confirmed an interaction between genotype and folate levels (Markus *et al.* 1997). Therefore the variant may be a risk factor in individuals with low folate intake, but further studies in this population are required.

7.4.5 Lipid Metabolism

Individuals with higher levels of plasma cholesterol, increased low density lipoprotein (LDL) and decreased HDL, have a higher risk of premature atherosclerosis. The phenotype can arise not only from single gene disorders but also from a number of genetic variants including polymorphic variants of genes encoding the apolipoproteins, lipoprotein receptors, and the key enzymes of plasma lipoprotein metabolism. Apolipoprotein E is a glycoprotein that mediates the binding of lipoprotein particles to specific lipoprotein receptors. Three major isoforms arising from different amino acid substitutions, and encoded by the different alleles $\epsilon2$, $\epsilon3$, $\epsilon4$, have been identified. The $\epsilon4$ variant has been associated with higher total serum cholesterol and LDL cholesterol levels and has been postulated as an important risk factor for ischaemic stroke, whilst the $\epsilon2$ allele may have a protective role. However, the situation is unclear as a number of prospective studies have found no influence of apolipoprotein E phenotype on stroke risk, whilst the there have also been reports that the $\epsilon2$ allele may itself also be associated with increased stroke risk (Table 7.3). In a recent meta-analysis the $\epsilon4$ was only a weak risk factor in patients with ischaemic stroke, and no association was reported for the $\epsilon2$ allele (McCarron *et al.* 1999).

As well as examining the role of apolipoproteins as stroke risk factors, several groups have examined the role of these variants in modulating the outcome of cerebral infarction, as these proteins are important regulators of lipid turnover within the brain and of neuronal maintenance and repair. Transgenic mice which carry different forms of the human apolipoprotein E alleles develop markedly different infarct volumes following experimental MCA occlusion, with $\epsilon4$ carriers developing the largest infarct size (Sheng *et al.* 1998). Studies of patients with head injury and intracerebral haemorrhage have also indicated that the $\epsilon4$ allele is a predictor of poor outcome in terms of both death and disability (Alberts *et al.* 1995, Teasdale *et al.* 1997). This is consistent with a report of cognitive decline in $\epsilon4$ carriers with cerebrovascular disease (Kalmijn *et al.* 1996). However, both favourable (MCarron *et al.* 1998), and poor outcomes (Corder *et al.* 2000), associated with the $\epsilon4$ allele have been reported post stroke. The conflicting reports may in part reflect the use of broad measures of outcome such as stroke mortality. In a study where more detailed measures of stroke outcome were used, no association with apolipoprotein E genotype was found (McCarron *et al.* 2000).

7.4.6 Pro-inflammatory genes

There has been considerable interest in the hypothesis that atherosclerotic conditions are inflammatory diseases. It is possible that conventional risk factors such as smoking and LDL cholesterol and other potential contributors to endothelial injury initiate an inflammatory cascade that leads to activation of monocytes and lymphocytes in the arterial wall contributing to smooth muscle cell proliferation and thickening of the arterial wall. Inflammatory processes may also be involved in the sequence of events leading to plaque rupture. It has been suggested that release of pro-inflammatory cytokines after cerebral ischaemia may be an important pathogenic mechanism determining infarct size and subsequent outcome. Chronic infection may be a risk factor for atherosclerosis via effects on inflammatory pathways. This has prompted some groups to examine the role of a variant in the CD14 (endotoxin) receptor following reports of association with ischaemic heart disease (Hubacek *et al.* 1999). This variant is associated with increased expression of CD14 receptors on monocytes. However, both a case–control study (Ito *et al.* 2000*b*) and a prospective evaluation (Zee *et al.* 2002) in stroke provided negative conclusions.

Many functional variants in pro-inflammatory genes have now been characterized including the different cytokines and their receptors. Whilst many of these polymorphisms have been tested in ischaemic heart disease (Andreotti *et al.* 2002), at present there are few large studies examining the role of these as risk factors in ischaemic stroke, although these variants are likely to be tested in the future.

7.5 Using intermediate phenotypes

As stroke is the end result of a number of pathologically different processes, it is possible that many genes each conferring a small amount of risk are involved in influencing the end phenotype. Conventional case–control studies may not be sufficiently powerful to detect the contribution of an individual disease allele and one logical step is to use intermediate phenotypes. Intermediate phenotypes represent specific components of the disease process. As the number of genes involved is likely to be less than that for ischaemic stroke, it is hypothesized that the overall contribution of each allele to the intermediate phenotype is greater and therefore easier to detect. A further advantage of intermediate phenotypes is that often it is possible to express the intermediate phenotype as a quantitative trait or continuous variable, rather than the presence or absence of disease. This greatly increases the statistical power of studies. Equally, importantly, the ability to detect 'subclinical disease' avoids the reduction in power due to incomplete penetrance in case–control studies. As well as using cross-sectional methods, it is also possible to follow progression of the intermediate phenotype longitudinally, thus providing a prospective element to the study.

A number of intermediate phenotypes have been used for human stroke. Common carotid artery intima medial thickness (IMT), determined by ultrasonography has been widely used as a marker for early carotid atherosclerosis, whilst the presence and size of carotid plaque has been used as an estimate of more advanced disease. Carotid ultrasound has been widely used in this context to determine the role of a variety of conventional risk factors and novel risk factors such as chronic infection and inflammation (Crouse and Thompson 1993). Estimates of IMT and extent of carotid plaque may therefore be useful intermediate phenotypes for large vessel stroke. Silent white matter hyperintensities on T2-weighted MRI can be considered as an intermediate phenotype for small vessel disease stroke (Kobayashi *et al.* 1997, Mantyla *et al.* 1999). Family and twin studies are consistent with the notion that genetic factors strongly influence these intermediate phenotypes (Duggirala *et al.* 1996, Carmelli *et al.* 1998, Zannad *et al.* 1998) and there have been several studies testing for association between these intermediate phenotypes and candidate genes. The use of intermediate phenotpyes in investigating the genetic basis of ischaemic stroke is covered in detail in Chapter 8.

Animal models, dealt with in detail in Chapter 5, have also been used to represent intermediate phenotypes of human stroke (Rubattu *et al.* 1996, Jeffs *et al.* 1997). For example, sensitivity to cerebral ischaemia can be determined by measuring infarct volumes following experimental MCA artery occlusion or stroke susceptibility estimated based on latency to stroke. The phenotypic variance of these traits have been found to be determined by relatively few genetic loci, and there are candidate genes relevant to human stroke which lie on syntenic chromosomes in man (Read *et al.* 2001). However, one should remain cautious about using these approaches as it may not be possible to extrapolate data from these highly inbred animal strains to complex human stroke.

7.6 Alternative approaches to studying polygenic ischaemic stroke

Traditional case–control, cross-sectional and cohort association studies are statistically powerful methods for characterizing stroke genes, and may be particularly powerful when combined with rigorous stroke subtyping and selection of appropriate pheno-type. However, there are a number of problems associated with these methods. One of the main problems is that because the frequency of genetic polymorphisms can differ quite markedly amongst different ancestral populations, spurious associations can arise as a consequence of mismatching of cases and controls. This is known as population stratification. A second major problem with case–control (or other strategies) relying on candidate genes is that they are based on existing knowledge of the pathophysiology of stroke and lack the ability to identify novel genes and potential new therapeutic targets. To some extent these difficulties can be overcome by adopting alternative genetic approaches, which include family based association and linkage studies. There application to ischaemic stroke is reviewed below; further more technical details about their implementation are covered in Section 2.7.

7.6.1 Family-based association studies

Family-based association studies have been used with some success in several late onset polygenic diseases (Rogus *et al.* 1998, Niu *et al.* 1999). These methods were originally developed to detect very close linkage between a marker and a disease, by comparing marker frequencies between affected and unaffected different family members. Subsequently these techniques have also been used in candidate gene studies. Genetic association in these circumstances cannot be explained by population stratification, and is most likely to be a result of the variant being either directly responsible for the disease or being in linkage disequilibrium with a variant that is. The transmission disequilibrium test (TDT) (Spielman *et al.* 1993) is one variant of this approach and relies on the availability of both living unaffected parents and an affected living offspring for genotyping. If one parent is heterozygous for a disease allele than we would expect this allele to be transmitted in 50 per cent of cases to the offspring simply by chance. If there is distortion of the transmission frequency to the offspring than the variant is associated with the disease. This method has a potential benefit in that it can allow the differential effects of maternal versus paternal transmission to be detected. However, in stroke and other late onset polygenic diseases it is rare to have both available parents who are alive (Hassan *et al.* 2002). Therefore recruitment of sufficient numbers of parent offspring trios would be extremely difficult. Variants of the TDT have been developed, which may facilitate recruitment. As individuals with stroke frequently have unaffected living siblings, one method which could be used is based on genotyping the affected individual and the unaffected living siblings. This is known as the sibling transmission disequilibrium test (S-TDT) (Spielman and Ewens 1998). If the allele in questions is associated with disease we would expect the frequency of a disease allele to be greater amongst affected siblings compared to unaffected siblings. Although families of this type can be easily recruited, they tend to be less genetically informative. Therefore this method is not as powerful as the case control approach or the transmission disequilibrium test. A further problem is that unaffected siblings may have subclinical disease. This leads to overmatching and additional loss of statistical power.

A recent study estimated sample sizes (Table 7.4) for the different approaches to investigating ischaemic stroke, and the number of patients that would need to be screened to obtain these sample sizes (Hassan *et al.* 2002). A sibling relative risk was obtained from analysis of family history data in an English Caucasian population, and found to be 3.08 for young stroke with onset at 65 years or younger. Assuming 5 loci play an equally important role in stroke, 1200 affected sibling pairs (both ≤65 years) would be required for a linkage study, and >140,000 ischaemic stroke patients would need screening to achieve this sample size. For association studies, assuming an odds ratio of 2 and allele frequency of 0.1, the following sample sizes would be required: case control methodology 820, TDT methodology 31,680, and s-TDT 3062. The sample size estimates would be much higher if strokes of all ages were included, or if more genes played a major role in the pathogenesis of ischaemic stroke. This emphasizes that for TDT and S-TDT approaches studies are likely to be multi-centre particularly

Table 7.4 Sample sizes estimates for different study designs (case–control, TDT, and S-TDT) in patients with ischaemic stroke (from Hassan *et al.* 2002)

Odds ratio associated with study of genetic variant	Case–control study		TDT		TDT	
	Sample size	Strokes needing screening	Sample size	Strokes needing screening	Sample size	Strokes needing screening
1.5	1727	3421	1727	132,160	2581	12,808
2	414	820	414	31,680	617	3062
2.5	219	433	219	16,758	327	1622
3	144	285	144	11,018	215	1066

These are based on limiting recruitment to stroke patients and relatives aged ≤65 years, and on the assumption that 50% of living parents and sibling can be recruited. Four levels of risk associated with the genetic variant under study are shown with odds ratios between 1.5 and 3.

if individual stroke subtypes are to be studied which will require even larger number of stroke patients to be screened.

7.6.2 Linkage approaches

Linkage based approaches rely on whether fragments of genome are transmitted within families along with the phenotype according to certain patterns of inheritance. If a marker is linked to the disease it will co-segregate accordingly. In most polygenic diseases the inheritance pattern is more complex and cannot be predicted. However, one would still expects alleles which are linked to the disease to be more frequently shared between related affected family members, than that predicted by chance. By using a framework of polymorphic markers spanning the genome and computational methods (genome-wide screening), it is possible to determine extent of allele sharing across the genome and locate a chromosomal region containing the gene responsible for disease.

Whilst linkage approaches have been very successful for monogenic diseases, there has been less success in the polygenic diseases. One reason for this is that linkage studies may have less power than association studies to detect genes of low relative risk (relative risk <3) (Risch 2000). If there are many genes each with small relative risk (locus heterogeneity), linkage studies may not be a suitable approach in ischaemic stroke. However, complex patterns of inheritance can be produced by disorders involving few genes with high relative risks but weak penetrance, and if this scenario is applicable to stroke a linkage study might be an efficient tool (Gulcher *et al.* 2001).

Currently the linkage-based method remains the only approach that is amenable to genome-wide screening strategies although genome-wide association studies (see below) may be implemented in the future. The advantage of genome-wide screening is that a hypothesis is not required concerning the identity of the gene, which is identified according to its physical position on genetic maps now becoming available (Lander *et al.* 2001, Venter *et al.* 2001). Therefore linkage techniques have the potential for novel gene discovery. Furthermore, population stratification is less of a problem with linkage studies than with conventional association studies. Linkage approaches which are currently being tested in stroke include the affected sibling pair approach and the genealogical approach. We will consider each of these approaches in turn.

The affected sibling-pair method

This is the simplest form of linkage study. It is based on the premise that under random segregation, two affected siblings would be expected to share an identical allele (identity by descent) 50 per cent of the time (Lander and Schork 1994). In the case of a marker being linked to the disease, we would expect the distribution of this marker to deviate significantly from that predicted by chance. The power of an affected sibling-pair methodology to detect linkage depends on several factors. The first is the relative risk conferred by the disease locus, which is in turn dependent on the overall genetic

Table 7.5 Estimated number of affected sib pairs (ASP) required for a linkage study based on an estimated sibling relative risk of 3.08 (Hassan *et al.* 2002) and different number of anticipated stroke genes

Predicted stroke loci	ASPs needed
1	208 (164–1157)
3	953 (512–8256)
5	2446 (1157–18,580)
10	6800 (4642–74,334)
20	61230 (18,580–351,310)

The numbers given are based on detecting significant linkage in a genome wide screen (LOD score 3.6). Figures in parenthesis are sample sizes based around the 95% confidence intervals for the estimate of sibling relative risk 1.45–6.54.

contribution in the disease (sibling relative risk), and the number of different disease loci (Risch 1990). The sibling relative risk ratio for stroke has been estimated at around 1.5–6.0, and for this level of sibling risk sample size estimates are provided in Table 7.5 (Hassan *et al.* 2002). It can be appreciated that affected sibling-pair studies are unlikely to be successful if there are many stroke genes each conferring small effects. However, there is some evidence from animal (Rubattu *et al.* 1996, Jeffs *et al.* 1997) and human studies (Gretarsdottir *et al.* 2002) which suggests that there may be a few major stroke genes and in this scenario an affected sibling approach seems practical. Another important consideration centres around the population prevalence of affected stroke sibling pairs. As stroke is a late onset disease, it may be that affected siblings are no longer alive. The authors own experience indicates that 9 per cent of stroke patients reported a sibling history of stroke (Hassan *et al.* 2002). However, in only one half was the affected sibling alive, and potentially available for genotyping. Another study using a similar interview based approach reported higher sibling concordance rates of 20 per cent, with 11 per cent alive at the time of sampling (Meschia *et al.* 2001). These findings suggest that large numbers of stroke cases would have to be screened even to obtain conservative sample size estimates for a sibling-pair approach. Such a large scale multicentre approach is now being adopted in the United States (SWISS study) with the aim of recruiting 300 affected sibling pairs from the United States and Canada from 50 centres (Meschia *et al.* 2002).

The genealogical approach

An alternative approach to the affected sibling-pair method involves tracking genetic information through large extended families with affected and unaffected members. This type of linkage approach is particularly suited to populations where there is extensive genealogical data, and to populations which have been isolated over many centuries. These populations are likely to be more genetically homogenous. There may be fewer different stroke genes within the gene pool, that is, reduced locus heterogeneity, leading to the possibility of variants with high relative risk. Furthermore over-representation of alleles amongst disease populations is more likely to be a causal phenomenon because of the possibility of a founder effect. Recently a genealogical approach was adopted in Iceland to provide strong evidence for the existence of a novel stroke gene (Gretarsdottir *et al.* 2002). Nearly all Icelanders are descendants from Norwegian Vikings and the Irish settlers of the ninth century. Iceland is also unique in that genealogical records exist including all 270,000 living Icelanders and most of their ancestors. A population-based list of all living stroke individuals was compared with genealogical data to construct 179 extended families containing multiply affected and unaffected individuals, who were asked to provide DNA following informed consent. Genome wide screening subsequently revealed strong evidence of linkage to chromosome 5q12 (Gretarsdottir *et al.* 2002) where a gene concerned with endothelial proliferation was found to account for much of the relative risk of stroke in this population (Steffansson, K., personal communication, 2001). Interestingly this locus was found to contribute equally to all stroke subtypes, with the possible exception of haemorrhagic stroke. This study would suggest that relatively few stroke genes may be present which account for the bulk of stroke genetic risk and which may be important in the expression of different disease subtypes. However, whilst this study may provide novel insights into stroke pathogenesis, it should be remembered that these findings apply to a unique population. Neither this approach nor its findings may be reproducible in other racial populations.

7.7 Genome-wide association studies

Because linkage studies have only had modest success in most polygenic diseases, some authors have proposed that a genome-wide single nucleotide polymorphism case–control study would provide a useful alternative to a linkage study (Risch and Merikangas 1996, Collins *et al.* 1997). It is predicted that association techniques have a better chance of finding disease causing alleles with low relative risk, but share the advantage of linkage studies in not requiring an *a priori* hypothesis. A screening approach would involve systematically comparing the frequency of bi-allelic markers (single nucleotide polymorphisms—SNPs) across the genome in order to find association (linkage disequilibrium) with disease. The power of genome-wide association studies depends on disease allele frequencies and the extent of linkage disequilibrium between marker and disease alleles. Typically linkage disequilibrium extends for short chromosomal distances, usually 5–500 kb, and it has been estimated that a useful marker framework would contain between 60,000–500,000 (Collins *et al.* 1997, Kruglyak 1999) evenly spaced SNPs. This approach requires much higher levels of significance to avoid type I error, typically 8.3×10^{-7} and 1×10^{-7} using a Bonferroni correction. At this level of marker density, there is still a possibility that a locus could go undetected because of weak or absent linkage disequilibrium between a disease allele and adjacent SNPs.

However, the power of genome-wide association studies could be increased by using more markers or focusing on coding polymorphisms which are more likely to be directly involved in disease pathogenesis (Risch 2000). Advances in identifying and cataloguing sequence variation (Syvanen 2001) have made genome-wide association studies a realistic prospect. However, with current technology, these techniques remain prohibitively expensive. Once these restraints are removed, genome-wide association studies could be applied to existing DNA stroke databases, which so far have been used exclusively for single gene association studies.

7.8 Conclusions

Ischaemic stroke is a major cause of death and disability throughout the world, but attempts to define the genetic basis of this condition have until now lagged behind studies of other polygenic disorders. The identification of individual causative mutations in stroke remains problematic and has in part been limited by the number of approaches available. Traditional association studies remain the mainstay of research, although the most valuable studies will be those which focus on large numbers of well characterized stroke phenotypes. Increasingly newer techniques utilizing linkage or combined linkage/association techniques will be implemented and there has been some very exciting early findings using these approaches. The ultimate goal of these endeavours will be not only to provide new avenues for prevention, but also to provide insights into factors that influence the outcome of stroke and new therapeutic targets for when preventative strategies have failed.

References

Adams, H.P., Bendixen, B.H., Kappelle, L.J., *et al.* (1993). Classification of subtype of acute ischemic stroke. Definitions for use in a multicenter clinical trial. TOAST. Trial of Org 10172 in Acute Stroke Treatment. *Stroke*, **24**, 35–41.

Alberts, M.J., Graffagnino, C., McClenny, C., *et al.* (1995). ApoE genotype and survival from intracerebral haemorrhage. *Lancet*, **346**, 575.

Andreotti, F., Porto, I., Crea, F., and Maseri, A. (2002). Inflammatory gene polymorphisms and ischaemic heart disease: review of population association studies. *Heart*, **87**, 107–12.

Bak, S., Gaist, D., Sindrup, S.H., Skytthe, A., and Christensen, K. (2002). Genetic liability in stroke: a long-term follow-up study of Danish twins. *Stroke*, **33**, 769–74.

Baker, R.I., Eikelboom, J., Lofthouse, E., *et al.* (2001). Platelet glycoprotein Ibalpha Kozak polymorphism is associated with an increased risk of ischemic stroke. *Blood*, **98**, 36–40.

Bamford, J., Sandercock, P., Dennis, M., Burn, J., and Warlow, C. (1991). Classification and natural history of clinically identifiable subtypes of cerebral infarction. *Lancet*, **337**, 1521–6.

Basun, H., Corder, E.H., Guo, Z., *et al.* (1996). Apolipoprotein E polymorphism and stroke in a population sample aged 75 years or more. *Stroke*, **27**, 1310–15.

Bird, T.D., Jarvik, G.P., and Wood, N.W. (2001). Genetic association studies, genes in search of diseases. *Neurology*, **57**, 1153–4.

Boers, G.H., Smals, A.G., Trijbels, F.J., *et al.* (1985). Heterozygosity for homocystinuria in premature peripheral and cerebral occlusive arterial disease. *New England Journal of Medicine*, **313**, 709–15.

Boerwinkle, E., Doris, P.A., and Fornage, M. (1999). Field of needs, the genetics of stroke. *Circulation*, **99**, 31–333.

Brass, L.M., Isaacsohn, J.L., Merikangas, K.R., and Robinette, C.D. (1992). A study of twins and stroke. *Stroke*, **23**, 221–3.

Brass, L.M., Page, W.F., and Lichtman, J.H. (1998). Stroke in Twins III, A Follow-up study. *Stroke*, **29** (Suppl), 256 (abstract).

Brattstrom, L., Wilcken, D.E., Ohrvik, J., and Brudin, L. (1998). Common methylenetetrahydrofolate reductase gene mutation leads to hyperhomocysteinemia but not to vascular disease, the result of a meta-analysis. *Circulation*, **98**, 2520–6.

Cambien, F., Poirier, O., Lecerf, L., *et al.* (1992). Deletion polymorphism in the gene for angiotensin-converting enzyme is a potent risk factor for myocardial infarction. *Nature*, **359**, 641–4.

Carlsson, L.E., Santoso, S., Spitzer, C., Kessler, C., and Greinacher, A. (1999). The alpha2 gene coding sequence T807/A873 of the platelet collagen receptor integrin alpha2beta1 might be a genetic risk factor for the development of stroke in younger patients. *Blood*, **93**, 3583–6.

Carmelli, D., DeCarli, C., Swan, G.E., *et al.* (1998). Evidence for genetic variance in white matter hyperintensity volume in normal elderly male twins. *Stroke*, **29**, 1177–81.

Carter, A.M., Catto, A.J., Bamford, J.M., and Grant, P.J. (1997). Gender-specific associations of the fibrinogen B beta 448 polymorphism, fibrinogen levels, and acute cerebrovascular disease. *Arteriosclerosis, Thrombosis and Vascular Biology*, **17**, 589–94.

Carter, A.M., Catto, A.J., Bamford, J.M., and Grant, P.J. (1998). Platelet GP IIIa PlA and GP Ib variable number tandem repeat polymorphisms and markers of platelet activation in acute stroke. *Arteriosclerosis, Thrombosis and Vascular Biology*, **18**, 1124–31.

Carter, A.M., Catto, A.J., Bamford, J.M., and Grant, P.J. (1999). Association of the platelet glycoprotein IIb HPA-3 polymorphism with survival after acute ischemic stroke. *Stroke*, **30**, 2606–11.

Carter, A.M., Ossei-Gerning, N., and Grant, P.J. (1996). Platelet glycoprotein IIIa PlA polymorphism in young men with myocardial infarction (letter). *Lancet*, **348**, 485–6.

Catto, A., Carter, A., Ireland, H., *et al.* (1995). Factor V Leiden gene mutation and thrombin generation in relation to the development of acute stroke. *Arteriosclerosis, Thrombosis and Vascular Biology*, **15**, 783–5.

Catto, A., Carter, A., and Grant, P.J. (1996*a*). Factor V Leiden mutation and completed stroke (letter). *Stroke*, **27**, 573–73.

Catto, A., Carter, A.M., Barrett, J.H., *et al.* (1996*b*). Angiotensin-converting enzyme insertion/deletion polymorphism and cerebrovascular disease. *Stroke*, **27**, 435–40.

Catto, A.J., Carter, A.M., Stickland, M., Bamford, J.M., Davies, J., and Grant, P.J. (1997). Plasminogen activator inhibitor-1 (PAI-1) 4G/5G promoter polymorphism and levels in subjects with cerebrovascular disease. *Thrombosis and Haemostasis*, **77**, 730–4.

Catto, A.J., Kohler, H.P., Bannan, S., Stickland, M., Carter, A., and Grant, P.J. (1998). Factor XIII Val 34 Leu, a novel association with primary intracerebral hemorrhage. *Stroke*, **29**, 813–16.

Catto, A.J., McCormack, L.J., Mansfield, M.W., *et al.* (2000). Apolipoprotein E polymorphism in cerebrovascular disease. *Acta Neurologica Scandanivia*, **101**, 399–404.

Clarke, R., Daly, L., Robinson, K., *et al.* (1991). Hyperhomocysteinemia, an independent risk factor for vascular disease. *New England Journal of Medicine*, **324**, 1149–55.

Collins, F.S., Guyer, M.S., and Charkravarti, A. (1997). Variations on a theme, cataloging human DNA sequence variation. *Science*, **278**, 1580–1.

Corder, E.H., Basun, H., Fratiglioni, L., *et al.* (2000). Inherited frailty. ApoE alleles determine survival after a diagnosis of heart disease or stroke at ages 85+. *Annals New York Academy Sciences*, **908**, 295–8.

Crouse, J.R. and Thompson C.J. (1993). An evaluation of methods for imaging and quantifying coronary and carotid lumen stenosis and atherosclerosis. *Circulation*, **87**, II17–II33.

De Lucia, D., Nina, P., Papa, M.L., *et al.* (1997). Activated protein C resistance due to a factor V mutation associated with familial ischemic stroke. *Journal of Neurosurgical Sciences*, **41**, 373–8.

De Stefano, V., Chiusolo, P., Paciaroni, K., *et al.* (1998). Prothrombin G20210A mutant genotype is a risk factor for cerebrovascular ischemic disease in young patients. *Blood*, **91**, 3562–5.

Doi, Y., Yoshinari, M., Yoshizumi, H., Ibayashi, S., Wakisaka, M., and Fujishima, M. (1997). Polymorphism of the angiotensin-converting enzyme (ACE) gene in patients with thrombotic brain infarction. *Atherosclerosis*, **132**, 145–50.

Duggirala, R., Gonzalez Villalpando, C., O'Leary, D.H., Stern, M.P., and Blangero, J. (1996). Genetic basis of variation in carotid artery wall thickness. *Stroke*, **27**, 833–37.

Editorial. (1999). Freely associating. *Nature Genetics*, **22**, 1–2.

Eikelboom, J.W., Hankey, G.J., Anand, S.S., Lofthouse, E., Staples, N., and Baker, R.I. (2000). Association between high homocyst(e)ine and ischemic stroke due to large- and small-artery disease but not other etiologic subtypes of ischemic stroke. *Stroke*, **31**, 1069–75.

Elbaz, A., Mallet, C., Cambien, F., Amarenco, P. on behalf of the GENIC investigators. (1998). Association between the ACE 4656 (CT)2/3 polymorphism and plasma ACE levels with lacunar stroke in the GENIC study. *Cerebrovascular Diseases*, **8** (Suppl. 4), 13 (abstract).

Elbaz, A., Poirier, O., Canaple, S., Chedru, F., Cambien, F., and Amarenco, P. (2000*a*). The association between the Val34Leu polymorphism in the factor XIII gene and brain infarction. *Blood*, **95**, 586–91.

Elbaz, A., Poirier, O., and Moulin, T. (2000*b*) Association between the Glu298Asp polymorphism in the endothelial constitutive nitric oxide synthase gene and brain infarction. The GENIC investigators. *Stroke*, **31**, 1634–9.

Fatah, K., Silveira, A., Tornvall, P., Karpe, F., Blomback, M., and Hamsten, A. (1996). Proneness to formation of tight and rigid fibrin gel structures in men with myocardial infarction at a young age. *Thrombosis and Haemostasis*, **76**, 535–40.

Ferrucci, L., Guralnik, J.M., Pahor, M., *et al.* (1997). Apolipoprotein E epsilon 2 allele and risk of stroke in the older population. *Stroke*, **28**, 2410–16.

Frank, M.B., Reiner, A.P., Schwartz, S.M., *et al.* (2001). The Kozak sequence polymorphism of platelet glycoprotein Ibalpha and risk of nonfatal myocardial infarction and nonfatal stroke in young women. *Blood*, **97**, 875–9.

Green, F., Kelleher, C., Wilkes, H., Temple, A., Meade, T., and Humphries, S. (1991). A common genetic polymorphism associated with lower coagulation factor VII levels in healthy individuals. *Arteriosclerosis and Thrombosis*, **11**, 540–6.

Gretarsdottir, S., Sveinbjornsdottir, S., Jonsson, H.H., *et al.* (2002). Localization of a susceptibility gene for common forms of stroke to 5q12. *American Journal of Human Genetics*, **70**, 593–603.

Gulcher, J.R., Kong, A., and Stefansson, K. (2001). The role of linkage studies for common diseases. *Current Opinion in Genetics and Development*, **11**, 264–7.

Hankey, G.J., Eikelboom, J.W., van Bockxmeer, F.M., Lofthouse, E., Staples, N., and Baker, R.I. (2001). Inherited thrombophilia in ischemic stroke and its pathogenic subtypes. *Stroke* **32**, 1793–9.

Hassan, A., Sham, P.C., and Markus, H.S. (2002). Planning genetic studies in human stroke: sample size estimates based on family history data. *Neurology*, **58**, 1483–8.

Heinrich, J., Balleisen, L., Schulte, H., Assmann, G., and van de, L.J. (1994). Fibrinogen and factor VII in the prediction of coronary risk. Results from the PROCAM study in healthy men *Arteriosclerosis and Thrombosis*, **14**, 54–9.

Heywood, D.M., Carter, A.M., Catto, A.J., Bamford, J.M., and Grant, P.J. (1997). Polymorphisms of the factor VII gene and circulating FVII:C levels in relation to acute cerebrovascular disease and poststroke mortality. *Stroke*, **28**, 816–21.

Hindorff, L.A., Schwartz, S.M., Siscovick, D.S., Psaty, B.M., Longstreth, W.T., and Reiner, A.P. (2002). The association of PAI-1 promoter 4G/5G insertion/deletion polymorphism with myocardial infarction and stroke in young women. *Journal of Cardiovascular Risk*, **9**, 131–7.

Hou, L., Osei-Hyiaman, D., Yu, H., *et al.* (2001). Association of a 27-bp repeat polymorphism in ecNOS gene with ischemic stroke in Chinese patients. *Neurology*, **56**, 490–96.

Hubacek, J.A., Rothe, G., Pit'ha, J., *et al.* (1999). C(-260)->T polymorphism in the promoter of the CD14 monocyte receptor gene as a risk factor for myocardial infarction. *Circulation*, **99**, 3218–20.

Iacoviello, L., Di Castelnuovo, A., De Knijff, P., *et al.* (1998). Polymorphisms in the coagulation factor VII gene and the risk of myocardial infarction. *New England Journal of Medicine*, **338**, 79–85.

Inoue, N., Kawashima, S., Kanazawa, K., Yamada, S., Akita, H., and Yokoyama, M. (1998). Polymorphism of the NADH/NADPH oxidase p22 phox gene in patients with coronary artery disease. *Circulation*, **97**, 135–7.

Ito, D., Murata, M., Watanabe, K., *et al.* (2000*a*). C242T polymorphism of NADPH oxidase p22 PHOX gene and ischemic cerebrovascular disease in the Japanese population. *Stroke*, **31**, 936–9.

Ito, D., Murata, M., Tanahashi, N., *et al.* (2000*b*). Polymorphism in the promoter of lipopolysaccharide receptor CD14 and ischemic cerebrovascular disease. *Stroke*, **31**, 2661–4.

Jeffs, B., Clark, J.S., Anderson, N.H., *et al.* (1997). Sensitivity to cerebral ischaemic insult in a rat model of stroke is determined by a single genetic locus. *Nature Genetics*, **16**, 364–7.

Jousilahti, P., Rastenyte, D., Tuomilehto, J., Sarti, C., and Vartiainen, E. (1997). Parental history of cardiovascular disease and risk of stroke. A prospective follow-up of 14371 middle-aged men and women in Finland. *Stroke*, **28**, 1361–6.

Kalmijn, S., Feskens, E.J., Launer, L.J., and Kromhout, D. (1996). Cerebrovascular disease, the apolipoprotein e4 allele, and cognitive decline in a community-based study of elderly men. *Stroke*, **27**, 2230–35.

Kang, S.S., Zhou, J., Wong, P.W., Kowalisyn, J., and Strokosch, G. (1988). Intermediate homocysteinemia: a thermolabile variant of methylenetetrahydrofolate reductase. *American Journal of Human Genetics*, **43**, 414–21.

Kessler, C., Spitzer, C., Stauske, D., *et al.* (1997). The apolipoprotein E and beta-fibrinogen G/A-455 gene polymorphisms are associated with ischemic stroke involving large-vessel disease. *Arteriosclerosis, Thrombosis and Vascular Biology*, **17**, 2880–4.

Kobayashi, S., Okada, K., Koide, H., Bokura, H., and Yamaguchi, S. (1997). Subcortical silent brain infarction as a risk factor for clinical stroke. *Stroke*, **28**, 1932–9.

Kokubo, Y., Chowdhury, A.H., Date, C., Yokoyama, T., Sobue, H., and Tanaka, H. (2000). Age-dependent association of apolipoprotein E genotypes with stroke subtypes in a Japanese rural population. *Stroke*, **31**, 1299–1306.

Kristensen, B., Malm, J., Nilsson, T.K., *et al.* (1999). Hyperhomocysteinemia and hypofibrinolysis in young adults with ischemic stroke. *Stroke*, **30**, 974–80.

Kruglyak, L. (1999). Prospects for whole-genome linkage disequilibrium mapping of common disease genes. *Nature Genetics*, **22**, 139–44.

Kuusisto, J., Mykkanen, L., Kervinen, K., Kesaniemi, Y.A., and Laakso, M. (1995). Apolipoprotein E4 phenotype is not an important risk factor for coronary heart disease or stroke in elderly subjects. *Arteriosclerosis, Thrombosis and Vascular Biology*, **15**, 1280–6.

Lander, E.S., Linton, L.M., Birren, B., *et al.* (2001). Initial sequencing and analysis of the human genome. *Nature*, **409**, 860–921.

Lander, E.S. and Schork, N.J. (1994). Genetic dissection of complex traits. (Review). *Science*, **265**, 2037–48.

Liao, D., Myers, R., Hunt, S., *et al.* (1997). Familial history of stroke and stroke risk. The Family Heart Study. *Stroke*, **28**, 1908–12.

Longstreth, W.T., Jr., Rosendaal, F.R., Siscovick, D.S., *et al.* (1998). Risk of stroke in young women and two prothrombotic mutations, factor V Leiden and prothrombin gene variant (G20210A). *Stroke*, **29**, 577–80.

Madonna, P., De, S., Coppola, A., *et al.* (2002). Hyperhomocysteinemia and other inherited prothrombotic conditions in young adults with a history of ischemic stroke. *Stroke*, **33**, 51–6.

Mantyla, R., Aronen, H.J., Salonen, O., *et al.* (1999). Magnetic resonance imaging white matter hyperintensities and mechanism of ischemic stroke. *Stroke*, **30**, 2053–8.

Margaglione, M., D'Andrea, G., Giuliani, N., *et al.* (1999). Inherited prothrombotic conditions and premature ischemic stroke, sex difference in the association with factor V Leiden. *Arteriosclerosis, Thrombosis and Vascular Biology*, **19**, 1751–6.

Markus, H.S., Ali, N., Swaminathan, R., Sankaralingam, A., Molloy, J., and Powell, J. (1997). A common polymorphism in the methylenetetrahydrofolate reductase gene, homocysteine, and ischemic cerebrovascular disease. *Stroke*, **28**, 1739–43.

Markus, H.S., Barley, J., Lunt, R., *et al.* (1995). Angiotensin-converting enzyme gene deletion polymorphism. A new risk factor for lacunar stroke but not carotid atheroma. *Stroke*, **26**, 1329–33.

Markus, H.S., Ruigrok, Y., Ali, N., and Powell, J.F. (1998). Endothelial nitric oxide synthase exon 7 polymorphism, ischemic cerebrovascular disease, and carotid atheroma. *Stroke*, **29**, 1908–11.

Martinelli, I., Sacchi, E., Landi, G., Taioli, E., Duca, F., and Mannucci, P.M. (1998). High risk of cerebral-vein thrombosis in carriers of a prothrombin-gene mutation and in users of oral contraceptives. *New England Journal of Medicine*, **338**, 1793–7.

McCarron, M.O., Delong, D., and Alberts, M.J. (1999). APOE genotype as a risk factor for ischemic cerebrovascular disease, a meta-analysis. *Neurology*, **53**, 1308–11.

McCarron, M.O., Muir, K.W., Weir, C.J., *et al.* (1998). The apolipoprotein E epsilon4 allele and outcome in cerebrovascular disease. *Stroke*, **29**, 1882–7.

McCarron, M.O., Muir, K.W., Nicoll, J.A., *et al.* (2000). Prospective study of apolipoprotein E genotype and functional outcome following ischemic stroke. *Archives of Neurology*, **57**, 1480–4.

Meade, T.W., Mellows, S., Brozovic, M., *et al.* (1986). Haemostatic function and ischaemic heart disease, principal results of the Northwick Park Heart Study. *Lancet*, **2**, 533–7.

Meschia, J.F., Brown, R.D., Jr., Brott, T.G., Hardy, J., Atkinson, E.J., and O'Brien, P.C. (2001). Feasibility of an affected sibling pair study in ischemic stroke, results of a 2-center family history registry. *Stroke*, **32**, 2939–41.

Meschia, J.F., Brown, R.D., Jr., Brott, T.G., Chukwudelunzu, F.E., Hardy, J., and Rich, S.S. (2002). The Siblings With Ischemic Stroke Study (SWISS) Protocol. *Biomedcentral Medical Genetics*, **3**, 1.

Mudd, S.H., Skovby, F, Levy, H.L., *et al.* (1985). The natural history of homocystinuria due to cystathionine beta-synthase deficiency. *American Journal of Human Genetics*, **37**, 1–31.

Nasreen, S., Nabika, T., Shibata, H., *et al.* (2002). T-786C polymorphism in endothelial NO synthase gene affects cerebral circulation in smokers, possible gene-environmental interaction. *Arteriosclerosis, Thrombosis and Vascular Biology*, **22**, 605–10.

Niu, T., Yang, J., Wang, B., *et al.* (1999). Angiotensinogen gene polymorphisms M235T/T174M, no excess transmission to hypertensive Chinese. *Hypertension*, **33**, 698–702.

Nowak-Gottl, U., Strater, R., Heinecke, A., *et al.* (1999). Lipoprotein (a) and genetic polymorphisms of clotting factor V, prothrombin, and methylenetetrahydrofolate reductase are risk factors of spontaneous ischemic stroke in childhood. *Blood*, **94**, 3678–82.

Poirier, J., Davignon, J,, Bouthillier, D., Kogan, S., Bertrand, P., and Gauthier, S. (1993). Apolipoprotein E polymorphism and Alzheimer's disease. *Lancet*, **342**, 697–9.

Polychronopoulos, P., Gioldasis, G., Ellul, J., *et al.* (2002). Family history of stroke in stroke types and subtypes. *Journal of the Neurological Sciences*, **195**, 117–22.

Read, S.J., Parsons, A.A., Harrison, D.C., *et al.* (2001). Stroke genomics: approaches to identify, validate, and understand ischemic stroke gene expression. *Journal of Cerebral Blood Flow and Metabolism*, **21**, 755–78.

Reiner, A.P., Kumar, P.N., Schwartz, S.M., *et al.* (2000). Genetic variants of platelet glycoprotein receptors and risk of stroke in young women. *Stroke*, **31**, 1628–33.

Reiner, A.P., Schwartz, S.M., Frank, M.B., *et al.* (2001). Polymorphisms of coagulation factor XIII subunit A and risk of nonfatal hemorrhagic stroke in young white women. *Stroke*, **32**, 2580–7.

Ridker, P.M., Henekens, C.H., and Miletich, J.P. (1999). G20210A mutation in prothrombin gene and risk of myocardial infarction, stroke, and venous thrombosis in a large cohort of US men. *Circulation*, **99**, 999–1004.

Risch, N. (1990). Linkage strategies for genetically complex traits. II. The power of affected relative pairs. *American Journal of Human Genetics*, **46**, 229–41.

Risch, N. and Merikangas, K. (1996). The future of genetic studies of complex human diseases. *Science*, **273**, 1516–17.

Risch, N.J. (2000). Searching for genetic determinants in the new millennium. *Nature*, **405**, 847–56.

Roest, M., van der Schouw, Y.T., Banga, J.D., *et al.* (2000). Plasminogen activator inhibitor 4G polymorphism is associated with decreased risk of cerebrovascular mortality in older women. *Circulation*, **101**, 67–70.

Rogus, J.J., Moczulski, D., Freire, M.B., Yang, Y., Warram, J.H., and Krolewski, A.S. (1998). Diabetic nephropathy is associated with AGT polymorphism T235: results of a family-based study. *Hypertension*, **31**, 627–31.

Rubattu, S., Volpe, M., Kreutz, R., Ganten, U., Ganten, D., and Lindpaintner, K. (1996). Chromosomal mapping of quantitative trait loci contributing to stroke in a rat model of complex human disease. *Nature Genetics*, **13**, 429–34.

Rudic, R.D. and Sessa, W.C. (1999). Nitric oxide in endothelial dysfunction and vascular remodeling: clinical correlates and experimental links. (Review). *American Journal of Human Genetics*, **64**, 673–77.

Russo, R., Vecchione, C., Cosentino, F., *et al.* (1998). Impaired vasorelaxant responses to natriuretic peptides in the stroke-prone phenotype of spontaneously hypertensive rats. *Journal of Hypertension*, **16**, 151–6.

Samdani, A.F., Dawson, T.M., and Dawson, V.L. (1997). Nitric oxide synthase in models of focal ischemia. (Review). *Stroke*, **28**, 1283–8.

Sharma, P. (1998). Meta-analysis of the ACE gene in ischaemic stroke. *Journal of Neurology, Neurosurgery and Psychiatry*, **64**, 227–30.

Sheng, H., Laskowitz, D.T., Bennett, E., *et al.* (1998). Apolipoprotein E isoform-specific differences in outcome from focal ischemia in transgenic mice. *Journal of Cerebral Blood Flow and Metabolism*, **18**, 361–6.

Smith, F.B., Lee, A.J., Fowkes, F.G., Price, J.F., Rumley, A., and Lowe, G.D. (1997). Hemostatic factors as predictors of ischemic heart disease and *Stroke* in the Edinburgh Artery Study. *Arteriosclerosis, Thrombosis and Vascular Biology*, **17**, 3321–5.

Soriente, L., Coppola, A., Madonna, P., *et al.* (1998). Homozygous C677T mutation of the 5,10 methylenetetrahydrofolate reductase gene and hyperhomocysteinemia in Italian patients with a history of early-onset ischemic stroke. *Stroke*, **29**, 869–71.

Spielman, R.S. and Ewens, W.J. (1998). A sibship test for linkage in the presence of association: the sib transmission/disequilibrium test. *American Journal of Human Genetics*, **62**, 450–8.

Spielman, R.S., McGinnis, R.E., and Ewens, W.J. (1993). Transmission test for linkage disequilibrium: the insulin gene region and insulin-dependent diabetes mellitus (IDDM). *American Journal of Human Genetics*, **52**, 506–16.

Syvanen, A.C. (2001). Accessing genetic variation: genotyping single nucleotide polymorphisms. *Nature Reviews Genetics*, **2**, 930–42.

Szolnoki, Z., Somogyvari, F., Kondacs, A., Szabo, M., and Fodor, L. (2001). Evaluation of the roles of the Leiden V mutation and ACE I/D polymorphism in subtypes of ischaemic stroke. *Journal of Neurology*, **248**, 756–61.

Teasdale, G.M., Nicoll, J.A., Murray, G., and Fiddes, M. (1997). Association of apolipoprotein E polymorphism with outcome after head injury. *Lancet*, **350**, 1069–71.

Ueda, S., Weir, C.J., Inglis, G.C., Murray, G.D., Muir, K.W., and Lees, K.R. (1995). Lack of association between angiotensin converting enzyme gene insertion/deletion polymorphism and stroke. *Journal of Hypertension*, **13**, 1597–1601.

Venter, J.C., Adams, M.D., Myers, E.W., *et al.* (2001). The sequence of the human genome. *Science*, **291**, 1304–51.

Wagner, K.R., Giles, W.H., Johnson, C.J., *et al.* (1998). Platelet glycoprotein receptor IIIa polymorphism P1A2 and ischemic stroke risk: the Stroke Prevention in Young Women Study. *Stroke*, **29**, 581–5.

Wang, X.L., Sim, A.S., Badenhop, R.F., McCredie, R.M., and Wilcken, D.E. (1996). A smoking-dependent risk of coronary artery disease associated with a polymorphism of the endothelial nitric oxide synthase gene. *Nature Medicine*, **2**, 41–5.

Weiss, E.J., Bray, P.F., Tayback, M., *et al.* (1996). A polymorphism of a platelet glycoprotein receptor as an inherited risk factor for coronary thrombosis. *New England Journal of Medicine*, **334**, 1090–4.

Wu, A.H. and Tsongalis, G.J. (2001). Correlation of polymorphisms to coagulation and biochemical risk factors for cardiovascular diseases. *American Journal Cardiology*, **87**, 1361–6.

Yahashi, Y., Kario, K., Shimada, K., and Matsuo, M. (1998). The 27-bp repeat polymorphism in intron 4 of the endothelial cell nitric oxide synthase gene and ischemic stroke in a Japanese population. *Blood Coagulation and Fibrinolysis*, **9**, 405–9.

Zannad, F., Visvikis, S., Gueguen, R., *et al.* (1998). Genetics strongly determines the wall thickness of the left and right carotid arteries. *Human Genetics*, **103**, 183–8.

Zee, R.Y., Bates, D., and Ridker, P.M. (2002). A prospective evaluation of the CD14 and CD18 gene polymorphisms and risk of stroke. *Stroke*, **33**, 892–5.

Zee, R.Y., Ridker, P.M., Stampfer, M.J., Hennekens, C.H., and Lindpaintner, K. (1999). Prospective evaluation of the angiotensin-converting enzyme insertion/deletion polymorphism and the risk of stroke. *Circulation*, **99**, 340–3.

Zhu, L., Fratiglioni, L., Guo, Z., *et al.* (2000). Incidence of dementia in relation to stroke and the apolipoprotein E epsilon4 allele in the very old. Findings from a population-based longitudinal study. *Stroke*, **31**, 53–60.

Zunker, P., Hohenstein, C., Plendl, H.J., *et al.* (2001). Activated protein C resistance and acute ischaemic stroke, relation to stroke causation and age. *Journal of Neurology*, **248**, 701–4.

Chapter 8

Investigating the genetics of polygenic ischaemic stroke using intermediate phenotypes

Paula Jerrard-Dunne, Ahamad Hassan, and Hugh S. Markus

8.1 Introduction

As stroke is the end result of a number of pathologically different processes, it is possible that many genes, each conferring a small amount of risk, are involved in influencing the end phenotype. Conventional case control studies may not be sufficiently powerful to detect the contribution of an individual disease allele. One logical step is to use intermediate phenotypes. Intermediate phenotypes represent specific components of the disease process. As the number of genes involved is likely to be less than that for ischaemic stroke, it is hypothesized that the overall contribution of each allele to the intermediate phenotype is greater and therefore easier to detect. A further advantage of intermediate phenotypes is that often it is possible to express the intermediate phenotype as a quantitative trait or continuous variable rather than the presence or absence of disease. This avoids the reduction in power due to incomplete penetrance in case control studies. As well as using cross-sectional methods, it is also possible to follow progression of the intermediate phenotype longitudinally, thus providing a prospective element to the study. The major limitation of intermediate phenotypes is that ultimately they may not translate into clinical risk. However, a number of intermediate phenotypes have been shown to be independent predictors of stroke and other cardiovascular event risk, and therefore, appear to be clinically relevant phenotypes. In this chapter, we will review some of the major intermediate phenotypes that have been used to investigate the pathogenesis of ischaemic stroke, particularly large artery disease and small vessel disease.

8.2 Intermediate phenotypes for large vessel ischaemic stroke

Carotid artery stenosis secondary to atherosclerosis accounts for approximately 15 per cent of ischaemic strokes (Sacco 1994). For large vessel stroke, different pathophysiological processes may be involved in early vessel remodelling, atherosclerotic plaque formation, plaque instability, and thromboembolism. Different candidate genes could influence each component of the pathway and therefore the use of stroke as an endpoint may be relatively insensitive for examining these complex pathways.

A further problem is that with increasing age, atherosclerotic arterial changes are essentially ubiquitous in humans (Zhdanov *et al.* 1999, Roger *et al.* 2001). Few case-control studies of ischaemic stroke take into account this problem of non-penetrance of asymptomatic disease (Hill 2001). A number of methods have been developed to detect the early stages of vessel remodelling and asymptomatic atherosclerosis, making them useful intermediate phenotypes for large vessel stroke.

Common carotid artery intima-media thickness (IMT) has been widely used as a marker for early carotid atherosclerosis, whilst carotid plaque has been used as an estimate of more advanced disease. These measures can be estimated non-invasively using ultrasound, and appear to reflect sub-clinical atherosclerosis (Geroulakos *et al.* 1994).

8.3 Carotid artery IMT

Carotid artery IMT measures the combined thickness of the intimal and medial layers of the carotid artery. The arterial wall has three layers: the intima, media and the adventitia. The intima consists of a continuous monolayer of endothelial cells resting on a basement membrane. The media consists mainly of vascular smooth muscle cells and extracellular matrix and the adventitia comprises fibroblasts, connective tissue, blood vessels and fat (Newby and Zaltsman 2000). Intimal thickening occurs as an early feature of atherosclerosis and is exacerbated with age, male sex, hypertension and local haemodynamic stresses, for example at arterial bifurcations (Newby and Zaltsman 2000). Longitudinal, two-dimensional images of the carotid artery are obtained using high-resolution brightness (B)-mode ultrasound. The distance between the lumen-intima and media-adventitia interfaces indicates the IMT (Fig. 8.1).

An important requirement of any intermediate phenotype is that it should translate into clinical risk. Cross-sectional studies have shown that increased common carotid IMT correlates with cardiovascular risk factors (Heiss *et al.* 1991, Salonen and Salonen 1991*a*), is a marker of atherosclerosis elsewhere in the arterial system (Geroulakos *et al.* 1994) and of prevalent cardiovascular disease (Ebrahim *et al.* 1999). In a number of prospective cohort studies, increased IMT has been shown to be an independent predictor of future stroke and myocardial infarction (MI) risk (Salonen and Salonen 1991*b*, Bots *et al.* 1997*a*, O'Leary *et al.* 1999, Chambless *et al.* 2000). The strongest correlations with IMT are seen for large vessel stroke. Associations with small vessel disease, cardioembolic stroke and stroke of undetermined aetiology, although significant, are considerably weaker (Touboul *et al.* 2000). There appears to be a graded relationship between common carotid IMT and stroke risk. An odds ratio for stroke per standard deviation increase in IMT of 1.4 was found in one prospective study (Bots *et al.* 1997*a*).

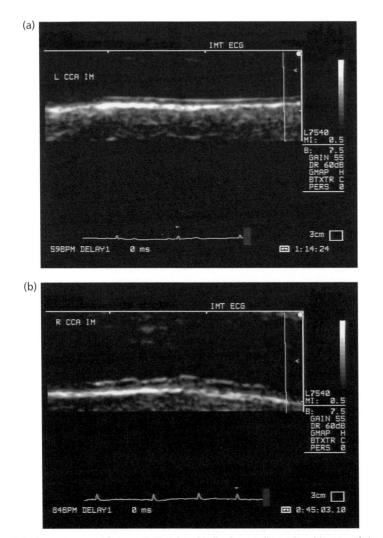

Fig. 8.1 Common carotid artery IMT. A longitudinal, two-dimensional image of the fall wall of the common carotid artery obtained using high-resolution brightness (B)-mode ultrasound. The distance between the lumen-intima and media-adventitia interfaces indicates the IMT (Copyright with author).

The Atherosclerosis Risk In Communities (ARIC) study also found a graded increase in stroke risk but with significant non-linearity, with hazards increasing more rapidly at lower IMT values than at higher ones (Chambless *et al.* 2000).

IMT measures have been shown to correlate strongly and consistently with a number of established vascular risk factors including increasing age, male sex, blood pressure, diabetes mellitus and body mass index. Correlations between IMT measurements and cholesterol levels have been less consistent (Salonen and Salonen 1991*a*,

Ebrahim *et al.* 1999, Davis *et al.* 2001). IMT also correlates with tobacco use, including years of cigarette smoking (Salonen and Salonen 1991*a*) and current smoking status (Ebrahim *et al.* 1999). A J-shaped relationship has been demonstrated between alcohol intake and IMT, with light to moderate intake being associated with reduced risk (Kiechl *et al.* 1998). Ethnicity is also an independent predictor of IMT, with subjects of African or African-Caribbean origin having significantly higher IMT compared with Caucasians (Markus *et al.* 2001).

These conventional risk factors together only explain an estimated 50 per cent of total IMT variability (Stensland-Bugge *et al.* 2001) and there is growing interest in the role of novel risk factors, particularly genetics, in the pathogenesis of atherosclerosis. Despite this the responsible genes remain largely unknown. Additionally, not all individuals with conventional risk factors will go on to develop disease and gene–environment interactions are also likely to play an important role in determining disease expression.

8.3.1 Evidence for the role of genetic factors in IMT

There is evidence for a strong genetic component to IMT variability. A family history of stroke was found to be an independent predictor of IMT in both sexes after controlling for traditional cardiovascular risk factors (Stensland-Bugge *et al.* 2001). In family studies using segregation analysis, genes were found to account for between 30 and 66 per cent of IMT variability (Duggirala *et al.* 1996, Zannad *et al.* 1998, Visvikis *et al.* 2000, Xiang *et al.* 2002). A recent study examining IMT in monozygotic and dizygotic twins found the heritability to be 36 per cent (Jartti *et al.* 2002).

8.3.2 Methods for measuring carotid artery IMT

A number of methods for measuring IMT have been described which vary in the arterial sites and number of points measured. Analysis can use either the mean or the maximum IMT and measurements can be performed either manually or using automated edge-tracking software.

Measurements from the far wall of the common carotid artery are easier to obtain and are more reproducible than at other sites (Kanters *et al.* 1997). Automated edge-tracking software can be used to determine the mean IMT over a large number of points with the advantage of reduced measurement error. A number of the major prospective outcome studies used mean IMT measurements in their analyses (Bots *et al.* 1997*a*, Chambless *et al.* 2000). A suggested drawback of using mean IMT measurements are that they assume uniform thickness throughout the blood vessel, and detect changes primarily in the media, whereas atherosclerosis is a focal phenomenon confined to the intima (Spence 2002). The carotid bifurcation and internal carotid artery are predilection sites for atherosclerotic plaque and IMT measures from these sites may be a better estimate of true atherosclerosis. The focal nature of atherosclerotic plaque formation is also the rationale for using maximum IMT measurements. Maximum IMT measurements may also correlate more strongly with vascular risk factors than those using the mean IMT (O'Leary *et al.* 1999).

A criticism of using IMT as a surrogate measure of atherosclerosis is that lower degrees of IMT thickening appear to reflect a non-atherosclerotic adaptive response to changes in shear and tensile stress rather than atherosclerosis *per se* (Bots *et al.* 1997*b*). This is consistent with previous studies suggesting that risk factors and future risk correlate better with an increased IMT above a certain value, rather than with IMT treated as a continuous variable (Salonen and Salonen 1991*b*, Chambless *et al.* 2000). One method used to overcome this is to look for associations with extreme values of IMT, for example >1 mm or above the 75th percentile. However, simplifying IMT measures as either present or absent loses significant data and therefore statistical power.

Atherosclerosis develops slowly over time. A further advantage of IMT measurements is that progression can be followed longitudinally, providing a prospective element to the study. A single measurement of IMT is likely to reflect past exposure to risk vascular factors whereas current risk may be influenced more by the current risk factor burden (Crouse 2001). Longitudinal measurement of IMT progression can provide prospective data and has been shown to correlate with incident vascular events (Hodis *et al.* 1998).

Each of these different methods of measuring IMT has its own particular advantages and limitations. Prospective outcome data is available for both mean and maximum IMT measurements and for measures from different arterial sites (O'Leary *et al.* 1999, Iglesias *et al.* 2002). In general these measures correlate well with one another and in practice many studies look for gene associations with more than one IMT measure.

There is some evidence that carotid bulb IMT may relate more specifically to stroke risk. In a large community study a family history of stroke, but not of MI, was an independent risk factor for carotid bulb IMT (Jerrard-Dunne *et al.* 2003). In contrast a family history of MI related more strongly to common carotid artery IMT. The carotid bulb is a predeliction site for carotid atherosclerosis and stenosis, a major cause of stroke. Atherosclerosis at this site develops both due to systemic factors, and local anatomic factors influencing flow dynamics. It is possible that these anatomic factors, which may include the angle of origin of the internal carotid artery (Sitzer *et al.* 2002), are under genetic control and this explain the association between bulb IMT and family history of stroke.

8.4 Carotid artery plaque

A complimentary approach to using IMT measurements is to determine the presence of established carotid plaque (Fig. 8.2). Study of plaque as well as IMT may be important for two reasons. First, small increases in wall thickness may reflect an adaptive vascular response to risk factors rather than atherosclerosis *per se*, and second the association of structural carotid artery changes with vascular risk appears to be stronger

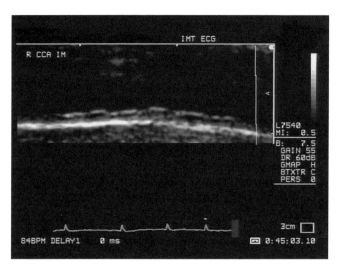

Fig. 8.2 Early carotid artery plaque. Visualized on the posterior wall of the common carotid artery using high-resolution ultrasound. A focal thickening of the intima with displacement of the arterial–wall interface can be seen. (Copyright with author).

for plaque than for IMT (Salonen and Salonen 1991*b*). The major disadvantage of using carotid plaque as an endpoint is reduced statistical power, first because the prevalence of plaque in a community population will be low and secondly because plaque represents a dichotomous outcome rather than a measurable quantitative trait.

A plaque is typically defined on ultrasound as a focal thickening of the intima with displacement of the arterial–wall interface. However, because IMT measurements do not correlate directly with the pathological features of atherosclerosis, the point at which localized intima-medial thickening becomes discreet plaque remains open to interpretation. Various studies have used cut-offs ranging from 1 to 1.7 mm, making comparison between studies difficult (Sitzer *et al.* 1993, Ebrahim *et al.* 1999, Spence 2002).

An alternative to dichotomizing plaque as present or absent is to quantify plaque area. Measures of two-dimensional plaque area appear to be a sensitive marker of atherosclerosis progression and a predictor of future vascular events (Spence 2002). Three-dimensional plaque volume measurements and qualitative features of carotid plaque morphology are also currently being evaluated as potential intermediate phenotypes (Pourcelot *et al.* 1999, Schminke *et al.* 2002, Spence 2002).

8.5 Alternative methods for assessing sub-clinical atherosclerosis

Other non-invasive measures of atherosclerosis include flow-mediated dilation (FMD), computed tomography measurement of coronary calcium and coronary magnetic resonance imaging (MRI).

Endothelial dysfunction is a very early feature of experimental models of atherosclerosis. FMD is a non-invasive method that assesses endothelial dysfunction using brachial artery ultrasound. Typically arterial dilatation is measured at rest, during reactive hyperaemia (endothelium-dependent dilatation), and after sub-lingual glyceryl trinitrate (endothelium-independent dilatation) (Celermajer *et al.* 1992). FMD correlates with vascular risk factors and has been associated with vascular disease in cross-sectional studies (Zhang *et al.* 2000). There are two major reasons why FMD may not be such a suitable intermediate phenotype for studying the genetic basis of atherothrombotic stroke. First, in contrast to IMT measurements, prospective outcome data are currently lacking. Second, a recent study examining the heritability of FMD measures found that measures did not correlate between twin pairs, suggesting that the genetic component to FMD is very modest (Jartti *et al.* 2002). In contrast asymptomatic family members of patients with stroke have been reported to have impaired endothelial function (Section 5.2).

Electron beam computed tomography could be used to determine the extent of coronary artery calcification (CAC). CAC is predictive of future MI and correlates well with vascular risk factors (Keelan *et al.* 2001). Outcome data relating to stroke are not currently available and exposure to radiation makes this method potentially more invasive than ultrasound techniques. Coronary calcification assessment assumes that the extent of atherosclerosis parallels the degree of calcification, when in fact soft plaques are more liable to rupture than stable calcified plaque. There is evidence for a strong genetic component to CAC, with one family study suggesting that as much as 42 per cent of CAC variability may be attributable to genetic factors (Peyser *et al.* 2002).

MRI shows promise as a method to identify plaque volume and morphology with high sensitivity and specificity (Choudhury *et al.* 2002). However, outcome measures are currently lacking and current costs are prohibitive for large-scale screening.

8.6 Association studies using intermediate phenotypes for large vessel ischaemic stroke

All studies to date investigating the genes underlying an increased IMT and the presence of carotid plaque have been candidate gene association studies. A large number of these have been published and a comprehensive review of these publications would be beyond the scope of this chapter. The results of some of the larger studies are presented here as examples. While a number of these studies do provide evidence that genetic variants influence atherosclerosis risk, the findings in some cases are conflicting or inconsistent. These conflicting results may arise from a number of factors. While they can overcome the problem of population stratification, association studies using intermediate phenotypes remain susceptible to the common errors that influence all genetic association studies, that is, small sample size; multiple hypothesis testing; random error; failure to independently replicate study results and positive publication bias

(Cardon and Bell 2001). Additional problems include failure to account for ethnic mix or to consider the confounding effects of gene–gene and gene–environment interactions.

Table 8.1 provides a summary of some of the larger association studies using IMT and carotid plaque. For clarity, these have been ordered into a number of major gene systems relating to lipid metabolism, endothelial function, homocysteine metabolism, inflammation, vascular remodelling and the renin-angiotensin system. It should be remembered, however, that in many cases there is overlap between these gene systems, with candidate genes having functional effects that relate to more than one system. Association studies between genetic variants in these gene-systems in relation to stroke are covered in Chapter 7 in detail.

8.6.1 Lipid metabolism

The enzyme paraoxonase (PON-1) can eliminate lipid peroxides and is believed to protect against oxidation of low-density lipoprotein (LDL) cholesterol. At position 54 of the PON-1 gene a methionine (M allele) to leucine (L allele) interchange has been identified. In a middle aged Austrian population ($n = 316$), the LL genotype was significantly associated with the presence and severity of carotid disease (Schmidt et al. 1998). A later study found similar results but also identified a significant interaction between this polymorphism and smoking status, with the effect confined to non-smokers (Malin et al. 2001). However, other studies have failed to demonstrate an association between IMT and paraxonase polymorphisms (Markus et al. 2001).

Apolipoprotein E (apoE) is a glycoprotein that mediates the binding of lipoprotein particles to specific receptors. The ε4 allele of apoE has been associated with increased LDL-cholesterol levels. Studies investigating the role of apoE in IMT and carotid plaque support a role for the ε4 allele in the pathogenesis of early atherosclerosis (Terry et al. 1996, Cattin et al. 1997).

8.6.2 Endothelial function

Decreased production of endothelial nitric oxide (NO) has been associated with athero-sclerosis. However, a study investigating the relationship between the Glu298Asp polymorphism of the NO gene and IMT in hypertensive subjects found no significant association (Karvonen et al. 2002).

8.6.3 Homocysteine metabolism

Serum homocysteine levels are an independent risk factor for vascular disease and the C677T polymorphism in the methylene tetrahydrofolate reductase (MTHFR) gene is associated with elevated homocysteine levels. In a large community population ($n = 1111$; 52 ± 13 years), no association was found between this polymorphism and IMT (McQuillan et al. 1999). A similar negative result was found in a community

Table 8.1 Association studies using intermediate phenotypes for large vessel ischaemic stroke

Gene system	Gene	Methodology	Polymorphism	Result	Comment
Lipid metabolism	**Paraoxonase 1**				
	(Schmidt et al. 1998)	Cross-sectional 316 subjects	Met54Leu	Positive	LL associated with carotid atheroma
	(Malin et al. 2001)	Cross-sectional 199 subjects	Met54Leu	Positive	LL associated with increased IMT in non-smokers
	(Markus et al. 2001)	Cross-sectional 292 subjects	Met54Leu	Negative	202 Caucasian men and 89 African Caribbean men
	ApoE				
	(Cattin et al. 1997)	Cross-sectional 260 subjects	Apoε2, ε3, ε4	Positive	ε4 allele associated with highest IMT
	(Terry et al. 1996)	Cross-sectional 260 subjects	Apoε2, ε3, ε4	Positive	ε2 protective, ε4 associated with increased IMT
Endothelial function	**ENOS**				
	(Karvonen et al. 2002)	Cross-sectional 600 hypertensives 600 controls	Glu298Asp	Negative	
Homocysteine	**MTHFR**				
	(McQuillan et al. 1999)	Cross-sectional 1111 subjects	C677T	Negative	T allele associated with homocysteine but not IMT
	(Kawamoto et al. 2001)	Cross-sectional 326 elderly subjects	C677T	Positive	T allele associated with increased IMT
	(Markus et al. 2001)	Cross-sectional 292 male subjects	C677T	Negative	202 Caucasian and 89 African Caribbean
Inflammation	**Toll-like receptor 4**				
	(Kiechl et al. 2002)	Cross-sectional 810 subjects	Asp299Gly	Positive	Gly299 associated with lower IMT and less progression

(continued)

Table 8.1 (continued)

Gene system	Gene	Methodology	Polymorphism	Result	Comment
	Interleukin-6				
	(Rauramaa et al. 2000)	Cross-sectional 92 subjects	-174G/C	Negative	
	(Rundek et al. 2002)	Cross-sectional 87 multiethnic subjects	-174G/C	Positive	GG associated with increased IMT
	(Brull et al. 2002)	Cross-sectional 248 subjects 20–28	-174G/C	Positive	CC associated with impaired FMD in smokers
Vascular remodelling	**Stromelysin-1**				
	(Rauramaa et al. 2000)	Cross-sectional 96 subjects	-1612 5A/6A	Positive	6A homozygotes had increased IMT
	(Rundek et al. 2002)	Cross-sectional 87 subjects	-1612 5A/6A	Positive	6A homozygotes had increased IMT
Renin-angiotensin	**ACE**				
	(Mannami et al. 2001)	Cross-sectional 4031 subjects	I/D	Negative	
	(Hung et al. 1999)	Cross-sectional 1111 subjects	I/D	Negative	
	(Arnett et al. 1998)	Cross-sectional 495 subjects	I/D	Negative	
	(Watanabe et al. 1997)	Cross-sectional 169 subjects	I/D	Positive	D allele associated with carotid plaque
	(Castellano et al. 1995)	Cross-sectional 199 subjects	I/D	Positive	DD genotype associated with increased IMT
	(Markus et al. 2001)	Cross-sectional 292 subjects	I/D	Negative	202 Caucasian men and 89 African Caribbean men
	Angiotensinogen				
	(Chapman et al. 2001)	Cross-sectional 1111 subjects	Promoter	Positive	-6A and -20C associated with increased IMT in women
	(Arnett et al. 1998)	Cross-sectional 475 subjects	M235T	Negative	
	(Schmidt et al. 2001)	Cross-sectional 431 subjects	M235T	Negative	

IMT, carotid artery intima-media thickness.

population of Caucasians and African Caribbeans in the United Kingdom (Markus *et al.* 2001). A subsequent study has suggested that the C677T polymorphism is a risk factor for carotid plaque in older individuals with vascular risk factors ($n = 326$; 73 ± 12 years) (Kawamoto *et al.* 2001).

8.6.4 Inflammation

Increasing evidence suggests that inflammation is important in the pathogenesis of atherosclerosis and ischaemic stroke (Ross 1999). Mutations in certain receptors that mediate the innate immune response have been shown to attenuate host response to pro-inflammatory stimuli. A good example is Toll-like receptor (TLR) polymorphisms. The TLR family are pathogen recognition receptors that mediate the innate immune response to infection. TLR-4 is a critical signal transducer for endotoxin, a lipopolysaccharide component of gram-negative bacterial cell walls (Kaisho and Akira 2002). Endotoxin is a potent mediator of inflammation and circulating levels of endotoxin independently predict incident atherosclerosis measured by carotid ultrasound (Wiedermann *et al.* 1999). A non-synonymous single nucleotide polymorphism (Asp299Gly) in the Toll-like receptor-4 (TLR-4) gene affects the responsiveness to lipopolysaccharide in humans (Arbour *et al.* 2000). In a prospective cohort of 810 individuals, subjects with the Asp299Gly TLR-4 allele were found to have lower levels of inflammatory markers, a lower risk of carotid plaque and a smaller IMT compared with the wild type (Kiechl *et al.* 2002).

Another good example of a candidate gene for atherosclerosis is the pro-inflammatory cytokine Interleukin-6 (IL-6). In prospective studies, elevated basal IL-6 levels are predictive of future vascular events (Ridker *et al.* 2000*a*) and both animal and *in vitro* studies support a direct role for this cytokine in atherogenesis (Moyer *et al.* 1991, Seino *et al.* 1994, Elhage *et al.* 1998, Huber *et al.* 1999, Ridker *et al.* 2000*b*). A genetic variant in the IL-6 gene (IL-6-174 G/C) has been associated with quantitative changes in inflammatory markers (Humphries *et al.* 2001, Vickers *et al.* 2002). Recent studies have found associations between the C allele of this polymorphism and both MI (Georges *et al.* 2001, Humphries *et al.* 2001), and prospective cardiovascular mortality in patients with abdominal aortic aneurysm (Jones *et al.* 2001). Two relatively small studies have looked at the role of the IL-6-174 polymorphism in IMT. In the first, which measured maximum IMT from the carotid bifurcation in 96 healthy male subjects, the IL-6 polymorphism was significantly associated with IMT univariately but no longer after covariate adjustment (Rauramaa *et al.* 2000). The second study measured the mean maximum IMT from three arterial sites in 87 multiethnic subjects. The GG genotype was found to be weakly associated with increased IMT (Rundek *et al.* 2002). However, the unusual ethnic mix of this population may have confounded the results. A further study looking at this polymorphism in relation to FMD found that CC homozygotes had significantly impaired FMD but only if they were smokers, highlighting the

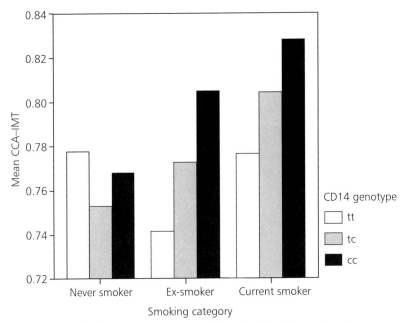

Fig. 8.3 The relationship between common carotid IMT and CD14 genotype by smoking status. A graded response was seen in current and ex-smokers but was absent in individuals who had never smoked. This emphasizes the importance of gene–environment interaction in the pathogenesis of carotid IMT (from Risley *et al.* 2003)

potential importance of gene–environment interactions in mediating atherosclerosis risk (Brull *et al.* 2002).

The importance of considering gene–environment interactions is further illustrated by association studies with endotoxin receptor CD14. Endotoxin is a potent mediator of inflammation and smokers have elevated plasma levels of endotoxin. The endotoxin-receptor, CD14, can enhance the endotoxin-neutralization capacity of plasma. Therefore one might expect an interaction between CD14 genotype as a risk factor and smoking and this was found to be the case in a large community study of 1000 middle aged individuals (Risley *et al.* 2003). A functional polymorphism in the promoter region of the CD14 gene (CD14–159 C/T) was studied. The CC genotype was associated with increased carotid IMT in the whole population. However this association was confined to current and ex-smokers in whom a graded response between gene-dose and IMT was found (Fig. 8.3).

8.6.5 Vessel remodelling

Vascular remodelling is an early phenomenon in the development of atherosclerosis. The matrix metalloproteinase (MMP) family regulate the accumulation of extracellular matrix during tissue injury and thus may influence the development and progression of atherosclerotic plaque (Woessner 1991). A functional promoter polymorphism-1612 (5A/6A) has been identified in the stromolysin-1 (MMP-3) gene. The 6A allele has been associated with reduced stromolysin-1, which would favour the development of atherosclerosis (Ye *et al.* 1996). Two independent studies have found significant associations between the 6A/6A genotype and increased IMT (Rauramaa *et al.* 2000, Rundek *et al.* 2002).

8.6.6 Renin-angiotensin system

The renin-angiotensin pathway is involved in the regulation of blood pressure, cellular growth and vascular remodelling. Polymorphisms of the renin-angiotensin system have been variably associated with ischaemic stroke (see Chapter 7). A number of studies have looked at the angiotensin converting enzyme (ACE) insertion/deletion polymorphism in relation to carotid IMT and plaque. A relatively small study ($n = 169$) in a Japanese population found an association between the D allele and the presence but not the extent of carotid plaque (Watanabe *et al.* 1997). Another study in Italian subjects ($n = 199$) found an association between DD genotype and increased IMT but not carotid plaque (Castellano *et al.* 1995). However, the three largest and most recent studies to date ($n = 495–4031$) have all been negative (Arnett *et al.* 1998, Hung *et al.* 1999, Mannami *et al.* 2001).

Variants in the angiotensinogen gene have also been studied in relation to IMT. Two studies investigating the M235T variant have been negative (Arnett *et al.* 1998, Schmidt *et al.* 2001). A large study ($n = 1111$) found an association between promoter variants -6G/A and -20A/C in the angiotensinogen gene and increased mean IMT but the effect was confined to women (Chapman *et al.* 2001).

8.7 The use of carotid IMT as an intermediate phenotype: future directions

Carotid IMT is a powerful technique to investigate the genetics of large vessel disease stroke for the reasons given in the introduction. However, from the examples above it can be appreciated that studies to date have often produced inconsistent results. How can this be improved? Improved experimental design of candidate gene association studies is required. Large samples providing sufficient statistical power are essential, and their selection needs to take into account ethnic heterogeneity. Account needs to be made of multiple hypothesis testing. Replication of positive associations in an independent population is essential. Association should also be examined in both cross-sectional study designs, and prospective studies with repeat IMT imaging at a later time-point. A number of the above examples emphasize the crucial importance of gene–environment interactions, and studies should be designed and statistically powered to allow both these and gene–gene interactions to be identified.

A number of other study designs could also be applied to carotid IMT. These are covered in detail in Chapter 2. Family association studies using IMT as a quantitative trait would be possible. Genome wide association studies are likely to become realistic in the near future and offer the advantage of allowing novel genes to be identified.

8.8 Intermediate phenotypes for small vessel disease

A quarter of ischaemic strokes are a consequence of cerebral small vessel disease, which leads to small lacunar infarcts in the deep parts of the brain or brain stem. Lacunar infarcts are caused by occlusion of one single deep penetrating artery. There is evidence to suggest a strong genetic component to small vessel disease. White matter hyper-intensities (WMH), determined using MRI have been used as an intermediate pheno-type for small vessel disease and newer phenotypes are being developed based on our current understanding of the pathophysiology of small vessel disease.

8.8.1 White matter hyperintensities

The development of MRI techniques has led to an increasing interest in the study of WMH. WMH represent high signal on T2-MRI and can include a spectrum of subcor-tical changes ranging from small focal lesions 5–15 mm in size, to more patchy or diffuse white matter changes which are seen in the periventricular regions and deep white matter, also referred to as leukoaraiosis (Fig. 8.4). WMH is a frequent finding amongst elderly subjects and its frequency increases with age (Breteler *et al.* 1994, Longstreth *et al.* 1996), although estimates for its prevalence vary according to the imaging method employed and the definition of WMH used. Individuals with WMH are frequently asymptomatic or may have overt evidence of cognitive impairment (Breteler *et al.* 1994, Longstreth Jr. *et al.* 1996, Kuller *et al.* 1998) or previous history of stroke (Awad *et al.* 1986*b*).

The measurement of WMH is a potentially useful intermediate phenotype for stroke genetic studies for several reasons which are discussed in more detail below, but which can be summarized as follows. First, WMH appears to have an ischaemic basis and represents a risk factor for stroke in later life. Therefore, it may be a useful substrate to study the early critical molecular events involved in the pathogenesis of stroke. Second, WMH have a strong genetic basis. Third, although methods of quantification are not as well developed as that of IMT, the amount of WMH can be quantified giving more statistical power for association studies than studies using the binary endpoint of stroke. In addition, progression of WMH has been shown to occur over several years allowing a prospective element to be incorporated into studies of genetic risk factors. Finally, WMH is particularly relevant to cerebral small vessel disease. Therefore, if we believe genetic influences are different according to stroke subtype, WMH may be a particularly useful intermediate phenotype for gaining insights into the genetics of lacunar or small vessel disease stroke.

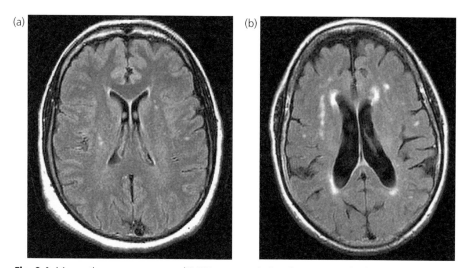

Fig. 8.4 Magnetic resonance scans (FLAIR sequence) showing WMH, which are used as an intermediate phenotype for cerebral small vessel disease. These images are from a community study of hypertensive individuals with no evidence of cerebral or cardiac symptoms. In the first subject (a) a few high intensity signals can be seen. In the second subject (b) more extensive and confluent WMH can be seen (Copyright with author).

8.8.2 **WMH has an ischaemic basis**

Autopsy studies are consistent with WMH having an underlying ischaemic basis with hyperintensities >5 mm likely to represent true lacunar infarcts associated with cerebral small vessel disease. However, the histological correlates of smaller focal lesions seen on T2 MRI are varied, particularly those lesions 1–2 mm in size. Lesions of this size may reflect dilated perivascular (Virchow Robin) spaces, gliosis and demyelination as well as focal lacunar infarcts (Fisher 1979, Awad *et al.* 1986*a*, Braffman *et al.* 1988).

The neuropathological appearance corresponding to leukoaraiosis is neuronal loss, ischaemic demyelination, and gliosis (Pantoni and Garcia 1997). In affected regions of white matter, arteriosclerosis is present in the small penetrating arterioles of the white matter. This refers to replacement of the smooth muscle cells by fibro-hyaline material and narrowing of the vascular lumen. Pathophysiologically it is believed that a diffuse arteriopathy of the cerebral small vessels results in hypoperfusion and impaired autoregulation, and subsequent ischaemia (Pantoni and Garcia 1997, Bakker *et al.* 1999, Terborg *et al.* 2000). If acute, this causes small focal regions of damage in perforating arteriole territories (lacunar infarction), while if it is more chronic it results in diffuse ischaemic injury (leukoaraiosis). Consistent with the notion of a common underlying vasculopathy, lacunar infarcts and leukoaraiosis frequently co-exist.

WMH is more common in individuals with vascular risk factors, which include aging, hypertension, diabetes mellitus and smoking (Breteler *et al.* 1994, Kuller *et al.* 1998) and is frequently encountered in patients with symptomatic stroke (Awad *et al.* 1986*b*). White matter lesions also appear to be feature in patients with Alzheimer's disease (Brun and Englund 1986). The patholophysiological basis of WMH in these cases is less clear. The white matter changes, however, may have an ischaemic basis because of structural changes in small blood vessels. In these cases, the pathology may predominantly reflect amyloid angiopathy rather than hypertensive arteriosclerosis (Mandybur 1975, Pantoni and Garcia 1997), although there may well be an overlap between the two vasculopathies.

It has been hypothesized that WMH in asymptomatic individuals is a marker for the development of stroke in later life. This hypothesis has been recently confirmed by a prospective study with evaluation of MRI findings in 933 neurologically normal adults. During a period of follow-up ranging from 1 to 7 years, it was demonstrated that silent lacunar infarction was a strong risk factor for subsequent clinical stroke (Kobayashi *et al.* 1997).

8.8.3 Evidence for a genetic involvement in WMH

Direct evidence for a role of genetic influences was provided by a twin study (Carmelli *et al.* 1998). Concordance rates for WMH volume were much higher in monozygotic 61 per cent versus dizygotic twins 38 per cent. It was estimated that 71 per cent of the variance in WMH volume was due to genetic factors. Interestingly the heritability for WMH was much higher than that for systolic hypertension in the same cohort suggesting that genetic influences were more important in this intermediate phenotype. Concordance rates for large amounts of WMH were much higher than those observed for stroke in the same twin registry (Brass *et al.* 1992).

8.8.4 Quantification and evolution of WMH

There have been many different approaches to both defining and quantifying WMH. Some studies have considered WMH as a dichotomous trait, defining the presence or absence of a minimum amount of WMH. A number of qualitative scales have been adopted to assess the severity of white matter changes (Mantyla *et al.* 1997). Scoring is performed by one or more raters with inter and intra-rater variability stated. In some studies, periventricular changes have been assessed separately from subcortical white matter changes. Based on pathological observations (Braffman *et al.* 1988), some studies have excluded small punctate lesions, for example, <3 mm, because of the increased likelihood of non-ischaemic aetiology (Kobayashi *et al.* 1997, Notsu *et al.* 1999). In some of these studies, the term silent lacunar infarction has been used exclusively for hyperintense focal lesions on T2 with corresponding focal hypointensity on T1, with other hyperintense lesions being separately rated.

Lack of standardization in defining or grading WMH has made comparison between epidemiological and risk factor studies difficult and this may also be an important issue for genetic studies. One approach may be to use more quantitative MRI volumetric techniques with WMH volume estimated using semi-automated software. An alternative approach to case–control or cross-sectional methods is based on the notion that WMH progresses gradually over time with the accumulation of vascular risk factors, ultimately resulting in stroke and or severe subcortical dementia. Therefore, it is possible to prospectively assess the role of risk factors on disease progression. This approach is a practical one as demonstrated by Schmidt and colleagues (Schmidt *et al*. 1999). It was found that there was evidence of WMH progression during a three-year follow up of 273 community dwelling elderly individuals, although during this short period of follow up, lesion progression was not associated with clinical measures of outcome such as cognitive decline.

8.8.5 **WMH and lacunar stroke**

Pathological studies and our understanding of underlying pathophysiology, suggest that WMH is associated closely with cerebral small vessel disease. MR studies have also been consistent with this notion with the presence of definite lacunar infarction being associated with more severe T2 hyperintensity (Mantyla *et al*. 1999). Further evidence for this hypothesis is provided by a prospective study of asymptomatic individuals with WMH. In this study, stroke due to lacunar infarction accounted for the vast majority of ischaemic strokes observed during follow up (Kobayashi *et al*. 1997). Comparison across clinical stroke subtypes has also been consistent, with WMH more frequently encountered in patients with lacunar stroke (Adachi *et al*. 2002). Therefore, WMH would seem to represent the intermediate phenotype of choice for genetic studies in lacunar stroke.

8.8.6 **Genetic studies of WMH**

To date there have been no genomic studies performed to identify genes in WMH, although in the future increasing availability of MRI to enable screening of sibs concordant for white matter changes may make this a feasible option. All studies have involved determining association with candidate genes. The range of candidate genes studied corresponds broadly with those outlined in Chapter 7. The main types of study design used have been case–control, comparing individuals with evidence of WMH and controls free of MRI disease, and cross-sectional or prospective follow up of community populations. Some representative studies are summarized in Table 8.2. As for IMT studies, future progress will depend upon carefully designed candidate gene studies with large samples, replication of positive association in independent populations, and accounting for ethnic heterogeneity and multiple hypothesis testing. Gene–environment interactions may be important, particularly interaction with hypertension.

Table 8.2 Association studies using intermediate phenotypes relevant to cerebral small vessel disease

Gene system	Gene	Methodology	Phenotypes	Polymorphism	Result	Comment
Lipid metabolism	**ApoE** (Schmidt et al. 1997)	Cross-sectional 280 subjects 50–75	MARCD defined as confluent or early confluent white matter hyperintensity or presence of lacunes on T2	Apoε2, ε3, ε4	Positive	ε2/ε3 genotype a risk factor for WMH
	Paraoxanase 1 (Schmidt et al. 2000)	Cohort 264 subjects 44–75	WMH = presence/absence and grade of disease at base line and follow up	Met54Leu glu191arg	Positive	LL genotype associated with WMH progression
Endothelial function	**ENOS** (Nasreen et al. 2002)	Cross-sectional 166 male non-smokers, 344 male smokers	Cerebral blood flow and CVR	T786C	Positive	TT genotype associated with increased CVR and decreased blood flow in smokers
Homocysteine	**MTHFR** (Notsu et al. 1999)	Case control 147 cases 214/176 controls	Presence/absence of silent LI = hyperintensity on T2 and hypointensity T1 MRI disease free controls	C677T	Negative	
	ACE (Notsu et al. 1999)	Case control 147 cases 214/176 controls	Presence/absence silent LI = hyperintensity on T2 and hypointensity T1 MRI disease free controls	I/D	Negative	

	Reference	Study	Phenotype	Polymorphism	Association	Comments
	(Watanabe et al. 1997)	Cross-sectional 169 cases	Presence/absence silent LI = hyperintensity on T2 and hypointensity T1	I/D	Negative	
Renin-angiotensin	**Angiotensinogen**					
	(Schmidt et al. 2001a)	Cross-sectional/cohort 396 subjects mean age 60	WMH = presence/absence and grade of disease at base line and follow up	M235T	Positive	TT genotype associated with progression of WMH
	(Schmidt et al. 2001b)	Cross-sectional 410 subjects 50–75	MARCD defined as confluent or early confluent white matter hyperintensity or presence of lacunes on T2	Promoter variants	Positive	BB/B/A− haplotypes associated with WMH

LI, lacunar infarction; WMH, white matter hyperintensity; CVR, cerebrovascular resistance; MARCD, microangiopathy related cerebral disease.

This is the major risk factor for both WMH and lacunar stroke, but a striking feature of the disease is that individuals with the same degree of hypertension may have either no WMH or many WMH, suggesting other modulating influences are important, and these are likely to include genetic factors.

8.8.7 Other small vessel disease intermediate phenotypes

WMH remains currently the most well validated of intermediate phenotypes relevant to small vessel disease, although alternative phenotypes have been proposed. Measurement of cerebral blood flow has been suggested, as a marker since cerebral hypoperfusion appears to be associated with the presence of cerebral small vessel disease (Markus *et al.* 2000). Recently this approach was used to report a possible interaction between a functional promoter polymorphism in the endothelial NO synthase gene and smoking, resulting in reduction of cerebral blood flow (Nasreen *et al.* 2002). This is an exciting finding and illustrates the role of intermediate phenotypes in improving our understanding of disease pathophysiology. However, the role of such genetic variants as important clinical risk factors, can only be determined by testing in symptomatic individuals with stroke.

8.9 Conclusions

In summary, carotid artery ultrasound is a safe, reproducible and non-invasive method for investigating the atherosclerotic nature of large vessel stroke. There is a large body of evidence to suggest that elevated IMT translates into clinical stroke risk and that IMT has a strong genetic component. WMH, determined using MRI also have a strong genetic component and may be a particularly useful intermediate phenotype for gaining insights into the genetics of lacunar stroke. New phenotypes are currently being developed based on our improved understanding of the pathophysiology of stroke and advances in imaging technology.

The use of intermediate phenotypes has a number of potential advantages. First, the numbers of genes involved in the intermediate phenotype are likely to be considerably less than those involved in ischaemic stroke. Second, the techniques can be readily applied to large-scale community-based populations, reducing selection bias. Third, the use of a continuous index of risk rather than a dichotomous variable such as stroke, and the related avoidance of non-penetrance of asymptomatic disease, markedly increases power. Finally, these measures provide the opportunity for prospective followup of disease progression.

As with candidate gene case–control studies, the interpretation of genetic association studies using intermediate phenotypes should take into account accuracy and reproducibility of the phenotype, sample size and characteristics, correction for multiple hypothesis testing, the ability to replicate the findings in an independent population and positive publication bias.

References

Adachi, T., Kobayashi, S., and Yamaguchi, S. (2002). Frequency and pathogenesis of silent subcortical brain infarction in acute first-ever ischemic stroke. *Internal Medicine*, **41**, 103–8.

Arbour, N.C., Lorenz, E., Schutte, B.C., *et al.* (2000). TLR4 mutations are associated with endotoxin hyporesponsiveness in humans. *Nature Genetics*, **25**, 187–91.

Arnett, D.K., Borecki, I.B., Ludwig, E.H., *et al.* (1998). Angiotensinogen and angiotensin converting enzyme genotypes and carotid atherosclerosis: the atherosclerosis risk in communities and the NHLBI family heart studies. *Atherosclerosis*, **138**, 111–16.

Awad, I.A., Johnson, P., Spetzler, R., and Hodak, J. (1986a). Incidental subcortical lesions identified on magnetic resonance imaging in the elderly. II. Postmortem pathological correlations. *Stroke*, **17**, 1090–7.

Awad, I.A., Spetzler, R.F., Hodak, J.A., Awad, C.A., and Carey, R. (1986b). Incidental subcortical lesions identified on magnetic resonance imaging in the elderly. I. Correlation with age and cerebrovascular risk factors. *Stroke*, **17**, 1084–9.

Bakker, S.L., de Leeuw, F.E., de Groot, J.C., *et al.* (1999). Cerebral vasomotor reactivity and cerebral white matter lesions in the elderly. *Neurology*, **52**, 578–83.

Bots, M.L., Hoes, A.W., Koudstaal, P.J., Hofman, A., and Grobbee, D.E. (1997a). Common carotid intima-media thickness and risk of stroke and myocardial infarction: the Rotterdam Study. *Circulation*, **96**, 1432–7.

Bots, M.L., Hofman, A., and Grobbee, D.E. (1997b). Increased common carotid intima-media thickness. Adaptive response or a reflection of atherosclerosis? Findings from the Rotterdam Study. *Stroke*, **28**, 2442–7.

Braffman, B.H., Zimmerman, R.A., Trojanowski, J.Q., *et al.* (1988). Brain MR: pathologic correlation with gross and histopathology. 1. Lacunar infarction and Virchow-Robin spaces. *American Journal of Roentgenology*, **151**, 551–8.

Brass, L.M., Isaacsohn, J.L., Merikangas, K.R., and Robinette, C.D. (1992). A study of twins and stroke. *Stroke*, **23**, 221–3.

Breteler, M.M., van Swieten, J.C., Bots, M.L., *et al.* (1994). Cerebral white matter lesions, vascular risk factors, and cognitive function in a population-based study: the Rotterdam Study. *Neurology*, **44**, 1246–52.

Brull, D.J., Lesson, C.P., Montgomery, H.E., *et al.* (2002). The effect of the Interleukin-6–174G > C promoter gene polymorphism on endothelial function in healthy volunteers. *European Journal of Clinical Investigation*, **32**, 153–7.

Brun, A. and Englund, E. (1986). A white matter disorder in dementia of the Alzheimer type: a pathoanatomical study. *Annals of Neurology*, **19**, 253–62.

Cardon, L.R. and Bell, J.I. (2001). Association study designs for complex diseases. *Nature Reviews Genetics*, **2**, 91–9.

Carmelli, D., DeCarli, C., Swan, G.E., *et al.* (1998). Evidence for genetic variance in white matter hyperintensity volume in normal elderly male twins. *Stroke*, **29**, 1177–81.

Castellano, M., Muiesan, M.L., Rizzoni, D., *et al.* (1995). Angiotensin-converting enzyme I/D polymorphism and arterial wall thickness in a general population. The Vobarno Study. *Circulation*, **91**, 2721–4.

Cattin, L., Fisicaro, M., Tonizzo, M., *et al.* (1997). Polymorphism of the apolipoprotein E gene and early carotid atherosclerosis defined by ultrasonography in asymptomatic adults. *Arteriosclerosis, Thrombosis and Vascular Biology*, **17**, 91–4.

Celermajer, D.S., Sorensen, K.E., Gooch, V.M., *et al.* (1992). Non-invasive detection of endothelial dysfunction in children and adults at risk of atherosclerosis. *Lancet*, **340**, 1111–15.

Chambless, L.E., Folsom, A.R., Clegg, L.X., *et al.* (2000). Carotid wall thickness is predictive of incident clinical stroke: the Atherosclerosis Risk in Communities (ARIC) study. *American Journal of Epidemiology*, **151**, 478–87.

Chapman, C.M., Palmer, L.J., McQuillan, B.M., *et al.* (2001). Polymorphisms in the angiotensinogen gene are associated with carotid intimal-medial thickening in females from a community-based population. *Atherosclerosis*, **159**, 209–17.

Choudhury, R.P., Fuster, V., Badimon, J.J., Fisher, E.A., and Fayad, Z.A. (2002). MRI and characterization of atherosclerotic plaque: emerging applications and molecular imaging. *Arteriosclerosis, Thrombosis and Vascular Biology*, **22**, 1065–74.

Crouse, J.R.I. (2001). Predictive value of carotid 2-dimensional ultrasound. *American Journal of Cardiology*, **88**, 27–30E.

Davis, P.H., Dawson, J.D., Riley, W.A., and Lauer, R.M. (2001). Carotid intimal-medial thickness is related to cardiovascular risk factors measured from childhood through middle age: the Muscatine Study. *Circulation*, **104**, 2815–19.

Duggirala, R., Gonzalez, V.C., O'Leary, D.H., Stern, M.P., and Blangero, J. (1996). Genetic basis of variation in carotid artery wall thickness. *Stroke*, **27**, 833–7.

Ebrahim, S., Papacosta, O., Whincup, P., *et al.* (1999). Carotid plaque, intima media thickness, cardiovascular risk factors, and prevalent cardiovascular disease in men and women: the British Regional Heart Study. *Stroke*, **30**, 841–50.

Elhage, R., Maret, A., Pieraggi, M.T., *et al.* (1998). Differential effects of interleukin-1 receptor antagonist and tumor necrosis factor binding protein on fatty-streak formation in apolipoprotein E-deficient mice. *Circulation*, **97**, 242–4.

Fisher, C.M. (1979). Capsular infarcts: the underlying vascular lesions. *Archives of Neurology*, **36**, 65–73.

Georges, J.L., Loukaci, V., Poirier, O., *et al.* (2001). Interleukin-6 gene polymorphisms and susceptibility to myocardial infarction: the ECTIM study. Etude Cas-Temoin de l'Infarctus du Myocarde. *Journal of Molecular Medicine*, **79**, 300–5.

Geroulakos, G., O'Gorman, D.J., Kalodiki, E., Sheridan, D.J., and Nicolaides, A.N. (1994). The carotid intima-media thickness as a marker of the presence of severe symptomatic coronary artery disease. *European Heart Journal*, **15**, 781–5.

Heiss, G., Sharrett, A.R., Barnes, R., *et al.* (1991). Carotid atherosclerosis measured by B-mode ultrasound in populations: associations with cardiovascular risk factors in the ARIC study. *American Journal of Epidemiology*, **134**, 250–6.

Hill, A.V. (2001). Immunogenetics and genomics. *Lancet*, **357**, 2037–41.

Hodis, H.N., Mack, W.J., LaBree, L., *et al.* (1998). The role of carotid arterial intima-media thickness in predicting clinical coronary events. *Annals of Internal Medicine*, **128**, 262–9.

Huber, S.A., Sakkinen, P., Conze, D., Hardin, N., and Tracy, R. (1999). Interleukin-6 exacerbates early atherosclerosis in mice. *Arteriosclerosis, Thrombosis and Vascular Biology*, **19**, 2364–7.

Humphries, S.E., Luong, L.A., Ogg, M.S., Hawe, E., and Miller, G.J. (2001). The interleukin-6-174 G/C promoter polymorphism is associated with risk of coronary heart disease and systolic blood pressure in healthy men. *European Heart Journal*, **22**, 2243–52.

Hung, J., McQuillan, B.M., Nidorf, M., Thompson, P.L., and Beilby, J.P. (1999). Angiotensin-converting enzyme gene polymorphism and carotid wall thickening in a community population. *Arteriosclerosis, Thrombosis and Vascular Biology*, **19**, 1969–74.

Iglesias, d.S., Bots, M.L., Grobbee, D.E., Hofman, A., and Witteman, J.C. (2002). Carotid intima-media thickness at different sites: relation to incident myocardial infarction. The Rotterdam Study. *European Heart Journal*, **23**, 934–40.

Jartti, L., Ronnemaa, T., Kaprio, J., *et al.* (2002). Population-based twin study of the effects of migration from Finland to Sweden on endothelial function and intima-media thickness. *Arteriosclerosis, Thrombosis and Vascular Biology*, **22**, 832–7.

Jerrard-Dunne, P., Markus, H.S., Steckel, D.A., Buchler, A., von Kogler, S., and Sitzer, M. (2003). Early carotid *arteriosclerosis* and family history of vascular disease. specific effects on arterial sites have implications for genetic studies. *Arteriosclerosis, Thrombosis and Vascular Biology*, **23**, 302–6.

Jones, K.G., Brull, D.J., Brown, L.C., *et al.* (2001). Interleukin-6 (IL-6) and the prognosis of abdominal aortic aneurysms. *Circulation*, **103**, 2260–5.

Kaisho, T. and Akira, S. (2002). Toll-like receptors as adjuvant receptors. *Biochimica et Biophysica Acta*, **1589**, 1–13.

Kanters, S.D., Algra, A., van Leeuwen, M.S., and Banga, J.D. (1997). Reproducibility of *in vivo* carotid intima-media thickness measurements: a review. *Stroke*, **28**, 665–71.

Karvonen, J., Kauma, H., Kervinen, K., *et al.* (2002). Endothelial nitric oxide synthase gene Glu298Asp polymorphism and blood pressure, left ventricular mass and carotid artery atherosclerosis in a population-based cohort. *Journal of Internal Medicine*, **251**, 102–10.

Kawamoto, R., Kohara, K., Tabara, Y., *et al.* (2001). An association of 5,10-methylenetetrahydrofolate reductase (MTHFR) gene polymorphism and common carotid atherosclerosis. *Journal of Human Genetics*, **46**, 506–10.

Keelan, P.C., Bielak, L.F., Ashai, K., *et al.* (2001). Long-term prognostic value of coronary calcification detected by electron-beam computed tomography in patients undergoing coronary angiography. *Circulation*, **104**, 412–17.

Kiechl, S., Lorenz, E., Reindl, M., *et al.* (2002). Toll-like receptor 4 polymorphisms and atherogenesis. *New England Journal of Medicine*, **347**, 185–92.

Kiechl, S., Willeit, J., Rungger, G., *et al.* (1998). Alcohol consumption and atherosclerosis: what is the relation? Prospective results from the Bruneck Study. *Stroke*, **29**, 900–7.

Kobayashi, S., Okada, K., Koide, H., Bokura, H., and Yamaguchi, S. (1997). Subcortical silent brain infarction as a risk factor for clinical stroke. *Stroke*, **28**, 1932–9.

Kuller, L.H., Shemanski, L., Manolio, T., *et al.* (1998). Relationship between ApoE, MRI findings, and cognitive function in the Cardiovascular Health Study. *Stroke*, **29**, 388–98.

Longstreth, W.T., Jr., Manolio, T., and Arnold, A. (1996). Clinical correlates of white matter findings on cranial magnetic resonance imaging of 3301 elderly people. The Cardiovascular Health Study. *Stroke*, **27**, 1274–82.

Malin, R., Loimaala, A., Nenonen, A., *et al.* (2001). Relationship between high-density lipoprotein paraoxonase gene M/L55 polymorphism and carotid atherosclerosis differs in smoking and nonsmoking men. *Metabolism*, **50**, 1095–101.

Mandybur, T.I. (1975). The incidence of cerebral amyloid angiopathy in Alzheimer's disease. *Neurology*, **25**, 120–6.

Mannami, T., Katsuya, T., Baba, S., *et al.* (2001). Low potentiality of angiotensin-converting enzyme gene insertion/deletion polymorphism as a useful predictive marker for carotid atherogenesis in a large general population of a Japanese city: the Suita study. *Stroke*, **32**, 1250–6.

Mantyla, R., Aronen, H.J., Salonen, O., *et al.* (1999). Magnetic resonance imaging white matter hyperintensities and mechanism of ischemic stroke. *Stroke*, **30**, 2053–8.

Mantyla, R., Erkinjuntti, T., Salonen, O., *et al.* (1997). Variable agreement between visual rating scales for white matter hyperintensities on MRI. Comparison of 13 rating scales in a poststroke cohort. *Stroke*, **28**, 1614–23.

Markus, H., Kapozsta, Z., Ditrich, R., *et al.* (2001). Increased common carotid intima-media thickness in UK African Caribbeans and its relation to chronic inflammation and vascular candidate gene polymorphisms. *Stroke*, **32**, 2465–71.

Markus, H.S., Lythgoe, D.J., Ostegaard, L., O'Sullivan, M., and Williams, S.C. (2000). Reduced cerebral blood flow in white matter in ischaemic leukoaraiosis demonstrated using quantitative exogenous contrast based perfusion MRI. *Journal of Neurology, Neurosurgery, and Psychiatry*, **69**, 48–53.

McQuillan, B.M., Beilby, J.P., Nidorf, M., Thompson, P.L., and Hung, J. (1999). Hyperhomocysteinemia but not the C677T mutation of methylenetetrahydrofolate reductase is an independent risk determinant of carotid wall thickening. The Perth Carotid Ultrasound Disease Assessment Study (CUDAS). *Circulation*, **99**, 2383–8.

Moyer, C.F., Sajuthi, D., Tulli, H., and Williams, J.K. (1991). Synthesis of IL-1 alpha and IL-1 beta by arterial cells in atherosclerosis. *American Journal of Pathology*, **138**, 951–60.

Nasreen, S., Nabika, T., Shibata, H., *et al.* (2002). T-786C polymorphism in endothelial NO synthase gene affects cerebral circulation in smokers: possible gene–environmental interaction. *Arteriosclerosis Thrombosis and Vascular Biology*, **22**, 605–10.

Newby, A.C. and Zaltsman, A.B. (2000). Molecular mechanisms in intimal hyperplasia. *Journal of Pathology*, **190**, 300–9.

Notsu, Y., Nabika, T., Park, H.Y., Masuda, J., and Kobayashi, S. (1999). Evaluation of genetic risk factors for silent brain infarction. *Stroke*, **30**, 1881–6.

O'Leary, D.H., Polak, J.F., Kronmal, R.A., *et al.* (1999). Carotid-artery intima and media thickness as a risk factor for myocardial infarction and stroke in older adults. Cardiovascular Health Study Collaborative Research Group. *New England Journal of Medicine*, **340**, 14–22.

Pantoni, L. and Garcia, J.H. (1997). Pathogenesis of leukoaraiosis: a review. *Stroke*, **28**, 652–9.

Peyser, P.A., Bielak, L.F., Chu, J.S., *et al.* (2002). Heritability of coronary artery calcium quantity measured by electron beam computed tomography in asymptomatic adults. *Circulation*, **106**, 304–8.

Pourcelot, L., Tranquart, F., De Bray, J.M., *et al.* (1999). Ultrasound characterization and quantification of carotid atherosclerosis lesions. *Minerva Cardioangiologica*, **47**, 15–24.

Rauramaa, R., Vaisanen, S.B., Luong, L.A., *et al.* (2000). Stromelysin-1 and interleukin-6 gene promoter polymorphisms are determinants of asymptomatic carotid artery atherosclerosis. *Arteriosclerosis, Thrombosis and Vascular Biology*, **20**, 2657–62.

Ridker, P.M., Hennekens, C.H., Buring, J.E., and Rifai, N. (2000*a*). C-reactive protein and other markers of inflammation in the prediction of cardiovascular disease in women. *New England Journal of Medicine*, **342**, 836–43.

Ridker, P.M., Rifai, N., Stampfer, M.J., and Hennekens, C.H. (2000*b*). Plasma concentration of interleukin-6 and the risk of future myocardial infarction among apparently healthy men. *Circulation*, **101**, 1767–72.

Risley, P., Jerrard-Dunne, P., Sitzer, M., Buehler, A., Von Kegler, S., and Markus, H.S. (2003) A promoter polymorphism in the endotoxin receptor (CD14) is associated with increased carotid atherosclerosis only in smokers: The Carotid Atherosclerosis Progression Study (CAPS). *Stroke*, **34**, online 10000055.

Roger, V.L., Weston, S.A., Killian, J.M., *et al.* (2001). Time trends in the prevalence of atherosclerosis: a population-based autopsy study. *American Journal of Medicine*, **110**, 267–73.

Ross, R. (1999). Atherosclerosis—an inflammatory disease. *New England Journal of Medicine*, **340**, 115–26.

Rundek, T., Elkind, M.S., Pittman, J., *et al.* (2002). Carotid intima-media thickness is associated with allelic variants of stromelysin-1, interleukin-6, and hepatic lipase genes: the Northern Manhattan Prospective Cohort Study. *Stroke*, **33**, 1420–3.

Sacco, R. (1994) Ischemic stroke. *Handbook of neuroepidemiology*, pp. 77–119. Marcel Decker Inc., New York.

Salonen, R. and Salonen, J.T. (1991*a*). Determinants of carotid intima-media thickness: a population-based ultrasonography study in eastern Finnish men. *Journal of Internal Medicine*, 229, 225–31.

Salonen, J.T. and Salonen, R. (1991*b*). Ultrasonographically assessed carotid morphology and the risk of coronary heart disease. *Arteriosclerosis and Thrombosis*, 11, 1245–9.

Schmidt, H., Fazekas, F., Kostner, G.M., van Duijn, C.M., and Schmidt, R. (2001*b*). Angiotensinogen gene promoter haplotype and microangiopathy-related cerebral damage: results of the Austrian Stroke Prevention Study. *Stroke*, 32, 405–12.

Schmidt, H., Schmidt, R., Niederkorn, K., *et al.* (1998). Paraoxonase PON1 polymorphism leu-Met54 is associated with carotid atherosclerosis: results of the Austrian Stroke Prevention Study. *Stroke*, 29, 2043–8.

Schmidt, R., Fazekas, F., Kapeller, P., Schmidt, H., and Hartung, H.P. (1999). MRI white matter hyperintensities: three-year follow-up of the Austrian Stroke Prevention Study. *Neurology*, 53, 132–9.

Schmidt, R., Schmidt, H., Fazekas, F., *et al.* (1997). Apolipoprotein E polymorphism and silent microangiopathy-related cerebral damage. Results of the Austrian Stroke Prevention Study. *Stroke*, 28, 951–6.

Schmidt, R., Schmidt, H., Fazekas, F., *et al.* (2000). MRI cerebral white matter lesions and paraoxonase PON1 polymorphisms: three-year follow-up of the Austrian stroke prevention study. *Arteriosclerosis, Thrombosis and Vascular Biology*, 20, 1811–16.

Schmidt, R., Schmidt, H., Fazekas, F., *et al.* (2001*a*). Angiotensinogen polymorphism M235T, carotid atherosclerosis, and small-vessel disease-related cerebral abnormalities. *Hypertension*, 38, 110–15.

Schminke, U., Hilker, L., Motsch, L., Griewing, B., and Kessler, C. (2002). Volumetric assessment of plaque progression with 3-dimensional ultrasonography under statin therapy. *Journal of Neuroimaging*, 12, 245–51.

Seino, Y., Ikeda, U., Ikeda, M., *et al.* (1994). Interleukin 6 gene transcripts are expressed in human atherosclerotic lesions. *Cytokine*, 6, 87–91.

Sitzer, M., Furst, G., Fischer, H., *et al.* (1993). Between-method correlation in quantifying internal carotid stenosis. *Stroke*, 24, 1513–18.

Sitzer, M., Puac, D., Buehler, A., Steckel, D.A., Von Kegler, S., Markus, H.S., and Steinmetz, S. (2003). Internal carotid artery angle of origin—a novel risk factor for early carotid atherosclerosis. *Stroke* (in press).

Spence, J.D. (2002). Ultrasound measurement of carotid plaque as a surrogate outcome for coronary artery disease. *American Journal of Cardiology*, 89, 10–15B.

Stensland-Bugge, E., Bonaa, K.H., and Joakimsen, O. (2001). Age and sex differences in the relationship between inherited and lifestyle risk factors and subclinical carotid atherosclerosis: the Tromso Study. *Atherosclerosis*, 154, 437–48.

Terborg, C., Gora, F., Weiller, C., and Rother, J. (2000). Reduced vasomotor reactivity in cerebral microangiopathy: a study with near-infrared spectroscopy and transcranial Doppler sonography. *Stroke*, 31, 924–9.

Terry, J.G., Howard, G., Mercuri, M., Bond, M.G., and Crouse, J.R., III (1996). Apolipoprotein E polymorphism is associated with segment-specific extracranial carotid artery intima-media thickening. *Stroke*, 27, 1755–9.

Touboul, P.J., Elbaz, A., Koller, C., *et al.* (2000). Common carotid artery intima-media thickness and brain infarction: the Etude du Profil Genetique de l'Infarctus Cerebral (GENIC) case-control study. The GENIC Investigators. *Circulation*, 102, 313–18.

Vickers, M.A., Green, F.R., Terry, C., *et al.* (2002). Genotype at a promoter polymorphism of the interleukin-6 gene is associated with baseline levels of plasma C-reactive protein. *Cardiovascular Research*, **53**, 1029–34.

Visvikis, S., Sass, C., Pallaud, C., *et al.* (2000). Familial studies on the genetics of cardiovascular diseases: the Stanislas cohort. *Clinical Chemistry and Laboratory Medicine*, **38**, 827–32.

Watanabe, Y., Ishigami, T., Kawano, Y., *et al.* (1997). Angiotensin-converting enzyme gene I/D polymorphism and carotid plaques in Japanese. *Hypertension*, **30**, 569–73.

Wiedermann, C.J., Kiechl, S., Dunzendorfer, S., *et al.* (1999). Association of endotoxemia with carotid atherosclerosis and cardiovascular disease: prospective results from the Bruneck Study. *Journal of the American College of Cardiology*, **34**, 1975–81.

Woessner, J.F., Jr. (1991). Matrix metalloproteinases and their inhibitors in connective tissue remodeling. *Federation of American Societies for Experimental Biology Journal*, **5**, 2145–54.

Xiang, A.H., Azen, S.P., Buchanan, T.A., *et al.* (2002). Heritability of subclinical atherosclerosis in Latino families ascertained through a hypertensive parent. *Arteriosclerosis, Thrombosis and Vascular Biology*, **22**, 843–8.

Ye, S., Eriksson, P., Hamsten, A., *et al.* (1996). Progression of coronary atherosclerosis is associated with a common genetic variant of the human stromelysin-1 promoter which results in reduced gene expression. *Journal of Biological Chemistry*, **271**, 13055–60.

Zannad, F., Visvikis, S., Gueguen, R., *et al.* (1998). Genetics strongly determines the wall thickness of the left and right carotid arteries. *Human Genetics*, **103**, 183–8.

Zhang, X., Zhao, S.P., Li, X.P., Gao, M., and Zhou, Q.C. (2000). Endothelium-dependent and -independent functions are impaired in patients with coronary heart disease. *Atherosclerosis*, **149**, 19–24.

Zhdanov, V.S., Sternby, N.H., Vikhert, A.M., and Galakhov, I.E. (1999). Development of atherosclerosis over a 25 year period: an epidemiological autopsy study in males of 11 towns. *International Journal of Cardiology*, **68**, 95–106.

Chapter 9

Genetics of intracerebral haemorrhage

Joost Haan

9.1 Cerebral haemorrhage: an overview and definitions

The worldwide incidence of haemorrhagic stroke (HS) ranges from 10 to 20 cases per 100,000 population, and increases with age (Qureshi *et al*. 2001). This figure is expected to double during the next 50 years as a result of the increasing age of the population and changes in racial demographics. HS accounts for 10–15 per cent of all cases of stroke.

In a patient with acute neurological signs and symptoms, the diagnosis of a HS is often straightforward, as cerebral CT- and MRI-scan are almost 100 per cent reliable in detecting or excluding the presence of intracranial haemorrhage. The cause of the HS is, however, very often not immediately clear. Sometimes there are clues that point to a certain cause, such as the previous medical history of the patient, use of medication, age of the patient, the localization size and form of the haemorrhage, and its association with other structural abnormalities seen on imaging. For example, a lobar haemorrhage (which is, by definition, located outside the basal ganglia), in combination with leukoencephalopathy, in an elderly patient, suggests the presence of cerebral amyloid angiopathy. A haemorrhage in the basal ganglia is often associated with hypertension.

When categorizing causes for HS, traditionally, a distinction between primary and secondary HS is made. A HS is called *primary* when it originates from the spontaneous rupture of a small vessel damaged by chronic hypertension or amyloid angiopathy, and *secondary* when the intracerebral haemorrhage occurs in association with vascular abnormalities, tumours, or coagulation disorders (Qureshi *et al*. 2001). This distinction, however, is rather artificial, as in the case of hypertension and amyloid angiopathy, the HS is also secondary to a known or presumed cause. Furthermore, in patients with HS, risk factors will usually be found, and therefore most cases of HS could be called secondary. An alternative approach is to classify HS based on risk factors, instead of using the designation primary or secondary. There are many possible risk factors associated with HS, sometimes acting alone, but most often in various combinations. Risk factors include blood vessel malformations, such as an arteriovenous malformation (AVM) or aneurysm, disorders of coagulation, or structural changes of the blood vessel wall due to hypertension or amyloid.

Many of the risk factors of HS have a genetic background. Family studies have shown an association between HS and a positive family history of HS, indicating an underlying genetic etiology (Alberts *et al.* 2002, Polychronopoulos *et al.* 2002). Data from twin studies, looking specifically at cerebral haemorrhage as opposed to stroke in general, is not available.

The genetic risk factors for HS are often divided into single-gene disorders (e.g. hereditary cerebral amyloid angiopathies), polygenic (where multiple genes act together to result in a certain phenotype), or multifactorial disorders in which genetic and environmental factors may interact such as in the case of hypertension. This distinction, however, is oversimplistic, in the case of single-gene disorders, as additional risk factors, genetic or environmental, often play a modifying role in the final phenotypic expression of the disease. For example, cerebral amyloid angiopathy is clearly a risk factor for HS, but there are many patients with amyloid angiopathy, who do not suffer from a HS at all. Furthermore, HS occurs in patients with cerebral amyloid angiopathy, with an enormous variety of clinical presentations (e.g. age at onset, age at death, occurrence of dementia). In amyloid angiopathy the co-occurrence with other risk factors such as an APOE genotype, the presence of hypertension, or head trauma, determines the presence or absence of a HS. Therefore, in this chapter, the genetics of risk factors for HS, such as hypertension, coagulation disorders, and amyloid angiopathy, will be summarized, without classifying them into primary or secondary, or single-gene or polygenic. The genetics of other risk factors for HS, such as AVMs, cavernous haemangiomas, aneurysms, and hereditary haemorrhagic telangiectasias will be discussed in the next chapters.

9.2 Epidemiological studies of risk factors in cerebral haemorrhage

The incidence of HS increases with age, although not as steeply as cerebral infarction. HS also varies by race and ethnicity, being more prevalent in Japanese, blacks and Hispanic individuals. A positive family history of HS is a risk factor for HS (Alberts *et al.* 2002, Polychronopoulos *et al.* 2002, Woo *et al.* 2002).

From large epidemiological studies, several aditional risk factors for HS have become evident (Juvela *et al.* 1995, Rastenyte *et al.* 1998, Gebel and Broderick 2000, Zodpey *et al.* 2000, Labovitz and Sacco 2001, Woo *et al.* 2002). In virtually all studies hypertension, heavy alcohol intake and anticoagulant treatment were shown to be independent risk factors. Other, but less frequent and convincingly proven, risk factors are: amphetamine or cocaine use, and a low serum cholesterol. Cerebral amyloid angiopathy is also a risk factor, but was not identified in epidemiological studies, as it is a histological diagnosis, that needs post-mortem or biopsy evidence. The genetic aspects of the various risk factors will be described separately.

9.3 Genetic risk factors for cerebral haemorrhage

9.3.1 Hypertension: genetic aspects

Hypertension is the single most significant risk factor for non-lobar HS (Gebel and Broderick 2000, Qureshi *et al.* 2001, Woo *et al.* 2002). It has been estimated that hypertension is present in 75 per cent of patients with HS (Gebel and Broderick 2000), and it appears that a dose-reponse curve exists; the higher the blood pressure, the higher the incidence of HS. Nevertheless, although hypertension clearly is a risk factor for HS, not every hypertensive individual develops a HS, nor can every case of non-lobar HS be ascribed to hypertension. The absence or presence of additional risk factors probably determines whether the patient will suffer from an ischaemic stroke, HS, or stroke at all (Bogousslavsky *et al.* 1996). Increasing age, cigarette smoking, hypercholesterolaemia, cardiac ischaemia, and diabetes mellitus are, in association with hypertension, associated with a increased risk of developing an ischaemic stroke. Dietary risk factors, amyloid angiopathy, and coagulopathy (see below) are probably additional risk factors for HS in hypertensive subjects, but this has not yet been proven epidemiologically.

Hypertensive HS mostly occurs in the putamen, external capsule, subcortical white matter, thalamus, internal capsule, cerebellum or brain-stem. The classic pathology underlying hypertensive HS is a small vessel vasculopathy, with complex pathological changes in arteries and arterioles, such as degeneration of the media and hyaline deposition in the intima, microaneurysms and microatheroma.

Hypertension is, at least partially, genetically determined (Svetkey *et al.* 1999, Doris 2002). It is estimated that about 30 per cent of blood pressure variance can be attributed to genetic factors. Hypertension represents the common endpoint of several pathophysiological pathways, and therefore may be due to an interacting family of genetic abnormalities (Svetkey *et al.* 1999). Some rare mendelian forms of hypertension in humans are known: Apparent mineralocorticoid excess, glucocorticoid-remediable aldosteronism, 17-alpha hydroxylase deficiency, pseudohypoaldosteronism type-I and type-II, early onset autosomal dominant hypertension with severe exacerbation in pregnancy, and Bardet–Biedl syndrome types 2 and 4 (Doris 2002). Studying these rare subtypes might elucidate some of the genetic factors responsible for HS. However, most hypertension is believed to be multifactorial. Many candidate genes for hypertension have been suggested including genes for renin, angiotensin converting enzyme, aldosterone, calmodulin, ion ATPases, phospholipase, kallikrein, endothelin, and adrenergic receptors. Genome-wide linkage surveys have found linkage for blood-pressure loci on almost all chromosomes (1, 2, 3, 5, 6, 7, 8, 11, 15, 16, 17, 18, 19, 22, and X) (Doris 2002). These associations and other aspects of the genetics of hypertension are reviewed in detail in Section 4.2.

9.3.2 Dietary risk factors: genetic aspects

In epidemiological studies, abuse of alcohol (Gill *et al.* 1991, Woo *et al.* 2002), cocaine and amphetamine were also associated with a higher incidence of HS. Genetic factors clearly play a role in these types of addiction, albeit a very complex one (Crabbe *et al.* 1999, Nestler 2001). A detailed summary of studies investigating these factors is outside the scope of this chapter.

9.3.3 Cerebral amyloid angiopathy

Pathogenesis

Cerebral amyloid angiopathy is an important risk factor for lobar HS. Amyloid is a term used to describe protein deposits with circumscript physical characteristics: beta-pleated sheet configuration, apple green birefringence under polarized light after Congo red staining, fibrillary structure and high insolubility (Castano and Frangione 1988). There are many different proteins that can accumulate as amyloid, and there are many different disease processes that can lead to amyloid formation (WHO-IUIS Nomenclature Subcommittee 1993). In hereditary amyloid diseases, a mutated variant protein or precursor protein is abnormally metabolized by proteolytic pathways and accumulates as amyloid (Castano and Frangione 1988). Very often amyloid deposition has a certain tissue affinity, leading to deposition in certain organs or at certain sites. In cerebral amyloid angiopathy, amyloid deposition occurs solely or predominantly in the cerebral blood vessels, with a preference for small cerebral arteries and arterioles (Fig. 9.1). Cerebral amyloid angiopathy can consist of amyloid-beta-protein, cystatin C, prion protein, ABri protein, transthyretin, or gelsolin (Yamada 2000) (Table 9.1). Amyloid deposition in cerebral blood vessels can have several clinical consequences (Vinters 1987, Haan *et al.* 1994, Yamada 2000). It can remain asymptomatic. For example during 'normal' ageing approximately 50 per cent of individuals over 80 years of age have cerebral amyloid angiopathy. Cerebral amyloid angiopathy can also weaken the vessel wall, causing rupture and lobar HS (Fig. 9.3). Finally, cerebral amyloid angiopathy can obliterate the vessel lumen, leading to ischaemia (cerebral infarction, 'incomplete' infarction, and leukoencephalopathy) (Fig. 9.4(a) and (b)). Through these vascular mechanisms,

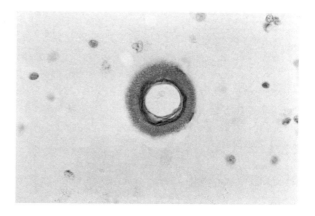

Fig. 9.1 Light microscopic specimen of patient with HCHWA-D, showing amyloid angiopathy.

Table 9.1 Hereditary cerebral amyloid angiopathy

Hereditary cerebral haemorrhage with amyloidosis—Dutch (HCHWA-D) (Bornebroek *et al.* 1999)
    Lobar haemorrhages, focal neurological deficits, dementia, and leukoencephalopathy
    Mean age at onset is 50 years
    Described in four families from the Netherlands
    Amyloid consists of beta A4
    APP gene mutation at codon 693 (chromosome 21) (Fig. 9.2)

Hereditary cerebral haemorrhage with amyloidosis—Italian (Bugiani *et al.* 1998)
    Lobar haemorrhages and dementia.
    Described in two Italian families
    Amyloid consists of beta A4
    APP-gene codon 693 mutation (chromosome 21), different from HCHWA-D (Fig. 9.2)

Hereditary cerebral haemorrhage with amyloidosis—Flemish (Hendriks *et al.* 1992, Roks *et al.* 2000)
    Progressive Alzheimer-like dementia, in some patients associated with a lobar haemorrhage
    Described in one single Dutch family (discovered in Belgium, therefore called 'Flemish')
    Amyloid consists of beta A4
    A codon 692 mutation in the APP-gene on chromosome 21 (Fig. 9.2)

Hereditary cerebral haemorrhage with amyloidosis—Icelandic type (Abrahamson *et al.* 1987)
    Lobar haemorrhages, focal neurological deficits, and dementia in a minority of cases
    Mean age at onset is 20 years
    Described in several families from two geographical areas in Iceland
    Amyloid consists of variant cystatin C
    Caused by a mutation at codon 68 in the cystatin gene at chromosome 20

Cerebral amyloid angiopathy in transthyretin amyloidosis (Vidal *et al.* 1996)
    Polyneuropathy is the main clinical symptom
    In a small number of patients ataxia, spasticity and dementia
    In some families, cerebral amyloid angiopathy, leading to HS (Sakashita *et al.* 2001)
    Various mutations in the chromosome 14 transthyretin gene

Cerebral amyloid angiopathy in prion disease (Ghetti *et al.* 1996)
    Creutzfeldt–Jakob disease, Gerstmann–Straussler–Scheinker disease and familial fatal insomnia
    Mutations in the chromosome 20 PRNP gene
    Cerebral amyloid angiopathy was found in one family with a PRNP gene codon 145 mutation
    In this family associated with AD-like dementia, not with HS

Cerebral amyloid angiopathy in gelsolin amyloidosis (Kiuri *et al.* 1999)
    Progressive corneal lattice dystrophy, cranial and peripheral neuropathy, and cutaneous amyloidosis
    Mutations in the gelsolin gene on chromosome 9
    Cerebral amyloid angiopathy described in several patients with dementia, ataxia and depression
    In these patients no HS

Cerebral amyloid angiopathy in Presenilin 1 (PS-1) and Presenilin 2 (PS-2) mutations
(Tandon *et al.* 2000)
    Progressive autosomal dominant Alzheimer dementia
    Mutations in the PS-1 gene on chromosome 14, or (less frequent) a chromosome 1 PS-2 mutation
    Associated with parenchymal beta-A4 amyloid deposits
    In some PS-1 and PS-2 kindreds abundant CAA
    Clinical features in these kindreds dominated by dementia, no HS

(continued)

Table 9.1 (continued)

Familial British dementia (Mead *et al.* 2000)

    Dementia, progressive spastic tetraparesis and cerebellar ataxia. HS occurs rarely

    Onset in the sixth decade

    One large family originating in the UK

    A stop codon mutation in the BRI gene on chromosome 13

Familial Danish dementia (Vidal et al. 2000)

    Also known as heredopathia ophthalmo-oto-encephalica

    Cataracts, deafness, progressive ataxia and dementia. No HS

    Decamer duplication in the BRI gene on chromosome 13

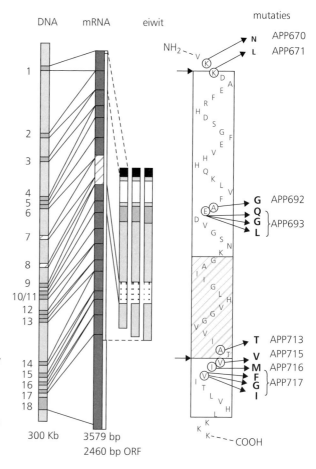

Fig. 9.2 The APP gene on chromosome 21 (left) and the gene product betaA4 (right) with various mutations. Only the APP 692 and 693 mutations frequently lead to HS, caused by cerebral amyloid angiopathy (see Table 9.1). The other mutations are associated with autosomal dominant Alzheimer's disease.

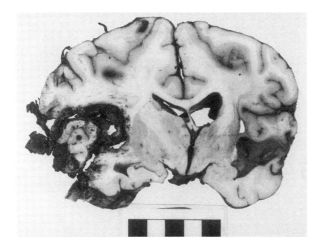

Fig. 9.3 Whole brain slice of the brain of a patient with HCHWA-D, showing bilateral lobar HSs, sparing the basal ganglia.

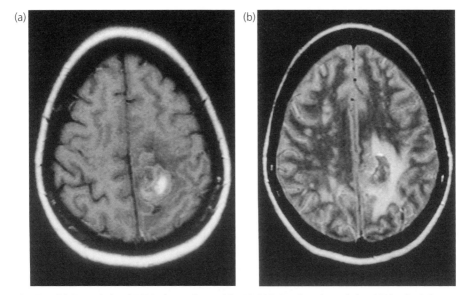

(a)   (b)

Fig. 9.4 (a) T1-weighted MRI of a patient with HCHWA-D, showing a lobar HS in the left hemisphere. (b) T2-weighted MRI of the same patient, showing (in addition to the HS) white matter lesions in both hemispheres.

focal neurological deficits, disturbances of consciousness, step wise dementia (mostly of the vascular type), and death can occur.

Genetic forms of amyloid angiopathy

All hereditary forms of cerebral amyloid angiopathy so far known have an autosomal dominant mode of inheritance (Haan 2002). Virtually all are very rare diseases

Table 9.2 Possible clinical presentations of (hereditary) cerebral amyloid angiopathy

Multiple lobar cerebral haemorrhages
Recurrent lobar cerebral haemorrhages
Lobar cerebral haemorrhage(-s) with leukoencephalopathy
Otherwise unexplained white matter lesions
Dementia and cerebral haemorrhages, with or without leukoencephalopathy
Lobar cerebral haemorrhages after coagulation-therapy or thrombolysis
All cerebral symptoms in a member of a family with known hereditary CAA
In some families, ataxia, spasticity, progressive dementia

described in a single family or a small number of families. The practical importance, therefore, is limited. Not all hereditary cerebral amyloid angiopathies are associated with HS. The different types of hereditary amyloid angiopathy are shown in Table 9.1, with the underlying genetic basis. HS is found as part of the phenotype for the Dutch, Italian, and Flemish types involving mutations in the amyloid precursor gene, and the Icelandic type which occurs secondary to a mutation in the cystatin gene. In hereditary cerebral amyloid angiopathy, there is a considerable phenotypic heterogeneity, with a large variation in presenting symptoms, age at onset, and course of the disease, which sometimes makes the diagnosis difficult. This phenotypic heterogeneity is probably partly caused by additional vascular risk factors, many of which are also genetically determined (Bornebroek *et al.* 1999). The spectrum of clinical features which can be found in hereditary amyloid angiopathy are shown in Table 9.2. The two main types associated with HS are HCHWA-D and HCHWA-I.

(i) Hereditary cerebral haemorrhage with amyloidosis Dutch type (HCHWA-D)
Hereditary cerebral haemorrhage with amyloidosis Dutch type is a rare disorder which originated from the Netherlands. Some HCHWA-D patients have been described in the United States but these are believed to originate from the Netherlands. In this disease, cerebral amyloid angiopathy is the predominant histopathological hallmark, although in addition parenchymal deposits that resemble diffuse and neuritic plaques are also present. (Maat-Schieman *et al.* 1996) The amyloid deposits are composed of the amyloid β protein which is also the major constituent of parenchymal and vascular deposits in both Alzheimer's disease and in sporadic cerebral amyloid angiopathy. However, in Alzheimer's disease neurofibrillary tangles and plaques are also important pathological hallmarks.

The clinical phenotype is of recurrent HSs and dementia. The first stroke usually occurs between the ages of 40 and 65 years and two-thirds of patients die as a direct consequence of it (Wattendorf *et al.* 1995). One-third of patients die within a year of the first stroke and half of them within 2 weeks. Those who survive suffer recurrent strokes which lead to severe disability. Dementia can develop after the first stroke, but sometimes it is the first or only symptom of HCHWA-D. Prominent neuropsychological features include constructional apraxia, agnosia and agraphia, and difficulties with calculation and language (Haan *et al.* 1990). The progression of dementia can be in a stepwise fashion related to the strokes, and the presence of dementia was found to correlate with the number of focal lesions on CT scan (Haan *et al.* 1990). In occasional patients a progressive cognitive decline has been documented in the absence of strokes, suggesting that dementia cannot be entirely ascribed to the effects of strokes (Haan *et al.* 1990). Some cases of HCHWA-D can be associated with multiple cerebral infarctions, which typically involve the deep cortical white matter although occasionally cortical infarctions can occur. One study found that 87 per cent of patients with the disease had intracerebral haemorrhage while 13 per cent had ischaemic stroke (Haan *et al.* 1990).

HCHWA-D is caused by a single base mutation at codon 693 of the amyloid β precursor protein located on chromosome 21 (Levy *et al.* 1990, van Broeckhoven *et al.* 1990). This is close to the middle of the β amyloid moiety, as compared to mutations causing Alzheimer's disease which are outside the β amyloid domain. The disease appears to have complete penetrance but the phenotypic expression is variable. The reasons for this are unclear, although one report has found the mortality rate in affected individuals was significantly higher in females than males, while it was lower when the disease was maternally transmitted (Bornebroek *et al.* 1997). The Italian and Flemish variants of HCHWA are caused by different mutations in the APP gene at codon 693, and 692 respectively. The Arctic variant is caused by a E693G mutation, and leads to Alzheimer's disease, and not to HS (Nilsberth *et al.* 2001). The Iowa variant (D694N) also does not lead to HS, but to dementia, cortical calcifications and leuko-encephalopathy (Grabowski *et al.* 2001, Van Nostrand *et al.* 2001).

(ii) Hereditary cerebral amyloid with amyloidosis—Icelandic type (HCHWA-I)
This is an autosomal dominant disorder causing intracerebral haemorrhage, usually with an onset of between 20 and 30 years (Gudmundsson *et al.* 1972). Although some patients may die from the disease as young as 15 years, one family has been reported with late onset dementia with some family members having intracerebral haemorrhage and others not (Greenberg *et al.* 1993) The amyloid angiopathy is more widely distributed in this type of amyloid angiopathy than in other types and involves arteries in the cerebrum, cerebellum and brainstem. The amyloid protein deposited is a mutant of cysteine protease inhibitor cystatin C, the gene for which is located on chromosome 20p. The underlying abnormality is point mutation is exon 2 of the gene with an A–T substitution resulting in amino acid change from leucine to glutamine (Levy *et al.* 1989). This abolishes an *Alu* I restriction site which allows mutation testing.

Diagnosis
The diagnosis of cerebral amyloid angiopathy can only be made with certainty after histologic investigation of affected brain tissue, obtained at autopsy or brain-biopsy.

In practice amyloid angiopathy is very often found unexpectedly at post-mortem investigation. Hereditary cerebral amyloid angiopathy can be suspected when there are several family members with signs and symptoms from Table 9.2. Diagnostic criteria (the Boston criteria) for amyloid angiopathy have been developed and are shown in Table 9.3. These categorize the diagnosis as definite, probable (with and without supporting pathological data), and possible. This classification has been validated against pathological data (Knudsen *et al.* 2001). Neuropathological confirmation from a full post-mortem is required for a definite diagnosis. The distribution and pattern of haemorrhage is a very useful pointer to the disease. Haemorrhages are lobar, cortical or cortico-subcortical. The presence of multiple haemorrhages is an important clue to diagnosis. In this respect gradient echo MRI is very useful. On CT imaging high signal due to acute blood disappears in the weeks following the bleed, leaving an area of low signal which may be indistinguishable from primary infarction. On conventional MRI it may also be difficult to differentiate old haemorrhage from infarction. Gradient echo MRI is sensitive to haemosiderin, a breakdown product from blood, which appears as low signal. Therefore, in an elderly patient with a first symptomatic cerebral haemorrhage, the presence of multiple areas of old haemorrhage is highly suspicious of amyloid angiopathy.

Table 9.3 Criteria for CAA (Case records of the Massachusetts general hospital, 1996)

Definite cerebral amyloid angiopathy

Full post-mortem examination demonstrating all three of the following:
    Lobar, cortical, or corticosubcortical haemorrhage
    Severe cerebral amyloid angiopathy*
    Absence of another diagnostic lesion

Probable cerebral amyloid angiopathy with supporting pathological evidence

Clinical data and pathological tissue (evacuated hematoma or cortical biopsy specimen)
  demonstrating all three of the following:
    Lobar, cortical, or corticosubcortical haemorrhage
    Some degree of vascular amyloid in tissue specimen
    Absence of another diagnostic lesion

Probable cerebral amyloid angiopathy

Clinical data and MRI findings demonstrating all three of the following:
    Age >60 years
    Multiple haemorrhages restricted to the lobar, cortical, or cortico-subcortical region
    Absence of another cause of haemorrhage

Possible cerebral amyloid angiopathy

Clinical data and MRI findings:
    Age >60 years
    Single lobar, cortical, or corticosubcortical haemorrhage without another cause, or multiple
    haemorrhages with a possible but not a definite cause or with some haemorrhages in an atypical
    location (e.g. brain stem)

Severity of CAA can be expressed as mild, moderate, or severe, based on (non-quantitative)
  pathological data (Vonsattel *et al.* 1991)

When one suspects a hereditary form of cerebral amyloid angiopathy, only a brain or leptomeningeal biopsy can prove this *in vivo*. Biopsies of other tissue (e.g. skin, peripheral nerve, liver) are only useful in amyloid diseases where systemic amyloid depositions can occur, in addition to the cerebral localization: hereditary cerebral haemorrhage with amyloidosis—Icelandic type, transthyretin amyloidosis, or gelsolin amyloidosis. When sporadic cerebral amyloid angiopathy is suspected as the cause of HS, DNA diagnosis is not routinely performed, but when one considers one of the hereditary forms of cerebral amyloid angiopathy (Tables 9.1–9.3), there are dedicated laboratories that are able to screen for a certain mutation. In such a case it is advised to contact one of the authors of publications describing a mutation associated with hereditary cerebral amyloid angiopathy (Table 9.1 and list of references).

Differential diagnosis

The differential diagnosis of hereditary cerebral amyloid angiopathy consists of all other hereditary diseases that can cause HS, such as familial AVMs, familial cerebral aneurysms, MELAS, familial cavernous hemangiomas, hereditary haemorrhagic telangiectasia, Von Hippel–Lindau disease, Moya–Moya disease, hypertension, and coagulation abnormalities. Cerebral amyloid angiopathy is, however, the most probable diagnosis when there are recurrent lobar haemorrhages (Fig. 9.5(a) and (b)), or

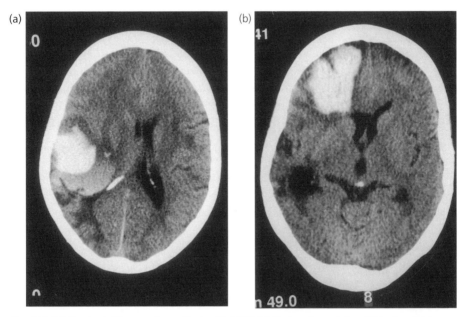

Fig. 9.5 (a) Cerebral CT-scan of a patient with HCHWA-D showing a lobar HS in the right hemisphere. (b) Cerebral CT-scan of the same patient showing a right parietal hypodense lesion due to the previous HS, and a recent right frontal HS.

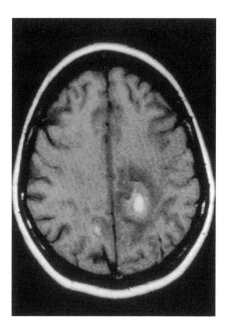

Fig. 9.6 T1-weighted MRI of a patient with HCHWA-D, showing 2 simultaneous lobar HSs, in both hemispheres.

multiple lobar haemorrhages (Fig. 9.6), or when lobar cerebral haemorrhages and leukoencephalopathy co-occur (Fig. 9.4(a) and (b)).

9.3.4 Coagulopathy: genetic aspects

Disturbances of coagulation—either as a result of medication, or due to hereditary disorders of haemostasis—are an important reason for HS, representing up to 8 per cent of all HS (del Zoppo and Mori 1992, Gebel and Broderick 2000). Of these, iatrogenic anticoagulation is the most frequent cause (Wintzen *et al.* 1984, Zodpey *et al.* 2000). It is not known whether a genetic susceptibility for anticoagulation-associated HS exists, but this is likely given the importance of genetic factors in anticoagulation in general (Highashi *et al.* 2002). Patients with cerebral amyloid angiopathy are at a higher risk for HS after anticoagulation or thrombolysis, especially when they are APOE epsilon 2 carriers (Nicoll and McCarron 2001).

Hereditary disorders of haemostasis are less common causes for HS (del Zoppo and Mori 1992, Ortel 1999). Among these are hereditary coagulopathies, such as various genetic clotting factor-deficiencies (Natowicz and Kelley 1987, Olson 1993). HS is the leading cause of death in patients with fibrinogen deficiencies, and the cause of death in many patients with haemophilia A (factor VIII deficiency), and haemophilia B (factor IX deficiency). Patients with factor VII, X, V, XI and XIII deficiencies can also suffer from HS, and HS has been described in patients with platelet disorders such as congenital megakaryocyte hypoplasia and the Wiskott-Aldrich syndrome (Ortel 1999). In sickle cell disease HS can occur in patients with prior infarction, due to

Moya–Moya disease or aneurysmal dilatation in the region of intimal hyperplasia (Prengler *et al.* 2002).

When a haematological cause for HS is suspected, it is important to take a history of previous haemorrhagic episodes, either spontaneous or associated with dental procedures. A detailed family history is also important, as is examination for the presence of petechiae, ecchymoses, and hepatosplenomegaly.

9.3.5 Polymorphisms and mutations associated with sporadic cerebral haemorrhage

Several genetic polymorphisms have been associated with an increased risk for apparently sporadic HS. Mutations in the endoglin gene are associated with hereditary haemorrhagic telangiectasia (see Chapter 11). In a recent study, it was shown that an endoglin gene polymorphism (a 6-base insertion in the intron between exons 7 and 8) in the homozygous state is a genetic risk factor for sporadic HS, independent from hypertension (Alberts *et al.* 1997). Other genetic risk factors for sporadic HS are polymorphisms in the genes for plasma platelet-activating factor acetylhydrolase (Yoshida *et al.* 1998), alpha1-antichymotrypsin (Obach *et al.* 2001), and factor XIII (Catto *et al.* 1998, Gemmati *et al.* 2001). In an unselected group of patients with sporadic HS, no APP or cystatin C gene mutations were found (Graffagnino *et al.* 1994, McCarron *et al.* 2000), but one patient with sporadic HS, in whom amyloid angiopathy was proven, had a cystatin C gene mutation (Graffagnino *et al.* 1995).

The influence of APOE genotype on sporadic cerebral amyloid angiopathy-related-HS has been studied intensively, with contradicting results. It is now accepted that the APOE epsilon 2 allele predisposes to rupture of beta A4 laden blood vessels, thus increasing the chance of HS of sporadic beta A4 cerebral amyloid angiopathy (McCarron and Nicoll 2000, Nicoll and McCarron 2001). A recent study found an overrepresentation of the APOE epsilon 2 and 4 alleles in patients with lobar HS (Woo *et al.* 2002), but as it was an epidemiological study, without histological investigation, the presence of cerebral amyloid angiopathy could be suspected, but was not proven.

9.3.6 Genetics of recurrent or multiple simultaneous cerebral haemorrhage

HS is generally a one-time event, but recurrences may occur (Neau *et al.* 1997, Gonzalez-Duarte *et al.* 1998, Hill *et al.* 2000). The frequency of recurrent HS in different studies varies between 2 an 24 per cent. A clearly established risk factor for recurrences is hypertension, with a recurrence-rate of up to 11 per cent, depending on blood pressure control (Arawaka *et al.* 1998). As expected, in hypertension the first as well as the second HS is likely to occur in the basal ganglia. Cerebral amyloid angiopathy causes a lobar–lobar pattern of recurrences, in up to 24 per cent of cases (Neau *et al.* 1997). In hereditary cerebral amyloid angiopathy, the recurrence-rate is almost 100 per cent, in patients who survive the first HS (Bornebroek *et al.* 1999) (Fig. 9.5(a) and (b)).

There are no studies of genetic factors on the recurrence of sporadic HS, except for the influence of APOE genotype on (presumed) cerebral amyloid angiopathy (O'Donnell *et al.* 2000). In a prospective, longitudinal cohort study of 71 patients with a lobar HS an overall 2-year cumulative incidence rate of 21 per cent was found, associated with APOE epsilon 2 and 4 alleles (O'Donnell *et al.* 2000).

Multiple simultaneous HS is rare, being reported in 1.7 and 2.8 per cent of cases, respectively in two separate series (Hill *et al.* 2000, Maurino *et al.* 2001). In one of the series hypertension seemed to be the major cause (Maurino *et al.* 2001), while in the other histologically proven cerebral amyloid angiopathy was (Hill *et al.* 2000). No specific genetic investigation was performed in these series. In HCHWA-D and HCHWA-I the multiple simultaneous occurrence of HS is common (Fig. 9.5).

9.4 **Microbleeds**

Microbleeds desribes small areas of haemosiderin deposition detected on MRI imaging which reflect old haemorrhage. Gradient-echo MRI is the most sensitive method to detect cerebral microbleeds (Greenberg *et al.* 1996, Fazekas *et al.* 1999). In patients with a HS, clinically silent ischaemic lesions and previous microbleeds are a common finding on MR imaging (Offenbacher *et al.* 1996). Microbleeds are also found in patients with ischaemic stroke, particularly due to small vessel disease (Nighoghossian *et al.* 2002, Senior 2002). As a consequence, all genetic risk factors for small vessel cerebral ischaemia may, indirectly, also be a genetic risk factors for HS. It has been

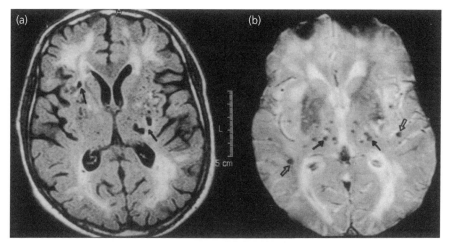

Fig. 9.7 (a) Fluid-attenuated inversion recovery image of a patient with CADASIL showing multiple lacunae and white matter lesions. (b) T2*-weighted gradient echo planar image (susceptibility) of the same CADASIL patient showing multiple microbleeds.

suggested that microbleeds occur secondary to a diffuse microangiopathy, and may reflect an increased risk for HS (Fazekas *et al.* 1999, Senior 2002). Microbleeds have also been found in sporadic patients with lobar HS, and attributed to probable cerebral amyloid angiopathy (Greenberg *et al.* 1999). So far, no investigation of microbleeds has been performed in patients with genetically determined HS, such as hereditary cerebral amyloid angiopathy. The only hereditary disease in which microbleeds were detected is CADASIL, a disease normally characterized by small vessel ischaemic stroke (see Section 6.2.1) (Lesnik Oberstein *et al.* 2001, Dichgans *et al.* 2002) (Fig. 9.7(a) and (b)). Here, microbleeds are also thought to be due to the microangiopathy, but it is not yet sure whether this finding has any clinical relevance, as HS only occurs rarely in CADASIL.

9.5 Practical consequences and treatment of genetic risk factors associated with cerebral haemorrhage

Genetic factors cannot be changed, but sometimes they can be modified. For this reason, there are some situations where it is important to consider the presence of genetic risk factors in a given patient with HS, and these may have implications for treatment. Establishing a diagnosis may also be important in order to offer genetic counselling to the patient, and inform his or her family-members about the risk they have to suffer from the same disease.

Of course, primary prevention to avoid the occurrence of first HS is the most desirable. In a patient who comes from a family in which members suffer from hypertension, rigorous control, and early treatment of the hypertension is likely to prevent complications such as HS. In families with bleeding disorders, treatment may also prevent haemorrhagic complications. When a patient is from a family known to have hereditary cerebral amyloid angiopathy, mutation analysis can be performed, to investigate whether the patient is carrier or not. If a mutation is discovered, no causal treatment is possible, but the elimination of additional risk factors for stroke (hypertension, hypercholesterolaemia, smoking, etc.) will probably have a beneficial effect on the course of the disease.

When a patient presents with HS, secondary prevention is needed similar to the primary prevention described above. It is not clinically indicated to routinely search for genetic factors associated with cerebral amyloid angiopathy, hypertension or bleeding disorders, unless one of the rare familial syndromes is suspected. Patients in whom genetic investigation should be considered are those with multiple or recurrent lobar cerebral haemorrhages, lobar cerebral haemorrhage with leukoencephalopathy, or dementia with cerebral haemorrhages. In these patients a search for mutations associated with hereditary cerebral amyloid angiopathy may be useful, especially when the symptoms occur at a relatively young age, and there is a positive family history of similar symptoms.

References

Abrahamson, M., Grubb, A., Olafsson, I., and Lundwall, A. (1987). Molecular cloning sequence analysis of cDNA coding for the precursor of the human cystatin protease inhibitor cystatin C. *FEBS Letters*, **216**, 228–33.

Alberts, M.J. (1999). Intracerebral hemorrhage and vascular malformations. In *Genetics of cerebrovascular disease* (ed. M.J. Alberts), pp. 209–36. Futura publishing, Armonk NY.

Alberts, M.J., Davis, J.P., Graffagnino, C., *et al.* (1997). Endoglin gene polymorphism as a risk factor for sporadic intracerebral hemorrhage. *Annals of Neurology*, **41**, 683–6.

Alberts, M.J., McCarron, M.O., Hoffmann, K.L., and Graffagnino, C. (2002). Familial clustering of intracerebral hemorrhage: A prospective study in North Carolina. *Neuroepidemiology*, **21**, 18–21.

Arawaka, S., Saku, Y., Inayashi, S., Nagao, T., and Fujishima, M. (1988). Blood pressure control and recurrence of hypertensive brain hemorrhage. *Stroke*, **29**, 1806–9.

Bornebroek, M., Westendorp, R.G.J., Haan, J., Bakker, E., Timmers, W.F., Van Broeckhoven, C., and Roos, R.A.C. (1997). Mortality from hereditary cerebral haemorrhage with amyloidosis—Dutch type. The impact of sex, parental transmission and year of birth. *Brain*, **120**, 2243–9.

Bogousslavsky, J., Castillo, V., Kumral, E., Henriques, I., and Van Melle, G. (1996). Stroke subtypes and hypertension. Primary hemorrhage vs infarction, large- vs small-artery disease. *Stroke*, **53**, 265–9.

Bornebroek, M., Haan, J., and Roos, R.A.C. (1999). HCHWA-D: a review of the variety in phenotypic expression. *Amyloid*, **6**, 215–24.

Bugiani, O., Padovani, A., Magoni, M., *et al.* (1998). An Italian type of HCHWA. *Neurobiology and Aging*, S238.

Case records of the Massachusetts General Hospital. (1996). *New England Journal of Medicine*, **335**, 189–96.

Castano, E.M. and Frangione, B. (1988). Human amyloidosis, Alzheimer disease and related disorders. *Laboratory Investigation*, **58**, 122–32.

Catto, A.J., Kohler, H.P., Bannan, S., Stickland, M., Carter, A., and Grant, P.J. (1998). Factor XIII Val 34 Leu. A novel association with primary intracerebral hemorrhage. *Stroke*, **29**, 813–6.

Crabbe, J.C., Philips, T.J., Buck, K.J., Cunningham, C.L., and Belknap, J.K. (1999). Identifying genes for alcohol and drug sensitivity: recent progress and future directions. *Trends in Neuroscience*, **22**, 173–9.

Del Zoppo, G.J. and Mori, E. (1992). Hematological causes of intracerebral hemorrhage and their treatment. *Neurosurgical Clinics of North America*, **3**, 637–58.

Dichgans, M., Holtmannspotter, M., Herzog, J., Peters, N., Bergmann, M., and Yousry, T.A. (2002). Cerebral microbleeds in CADASIL: a gradient-echo magnetic resonance imaging and autopsy study. *Stroke*, **33**, 67–71.

Doris, P.A. (2002). Hypertension genetics, single nucleotide polymorphisms, and the common disease: common variant hypothesis. *Hypertension*, **39**, 323–31.

Fazekas, F., Kleinert, R., Roob, G., *et al.* (1999). Histopathological analysis of foci of signal loss on gradient-echo T2*-weighted MR images in patients with spontaneous intracerebral hemorrhage: evidence of microangiopathy-related microbleeds. *American Journal of Neuroradiology*, **20**, 637–42.

Gebel, J.M. and Broderick, J.P. (2000). Intracerebral hemorrhage. *Neurologic Clinics*, **19**, 419–38.

Gemmati, D., Serino, M.L., Ongaro, A., *et al.* (2001). A common mutation in the gene for coagulation factor XIII-A (val34Leu): a risk factor for primary intracerebral hemorrhage is protective against atherothrombotic disease. *American Journal of Hematology*, **67**, 183–8.

Ghetti, B., Piccardo, P., Spillanti, M.G., *et al.* (1996). Vascular variant of prion protein cerebral amyloidosis with tau-positive neurofibrillary tangles: the phenotype of the stop codon 145 mutation in PRNP. *Proceedings of the National Academy of Sciences USA*, **93**, 744–8.

Gill, J.S., Shipley, M.J., Tsementizis, S.A., *et al.* (1991). Alcohol consumption—A risk factor for haemorrhagic and non-haemorrhagic stroke. *American Journal of Medicine*, **90**, 489–97.

Gonzalez-Duarte, A., Cantu, C., Ruiz-Sandoval, J.L., and Barinagarrementeria, F. (1998). Recurrent primary cerebral hemorrhage. Frequency, mechanisms, and prognosis. *Stroke*, **29**, 1802–5.

Grabowski, T.J., Cho, H.S., Vonsattel, J.P.G., Rebeck, G.W., and Greenberg, S.M. (2001). Novel amyloid precursor protein mutation in an Iowa family with dementia and severe amyloid angiopathy. *Annals of Neurology*, **49**, 697–705.

Graffagnino, C., Herbstreith, M.H., Roses, A.D., and Alberts, M.J. (1994). A molecular genetic study of intracerebral hemorrhage. *The Archives of Neurology*, **51**, 981–4.

Graffagnino, C., Herbstreith, M.H., Schmechel, D.E., Levy, E., Roses, A.D., and Alberts, M.J. (1995). Cystatin C mutation in an elderly man with sporadic amyloid angiopathy and intracerebral hemorrhage. *Stroke*, **26**, 2190–3.

Greenberg, S.M., Finklestein, S.P., and Schaefer, P.W. (1996). Petechial hemorrhages accompanying lobar hemorrhage: detection by gradient-echo MRI. *Neurology*, **46**, 1751–4.

Greenberg, S.M., O'Donnell, H.C., Schaefer, P.W., and Kraft, E. (1999). MRI detection of new hemorrhages: potential marker of progression in cerebral amyloid angiopathy. *Neurology*, **53**, 1135–8.

Greenberg, S.M., Vonsattel, J.P., Stakes, J.W., Gruber, M., and Finklestein, S.P. (1993). The clinical spectrum of cerebral amyloid angiopathy: presentations without lobar hemorrhage. *Neurology*, **43**, 2073–9.

Gudmundsson, G., Hallgrimsson, J., Jonasson, T., and Bjarnason, O. (1972). Hereditary cerebral haemorrhage with amyloidosis. *Brain*, **95**, 387–404.

Haan, J. (2002). Hereditary cerebral amyloid angiopathies. In *Stroke: predisposing conditions* (ed. D. Leys), pp. 79–88. Remedica Publishing, London.

Haan, J., Algra, P.R., and Roos, R.A. (1990). Hereditary cerebral haemorrhage with amyloidosis-Dutch type: clinical and computed tomographic analysis of 24 cases. *Archives of Neurology*, **47**, 649–53.

Haan, J., Lanser, J.B., Zijderveld, I., van der Does, I.G., and Roos, R.A. (1990). Dementia in hereditary cerebral hemorrhage with amyloidosis—Dutch type. *Archives of Neurology*, **47**, 965–7.

Haan, J., Maat-Schieman, M.L.C., and Roos, R.A.C. (1994). Clinical effects of cerebral amyloid angiopathy. *Dementia*, **5**, 210–13.

Hendriks, L., van Duijn, C.M., Cras, P., *et al.* (1992). Presenile dementia and cerebral haemorrhage linked to a mutation at codon 692 of the beta-amyloid precursor protein gene. *Nature Genetics*, **1**, 18–221.

Higashi, M.K., Veenstra, D.L., Kondo, L.M., *et al.* (2002). Associations between CYP2C9 genetic variants and anticoagulation-related outcomes during warfarin therapy. *Journal of the American Medical Association*, **287**, 1690–8.

Hill, M.D., Silver, F.L., Austin, P.C., and Tu, J.V. (2000). Rate of stroke recurrence in patients with primary intracerebral hemorrhage. *Stroke*, **31**, 123–7.

Juvela, S., Hillbom, M., and Palomaki, H. (1995). Risk factors for spontaneous intracerebral hemorrhage. *Stroke*, **26**, 1558–64.

Kiuri, S., Salonen, O., and Haltia, M. (1999). Gelsolin-related spinal spinal and cerebral amyloid angiopathy. *Annals of Neurology*, **45**, 305–11.

Knudsen, K.A., Rosand, J., Karluk, D., and Greenberg, S.M. (2001). Clinical diagnosis of cerebral amyloid angiopathy: validation of the Boston criteria. *Neurology*, 56, 537–9.

Labovitz, D.L. and Sacco, R.L. (2001). Intracerebral hemorrhage: update. *Current Opinion in Neurology*, 14, 103–8.

Levy, E., Lopez, O.C., Ghiso, J., Geltner, D., and Frangione, B. (1989). Stroke in Icelandic patients with hereditary amyloid angiopathy is related to a mutation in the cystatin C gene, an inhibitor of cysteine proteases. *Journal of Experimental Medicine*, 169, 1771–8.

Lesnik Oberstein, S.A.J., van den Boom, R., van Buchem, M.A., *et al.* (2001). Cerebral microbleeds in CADASIL. *Neurology*, 57, 1066–70.

Maat-Schieman, M.L., van Duinen, S.G., Bornebroek, M., Haan, J., and Roos, R.A. (1996). Hereditary cerebral hemorrhage with amyloidosis- Dutch type (HCHWA-D): II- A review of histopathological aspects. *Brain Pathology*, 6, 115–20.

Maurino, J., Saposnik, G., Lepera, S., *et al.* (2001). Multiple simultaneous intracerebral hemorrhages: clinical features and outcome. *Archives of Neurology*, 58, 629–32.

McCarron, M.O. and Nicoll, J.A.R. (2000). Apolipoprotein E genotype and cerebral amyloid angiopathy-related hemorrhage. *Annals of the New York Academy of Sciences*, 903, 176–9.

McCarron, M.O., Nicoll, J.A.R., Stewart, J., *et al.* (2000). Absence of cystatin C mutation in sporadic cerebral amyloid angiopathy-related hemorrhage. *Neurology*, 54, 242–4.

Mead, S., James-Galton, M., Revesz, T., *et al.* (2000). Familial British dementia with amyloid angiopathy. Early clinical, neuropsychological and imaging findings. *Brain*, 123, 975–91.

Natowicz, M. and Kelley, R.I. (1987). Mendelian etiologies of stroke. *Annals of Neurology*, 22, 175–92.

Neau, J.P., Ingrand, P., Couderq, C., *et al.* (1997). Recurrent intracerebral hemorrhage. *Neurology*, 49, 106–13.

Nestler, E.J. (2001). Molecular neurobiology of addiction. *American Journal of Addiction*, 10, 201–17.

Nicoll, J.A. and McCarron, M.O. (2001). APOE gene polymorphism as a risk factor for cerebral amyloid angiopathy-related hemorrhage. *Amyloid*, 8(Suppl. I), 51–5.

Nighoghossian, N., Hermier, M., Adeleine, P., *et al.* (2002). Old microbleeds are a potential risk factor for cerebral bleeding after ischemic stroke: a gradient-echo T2*-weighted brain MRI study. *Stroke*, 33, 735–42.

Nilsberth, C., Westlind-Danielsson, A., Eckman, C.B., *et al.* (2001). The Ártctic APP-mutation (E693G) causes Alzheimer's disease by protofibril formation. *Nature Neuroscience*, 4, 887–93.

Obach, V., Revilla, M., Vila, N., Cervera, A., and Chamorro, A. (2001). Alpha 1-antichymotrypsin polymorphism. A risk factor for hemorrhagic stroke in normotensive subjects. *Stroke*, 32, 2588–91.

O'Donnell, H.C., Rosand, J., Knudsen, K.A., *et al.* (2000). Apolipoprotein E genotype and the risk of recurrent lobar intracerebral hemorrhage. *New England Journal of Medicine*, 342, 240–5.

Offenbacher, H., Fazekas, F., Schmidt, R., Koch, M., Fazekas, G., and Kapeller, P. (1996). MR of cerebral abnormalities concomittnt with primary intracerebral hematomas. *American Journal of Neuroradiology*, 17, 573–8.

Olson, J.D. (1993). Mechanisms of hemostasis. Effect on intracerebral hemorrhage. *Stroke*, 24(Suppl 12), I109-I14.

Ortel, T.L. (1999). Genetics of coagulation disorders. In *Genetics of cerebrovascular disease* (ed. M.J. Alberts), pp. 129–56. Futura Publishing Company, New York.

Polychronopoulos, P., Gioldasis, G., Ellul, J., *et al.* (2002). Family history of stroke in stroke types and subtypes. *Journal of the Neurological Sciences*, 195, 117–22.

Prengler, M., Pavlakis, S.G., Prohovnik, I., and Adams, R.J. (2002). Sickle cell disease: the neurological complications. *Annals of Neurology*, **51**, 543–52.

Qureshi, A.I., Tuhrim, S.T., Broderick, J.P., Batjer, H.H., Hondo, H., and Hanley, D.F. (2001). Spontaneous intracerebral hemorrhage. *New England Journal of Medicine*, **344**, 1450–60.

Roks, G., Van Harskamp, F., de Koning, I., *et al.* (2000). Presentation of amyloidosis in carriers of the codon 692 mutation in te amyloid precursor protein gene (APP692). *Brain*, **123**, 2130–40.

Rastenyte, D., Tuomilehto, J., and Sarti, C. (1998). Genetics of stroke—A review. Journal of *Neurological Sciences*, **153**, 132–45.

Sakashita, N., Ando, Y., Jinnouchi, K., *et al.* (2001). *Pathology International*, **51**, 476–80.

Senior, K. (2002). Microbleeds may predict cerebral bleeding after stroke. *The Lancet*, **359**, 769.

Svetkey, L.P., O'Riordan, E., Conlon, P.J., and Emovon, O. (1999). Genetics of hypertension. In *Genetics of cerebrovascular disease* (ed. M.J. Alberts), pp. 57–80. Futura Publishing Company, New York.

Tandon, A., Rogaeva, E., Mullan, M., and St George-Hyslop, P.H. (2000). Molecular genetics of Alzheimer's disease: The role of beta-amyloid and the presenilins. *Current Opinion in Neurology* **13**, 377–84.

Van Nostrand, W.E., Melchor, J.P., Cho, H.S., Greenberg, S.M., and Rebeck, G.W. (2001). Pathogenic effects of D23N Iowa mutant amyloid beta-protein. *The Journal of Biological Chemistry*, **276**, 32860–6.

Vidal, R., Garzuly, F., and Budka, H., *et al.* (1996). Meningocerebrovascular amyloidosis associated with a novel transthyretin mis-sense mutation at codon 18 (TTRD18G). *American Journal of Pathology*, **148**, 361–6.

Vidal, R., Revesz, T., Rostagno, A., *et al.* (2000). A decamer duplication in the 3′ region of the BRI gene originates an amyloid peptide that is associated with dementia in a Danish kindred. *Proceedings of the National Academy of Sciences USA*, **97**, 4920–5.

Vinters, H.V. (1987). Cerebral amyloid angiopathy. A critical review. *Stroke*, **18**, 311–24.

Vonsattel, J.P.G., Myers, R.H., Hedley-White, E.T., Ropper, A.H., Bird, E.D., and Richardson, E.P. (1991). Cerebral amyloid angiopathy without and with cerebral hemorrhages: a comparative histological study. *Annals of Neurology*, **30**, 637–49.

Wattendorf, A.R., Frangione, B., Luyendijk, W., and Bots, G.T. (1995). Hereditary cerebral haemorrhage with amyloidosis, Dutch type (HCHWA-D): clinicopathological studies. *Journal of Neurology Neurosurgery and Psychiatry*, **58**, 699–705.

WHO-IUIS Nomenclature Subcommittee. (1993). Nomenclature of amyloid and amyloidosis. *Bulletin of the World Health Organization*, **71**, 105–8.

Wintzen, A.R., de Jonge, H., Loeliger, E.A., and Bots, G.T. (1984). The risk of intracerebral haemorrhage during oral anticoagulant treatment—A population study. *Annals of Neurology*, **16**, 553–8.

Woo, D., Sauerbeck, L.R., Kissela, B.M., *et al.* (2002). Genetic and environmental risk factors for intracerebral hemorrhage. Preliminary results of a population-based study. *Stroke*, **33**, 1190–6.

Yamada, M. (2000). Cerebral amyloid angiopathy: an overview. *Neuropathology*, **1**, 8–22.

Yoshida, H., Imaizumi, T., Fujimoto, K., *et al.* (1998). A mutation in plasma-activating factor acetylhydrolase (Val279Phe) is a genetic risk factor for cerebral hemorrhage but not for hypertension. *Thrombosis and Haemostasis*, **80**, 372–5.

Zodpey, S.P., Tiwari, R.R., and Kulkarni, H.R. (2000). Risk factors for haemorrhagic stroke: a case control study. *Public Health*, **114**, 177–82.

Chapter 10

Genetics of subarachnoid haemorrhage and intracranial aneurysms

Wouter I. Schievink

10.1 Introduction

About 85 per cent of cases of subarachnoid haemorrhage are caused by intracranial aneurysms (see section 'subarachnoid haemorrhage'). The exact etiology and pathogenesis of intracranial aneurysms remain unclear (Schievink 1997). Several lines of evidence implicate genetic factors, whereas others support the role of acquired risk factors such as smoking or hypertension. The two main lines of evidence supporting the role of genetic factors are the association of intracranial aneurysms with heritable connective tissue disorders and the familial occurrence of intracranial aneurysms.

10.2 Heritable connective tissue disorders

Numerous heritable connective tissue disorders have been associated with intracranial aneurysms, including polycystic kidney disease, Ehlers–Danlos syndrome type IV, Marfan's syndrome, neurofibromatosis type 1, and α_1-antitrypsin deficiency (Table 10.1) (Schievink *et al.* 1994c, Schievink 1998). To what extent these specific heritable disorders contribute to the entire population of patients with intracranial aneurysms is unknown. In one series of 100 consecutive hospitalized patients with intracranial aneurysms, five had an identifiable heritable connective tissue disorder (Schievink *et al.* 1996). The true frequency of heritable connective tissue disorders in patients with aneurysms is probably higher because these disorders often remain undiagnosed, reflecting the substantial variability in their phenotypic expression. Family history also may be negative because the disease can be caused by a new mutation. Nevertheless, identifiable heritable connective tissue disorders contribute to a relatively small percentage of intracranial aneurysms.

10.2.1 Autosomal dominant polycystic kidney disease

Autosomal dominant polycystic kidney disease (ADPKD) affects about 1 in 400–1000 persons and is the most common monogenic disease in humans (Fick and Gabow 1994).

Table 10.1 Heritable disorders associated with intracranial aneurysms

Disorder	MIM no.[a]	Inheritance pattern[b]	Locus	Gene	Gene product
Achondroplasia	100800	AD	4p16.3	FGFR3	Fibroblast Growth Factor Receptor 3
Alagille syndrome	118450	AD	20p12	JAG1	?
Alkaptonuria	203500	AR	3q2	AKU	?
Autosomal dominant-polycystic kidney disease	173900 173910	AD	16p13.3 4q21	PKD1 PKD2	Polycystin-1 Polycystin-2
Autosomal dominant-polycystic liver disease	174050	AD	19p13.2	?	?
Cohen syndrome	216550	AR	8q22	CHS1	?
Ehlers–Danlos syndrome type I	130000	AD	9q34.2	COL5A1	Collagen type V[c]
Ehlers–Danlos syndrome type IV	130050	AD	2q31	COL3A1	Collagen type III[c]
Fabry disease	301500	XL-R	Xq22.1	GLA	α-Galactosidase A
Kahn syndrome[d]	210050	AR	?	?	?
Marfan's syndrome	154700	AD	15q21.1	FBN1	Fibrillin-1
Neurofibromatosis type 1	162200	AD	17q11.2	NF1	Neurofibromin
Noonan syndrome	163950	AD	12q22	NS1	?
Osler–Rendu–Weber disease	187300	AD	9q34.1 12q	HHT1 HHT2	Endoglin ?
Osteogenesis imperfecta type 1	166200	AD	17q22.1 7q22.1	COL1A1 COL1A2	Collagen type 1[c] Collagen type I[e]

Disease					
Pompe disease	232300	AR	17q23	GAA	α-Glucosidase
Pseudoxanthoma elasticum	177850 264800	AD and AR	16p13.1	?	?
Rambaud syndrome[d]	277175	AR	?	?	?
Seckel syndrome	210600	AR	?	?	?
Tuberous sclerosis	191100 191092	AD	9q34 16p13.3	TSC1 TSC2	? Tuberin
Wermer syndrome	131100	AD	11q13	MEN1	?
3M syndrome	273750	AR	?	?	?
α₁-Antitrypsin deficiency	107400	ACoD	14q32.1	PI	α₁-Antitrypsin

[a]Mckusick VA: Mendelian Inheritance in Man: Catalogs of Human Genes and Genetic Disorders. Baltimore, Johns Hopkins University Press, 1994, edn 11. *Online Mendelian Inheritance in Man*. Center for Medical Genetics, Johns Hopkins University (Baltimore, MD), and National Center for Biotechnology Information, National Library of Medicine (Bethesda, MD). World Wide Web URL:http://www.ncbi.nlm.nih.gov/omim/.

[b]AD, autosomal dominant; AR, autosomal recessive; XL-R, X-linked recessive; ACoD, autosomal codominant.

[c]α1-Polypeptide.

[d]Syndromes associated with idiopathic nonarteriosclerotic cerebral calcifications.

[e]α2-Polypeptide.

It is inherited as an autosomal dominant trait with almost complete penetrance but with variable expression. Family history is negative in about 20 per cent of patients, suggesting a fairly high spontaneous mutation rate.

ADPKD is a systemic disease, and cysts are present in the kidneys, liver, pancreas, spleen, ovaries, and seminal vesicles (Fick and Gabow 1994). Moreover, ADPKD should be included among the heritable connective tissue disorders (Schievink *et al.* 1994c). A wide variety of connective tissues may be involved (Fick and Gabow 1994), including the heart valves (mitral valve prolapse), vasculature (aneurysms and dissections), and meninges (arachnoid cysts). Patients with ADPKD are at increased risk for the development of gastrointestinal diverticula and inguinal hernias (Fick and Gabow 1994).

Neurosurgical disorders that have been associated with ADPKD include intracranial aneurysms, cervicocephalic arterial dissections, intracranial dolichoectasia, intracranial arachnoid cysts, and spinal meningeal diverticula (Schievink *et al.* 1992, 1995, 1997c, Fick and Gabow 1994, Schievink and Torres 1997). Intracranial aneurysms have long been known to be associated with ADPKD. Until the underlying connective tissue defect of the disease became well known, however, aneurysms frequently were attributed to the arterial hypertension that usually accompanies ADPKD. Intracranial aneurysms are detected in approximately one fourth of patients with ADPKD at autopsy; in most of these patients, aneurysmal rupture was the cause of death (Schievink *et al.* 1992). Conversely, ADPKD accounts for 2–7 per cent of all patients with intracranial aneurysms (Suter 1949, Schievink *et al.* 1992, 1997c). Using MR angiography or, less commonly, catheter angiography in patients with good renal function, several groups have screened adult ADPKD patients for asymptomatic intracranial aneurysms. The detection rate has ranged between 5 and 10 per cent (Chapman *et al.* 1992, Huston *et al.* 1993, 1996, Ruggieri *et al.* 1994, Huges *et al.* 1996, Ronkainen *et al.* 1997, Iida *et al.* 1998, Nakajima *et al.* 2000). Familial clustering of intracranial aneurysms occurs in ADPKD; the yield of screening increases to 10–25 per cent in such families (Huston *et al.* 1993, 1996, Ronkainen *et al.* 1997, Belz *et al.* 2001). The presence of polycystic liver disease in ADPKD patients may also increase the development of intracranial aneurysms (Huston *et al.* 1993).

Screening patients with ADPKD for asymptomatic aneurysms remains controversial but should certainly be considered for those with a family history of intracranial aneurysms. Most asymptomatic intracranial aneurysms detected with screening are less than 6 mm in diameter. In one study, none of these small aneurysms ruptured during 500 months of cumulative follow-up (Huston *et al.* 1996). It has been suggested that ADPKD patients are at an increased risk of developing *de novo* aneurysms some time after their first intracranial aneurysm is discovered, but the exact significance of this risk remains to be determined (Huges *et al.* 1996, Huston *et al.* 1996, Nakajima *et al.* 2000). Compared with the general population, aneurysmal SAH in patients with ADPKD occurs at an earlier age but the mortality rate is similar (Schievink *et al.* 1992).

ADPKD is a genetically heterogeneous disease. Several loci are involved, and mutations, which are responsible for at least 85 per cent of cases, have been identified on a gene on chromosome 16 (PKD1) as well as on a gene on chromosome 4 (PDK2) (Kimberling *et al.* 1988, Harris 1999, Peters and Breuning 2001). In general, patients with mutations in the PKD1 gene are more severely affected than those with mutations in the PKD2 gene, but intracranial aneurysms are a manifestation of both types of ADPKD as well as of ADPKD unlinked to the PKD1 and PKD2 loci (Kimberling *et al.* 1988, van Dijk *et al.* 1995, McConnell *et al.* 2001). Polycystin-1 and polycystin-2 are the proteins encoded by the PKD1 and PKD2 genes, respectively (Harris 1999, Peters and Breuring 2001). Both proteins are integral membrane proteins with large extracellular domains, which probably play a role in maintaining the structural integrity of the connective tissue extracellular matrix (Harris 1999, Peters and Breuning 2001).

Autosomal dominant polycystic liver disease (ADPLD) is a familial form of isolated polycystic liver disease that is distinct from ADPKD (Schievink and Spetzler 1998, Reynolds *et al.* 2000). In patients with ADPLD multiple cysts are found in the liver but not in the kidneys. The locus for ADPLD has been identified on chromosome 19 (Reynolds *et al.* 2000). Patients with ADPLD also may be at high risk for the development of intracranial aneurysms (Schievink and Spetzler 1998).

10.2.2 Ehlers–Danlos syndrome type IV

Ehlers–Danlos syndrome type IV is potentially one of the most deadly heritable connective tissue disorders that neurosurgeons may encounter. It is uncommon, with a prevalence of approximately 1 in 50,000–500,000 persons (Byers 1995). It is inherited in an autosomal dominant fashion, but family history frequently is noncontributory because of the high spontaneous mutation rate (approximately 50%).

Ehlers–Danlos syndrome type IV can be life threatening because spontaneous rupture, dissection (most commonly causing ischaemic stroke, Section 6.3.2), or aneurysmal formation on large and medium-sized arteries occur in all areas of the body (Pope *et al.* 1991, 1996, Schievink *et al.* 1994c, Byers 1995, Pepin *et al.* 2000). These arterial complications cause death in most patients. Other well-described life-threatening complications of Ehlers–Danlos syndrome type IV are spontaneous rupture of the bowel or gravid uterus and spontaneous pneumothorax (Pope *et al.* 1991, 1996, Schievink *et al.* 1994c, Byers 1995, Pepin *et al.* 2000).

An intracranial aneurysm may be the initial manifestation of Ehlers–Danlos syndrome type IV. Consequently, neurosurgeons may be the first physicians involved in these patients' medical care. The syndrome often is difficult to recognize because external features can be subtle (Schievink *et al.* 1994c, Byers 1995, Pope *et al.* 1996). The characteristic facial appearance was first described by Graf, a neurosurgeon (Graf 1965); many striking examples have since been published (Pope *et al.* 1991, 1996). The facial features consist of (1) large expressive eyes with the sclera clearly visible around the iris,

(2) a thin nose, (3) thin lips, and (4) lobeless ears. Many patients with Ehlers–Danlos syndrome type IV, however, do not exhibit this facial appearance. The characteristic cutaneous features include thin and fragile skin that is almost transparent, allowing the subcutaneous veins to be clearly visible. Patients bruise easily, and multiple ecchymoses are common. Scars are often papyraceous and wide or they may be complicated by keloid formation. The skin of some patients with Ehlers–Danlos syndrome type IV, however, appears normal. The joint hypermobility is often mild and limited to the fingers and toes. Identifying Ehlers–Danlos syndrome type IV in any patient with an intracranial aneurysm is important because vascular fragility can make any invasive procedure a hazardous undertaking.

Intracranial aneurysms and spontaneous carotid-cavernous fistulae are well-described vascular complications of Ehlers–Danlos syndrome type IV (Graf 1965, Pope *et al.* 1991, 1996, Schievink *et al.* 1994c, North *et al.* 1995, Pepin *et al.* 2000). In some patients, the carotid-cavernous fistula is due to the rupture of a cavernous-carotid aneurysm although the fistula may be caused by a simple tear in the artery in other patients. The importance of intracranial aneurysmal disease in this group of patients is well described. For example, in a cohort of 202 patients with Ehlers–Danlos syndrome type IV, four had ruptured intracranial aneurysms, four suffered an intracranial haemorrhage of undetermined cause, and six had carotid-cavernous fistulae (North *et al.* 1995). The exact incidence of intracranial aneurysms in Ehlers–Danlos syndrome type IV is unknown because screening for asymptomatic intracranial aneurysms is limited and systematic autopsy studies are unavailable. I generally do not recommend screening for asymptomatic intracranial aneurysms in these patients because safe treatment options are limited; arteriography, endovascular intervention, and surgical treatment are all associated with high complication rates. However, some patients with Ehlers–Danlos syndrome type IV tolerate neurosurgical procedures quite well and screening in these families should be considered (Schievink *et al.* 2002).

Mutations in the gene encoding the pro-α_1-(III) chain of collagen type III (COL3A1) on chromosome 2 are the cause of Ehlers–Danlos syndrome type IV (Pope *et al.* 1991, 1996, Byers 1995, Pepin *et al.* 2000, Schwarze 2001). This type of collagen is the major structural component of distensible tissues, including arteries, veins, hollow viscera, and the uterus. In addition, collagen type III may play an important role in the fibrillo-genesis of collagen type I (Liu *et al.* 1997). Several studies have reported evidence of abnormal collagen type III metabolism in up to 50 per cent of patients with intracranial aneurysms who do not have Ehlers–Danlos syndrome type IV (Pope *et al.* 1981, 1990, Neil-Dwyer *et al.* 1983, Østergaard and Oxlund 1987, Majamaa *et al.* 1992, Brega *et al.* 1996, van den Berg *et al.* 1999). Mutations in the COL3A1 gene, however, are rare. For example, in a study of 40 patients with intracranial aneurysms, COL3A1 mutations were found in only two patients, and the functional consequences of these mutations were considered insignificant (Kuivaniemi *et al.* 1993). The reasons for these conflicting data are unclear.

10.2.3 α_1-antitrypsin deficiency

The structural integrity of the arterial wall depends on a wide variety of interrelated extracellular matrix proteins such as collagen and elastin. The degradation of these proteins by proteolytic enzymes (proteases) is regulated by protease inhibitors (antiproteases). Recently, several studies have focused on an imbalance between proteases and antiproteases as a possible risk factor for the development of intracranial aneurysms (Schievink *et al.* 1994*d*, 1996, Baker *et al.* 1995, Connolly *et al.* 1997, Chyatte *et al.* 1999, Sakai *et al.* 1999). α_1-Antitrypsin, a powerful and abundant circulating antiprotease, is a small glycoprotein that is synthesized in the liver (Cox 1995). The primary target of a α_1-antitrypsin is not trypsin but neutrophil elastase. Consequently, α_1-antitrypsin deficiency (a codominantly inherited disorder) is characterized by damage of elastic tissues such as the lungs, resulting in emphysema (Cox 1995). α_1-Antitrypsin deficiency may also cause a breakdown of subcutaneous septae, resulting in cutis laxa (Corbet *et al.* 1994). Several vascular disorders have been associated with α_1-antitrypsin deficiency, including arterial aneurysms, spontaneous arterial dissections, and arterial fibromuscular dysplasia (Cohen *et al.* 1990, Mitchell *et al.* 1993, Cox 1994, Schievink *et al.* 1994*a,d*, 1996, 1998, St. Jean *et al.* 1996, Gaglio *et al.* 2000). Patients with α_1-antitrypsin deficiency are at increased risk for the development of intracranial aneurysms, but it remains to be determined how clinically significant this risk is. Among 362 consecutive patients with α_1-antitrypsin deficiency seen at the Mayo Clinic in Rochester, Minnesota, three had suffered an aneurysmal SAH, a considerably higher number than would be expected by chance (Schievink *et al.* 1994*d*). Some studies have shown that α_1-antitrypsin deficiency is more common in patients with intracranial aneurysms than in the general population (Schievink *et al.* 1996, St Jean *et al.* 1996). By contrast, other smaller studies have not found a statistically significant excess of α_1-deficiency in patients with intracranial aneurysms (St. Jean *et al.* 1996, Kissella *et al.* 2002). Typically, screening for asymptomatic intracranial aneurysms in patients with α_1-antitrypsin deficiency is not advocated.

The α_1-antitrypsin gene is located on chromosome 14 (Cox 1995). It is a highly polymorphic gene, and more than 75 allelic variants have been identified. The locus has been designated 'Pi' for protease inhibitor. The most common allele is PiM, and more than 95 per cent of the Caucasian population carry the homozygous PiMM phenotype. Patients who are homozygous for the deficient PiZ phenotype have low serum levels of α_1-antitrypsin (approximately 15% of normal), whereas only moderately reduced levels of α_1-antitrypsin are found in individuals with the heterozygous PiMZ phenotype (approximately 65%) or PiMS phenotype (approximately 80%). Patients who are homozygous for PiZ usually develop pulmonary emphysema; in our experience, this occurs before they present with an intracranial aneurysm. Heterozygous patients tend to remain asymptomatic if they refrain from smoking cigarettes. Although the Pi phenotype is the major contributor to α_1-antitrypsin levels, α_1-antitrypsin is also an acute phase protein and its levels increase after injury (e.g., SAH and craniotomy) or infection. Thus, quantification of the serum α_1-antitrypsin level in isolation may give a false-negative result. Cigarette smoking has been observed to lower the inhibitory capacity of α_1-antitrypsin, but it does not affect α_1-antitrypsin levels.

10.2.4 Marfan's syndrome

Marfan's syndrome affects approximately 1 in 10,000–20,000 people and is character-ized by abnormalities of the skeleton, cardiovascular system, eye, and spinal meninges (Godfrey 1993, Pyeritz et al. 1993). Aortic and mitral valve insufficiency are the most frequent causes of death in children with Marfan's syndrome, and spontaneous aortic rupture and dissection are the most frequent causes of death in adults with the syn-drome (Godfrey 1993, Pyeritz et al. 1993). Dissections of medium-sized arteries, how-ever, are much less common (Schievink et al. 1994b). Although Marfan's syndrome is easily recognized in patients who display the main features of the syndrome (particu-larly the skeletal manifestations of tall stature, dolichostenomelia, arachnodactyly, and anterior chest deformity), the variability of phenotypic expression is great and the diagnosis is seldom straightforward (Godfrey 1993, Pyeritz et al. 1993). For example, if the parents of a patient with Marfan's syndrome are short, the affected person's habitus may be comparatively normal (Godfrey 1993). Ectopia lentis, the classic ocular mani-festation of Marfan's syndrome, is observed in only about half the cases (Godfrey 1993). Dural ectasia, another major diagnostic criterion of the syndrome, is usually asymptomatic and requires CT or magnetic resonance imaging (MRI) for diagnosis (Pyeritz et al. 1988, Fattori et al. 1999). Other manifestations of Marfan's syndrome include spontaneous pneumothorax, striae distensae, and retinal detachment (Godfrey 1993, Pyeritz et al. 1993).

Intracranial aneurysms in patients with Marfan's syndrome may be saccular or fusiform, and intracranial dissecting aneurysms have also been described (Rose et al. 1991, Schievink et al. 1994c, 1997a, Sekhar et al. 1999). Similar to Ehlers–Danlos syndrome Type IV, there is a propensity for proximal intracranial carotid artery involvement although carotid-cavernous fistulae seem to be rare (Schievink et al. 1994c). Connective tissue fragility is seldom a major problem in the neurosurgical treatment of patients with Marfan's syndrome. The frequently observed ectasia and tortuosity of the extracranial carotid and vertebral arteries, however, may render endovascular treatment of intracranial aneurysms impossible. The association of Marfan's syndrome and intracranial aneurysms has not been firmly established. In an autopsy series of seven patients with Marfan's syndrome collected during a 25-year period at the Mayo Clinic, intracranial aneurysms, one ruptured and one unruptured, were observed in two patients (Schievink et al. 1997a). Combining this autopsy study with one performed at Johns Hopkins University (Conway et al. 1999), but excluding the one ruptured aneurysm, incidental aneurysms were found in two (6.5%) of

31 patients (Schievink, in press). This frequency is higher than would be expected in the general population, particularly considering the young age of the patients (Schievink, in press). Results of screening for asymptomatic intracranial aneurysms in patients with Marfan's syndrome have not been reported.

Mutations in the gene encoding fibrillin-1 (FBN-1) cause Marfan's syndrome (Ramirez *et al.* 1999). Fibrillin-1 is a recently diagnosed glycoprotein that is one of the major components of microfibrils (Sakai *et al.* 1986, Ramirez *et al.* 1999). These microfibrils are important constituents of the extracellular matrix and are distributed throughout the body in elastic tissues (e.g., skin, aorta, nonelastic tissues (e.g., the ciliary zonules of the ocular lens)). In elastic arteries, such as the aorta, fibrillin-1 is found in all three layers of the arterial wall. It is thought that fibrillin-1 plays an important role in maintaining the structural integrity of connective tissues, in part by providing a scaffolding for elastic fibers. Mutations in the FBN1 gene or abnormal fibrillin metabolism ('fibrillinopathy') have also been detected in patients with isolated features of Marfan's syndrome but without the classical syndrome (Aoyama *et al.* 1995, Francke *et al.* 1995, Milewicz *et al.* 1995, Schrijver *et al.* 2002).

10.2.5 Neurofibromatosis type 1

Neurofibromatosis type 1 is a progressive systemic disease affecting approximately 1 in 3000–5000 persons (Riccardi 1992). The principal clinical features of neurofibromatosis type 1 are café-au-lait spots, neurofibromas, axillary freckling, and Lisch nodules (hamartomas) of the iris (Riccardi 1992). Although these features each occur in more than 90 per cent of adults with neurofibromatosis type 1, the number of lesions is variable. Patients with neurofibromatosis type 1 are also at increased risk of developing optic glioma, phaeochromocytoma, dural ectasia, and skeletal abnormalities such as scoliosis and sphenoid wing dysplasia (Riccardi 1992). Vascular complications of neurofibromatosis type 1 have been recognized since 1945 and are characterized by stenosis (resulting in ischaemic stroke, see Section 6.3.5), rupture, and aneurysm or fistula formation of large and medium-sized arteries (Reubi 1945, Greene *et al.* 1974, Schievink and Piepgras 1991, Riccardi 1992).

Intracranial aneurysms in patients with neurofibromatosis type 1 may be saccular or fusiform, and some have the appearance of dissecting aneurysms (Benatar 1994, Poli *et al.* 1994, Sasaki *et al.* 1995, Urashini *et al.* 1995, Schievink 1997, Zhao and Han 1998, Mitsui *et al.* 2001). Surgical repair of these aneurysms may be complicated by excessive vascular fragility or distortion of anatomic landmarks caused by sphenoid wing dysplasia (Schievink 1997). The intracranial aneurysms associated with neurofibromatosis type 1 often coexist with intracranial arterial occlusive disease (Sobata *et al.* 1988), increasing the risks of their surgical and particularly endovascular treatment. An increased probability of developing intracranial aneurysms has not been clearly established for patients with neurofibromatosis type 1, but the number of reported cases continues to increase and some have advocated screening patients with neuro-fibromatosis for asymptomatic intracranial aneurysms (Poli *et al.* 1994). Among a group of 100 consecutive patients with intracranial aneurysms, one patient was revealed to have neurofibromatosis type 1 (Schievink *et al.* 1996). We recently reviewed MRI scans of 22 patients with neurofibromatosis and noted incidental aneurysms in two patients (9%).

Neurofibromatosis type 1 is caused by mutations in the gene (NF1) encoding neuro-fibromin, a protein with a centrally located domain homologous to GTPase-activating protein (GAP) that is similar to other tumor suppressor gene products (Gutmann and Collins 1993, Shen and Harper 1996). The GAP domain of neurofibromin colocalizes with cytoplasmatic microtubules, and it has been postulated that neuro-fibromin may have a regulatory role in the development of various connective tissues, including vascular connective tissue, through an effect on microtubular function. In a mouse model of mutations in GAP and NF1 genes, Henkemeyer *et al.* (1995) demon-strated thinning and rupture of large and medium-sized arteries during embryonic development. The GAP domain of neurofibromin, however, encompasses only about 10 per cent of the protein and neurofibromin may have a variety of undiscovered functions.

10.3 **Familial intracranial aneurysms**

With the exception of ADPKD and, rarely, Ehlers–Danlos syndrome type IV, Pompe disease, or syndromes associated with idiopathic nonarteriosclerotic cerebral calcifica-tions, familial intracranial aneurysms have not been associated with any of the known heritable connective tissue disorders. The familial aggregation of intracranial aneurysms was first described by Chambers *et al.* (1954). Since then hundreds of fam-ilies have been reported. During the past decade, interest in familial intracranial aneurysms has been renewed. Several studies have been focused on their epidemiolog-ical features, clinical characteristics, and presymptomatic detection with noninvasive screening methods.

10.3.1 **Epidemiology**

Familial intracranial aneurysms are much more common than has generally been appre-ciated. Four epidemiological studies have examined the frequency of familial intracranial aneurysms and revealed that 7–20 per cent of patients with aneurysmal SAH had first- or second-degree relatives with intracranial aneurysms (Norrgård *et al.* 1987, Ronkainen *et al.* 1993, Schievink *et al.* 1995, De Braekeleer *et al.* 1996) (Fig. 10.1). However, this familial aggregation could have been fortuitous because at least 1 per cent of adults harbors intracranial aneurysms and most of the reported families have included only two affected members. Whether relatives of patients with intracranial aneurysms have an increased risk of developing SAH was therefore unknown.

To address these issues, five independently conducted studies examined the risk of SAH in relatives of patients with SAH and have reported comparable results despite widely

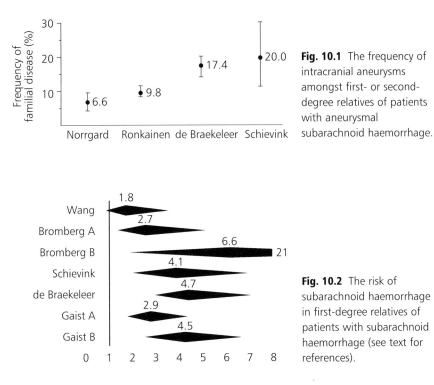

Fig. 10.1 The frequency of intracranial aneurysms amongst first- or second-degree relatives of patients with aneurysmal subarachnoid haemorrhage.

Fig. 10.2 The risk of subarachnoid haemorrhage in first-degree relatives of patients with subarachnoid haemorrhage (see text for references).

differing analytical methods and patient populations (Bromberg *et al.* 1995*a*, Schievink *et al.* 1995, Wang *et al.* 1995, De Braekeleer *et al.* 1996, Gaist *et al.* 2000) (Fig. 10.2). Among the population of King County, Washington, Wang *et al.* (1995) compared the frequency of familial SAH in patients with SAH to that of a control population. Patients with SAH were almost twice as likely to have an affected first-degree relative. However, this difference did not reach statistical significance and a family history of SAH was never verified. Bromberg *et al.* (1995) compared the frequency of SAH in first-degree relatives to that of second-degree relatives of patients with SAH who were admitted to several hospitals in the Netherlands. Depending on how well certain diagnostic criteria for SAH were met, they observed a three- to sevenfold increased risk. Among a group of patients with aneurysmal SAH from Rochester, Minnesota, colleagues and I (Schievink *et al.* 1995) compared the observed and expected number of first-degree relatives with aneurysmal SAH using the well-established incidence rates of SAH in this community and observed about a fourfold increased risk. Despite this significantly increased risk, we observed that the overall absolute risk of first-degree relatives for developing aneurysmal SAH did not reach 2 per cent until the age of 70 years. Among the inhabitants of the Saguenay Lac–Saint–Jean region of Quebec, Canada, De Braekeleer *et al.* (1996) compared the frequency of familial intracranial aneurysms in patients with ruptured and unruptured intracranial aneurysms to that of a control population and observed an approximately fivefold increased risk for first-degree relatives. In a Danish study, Gaist *et al.* (2000) found that first-degree relatives of patients with subarachnoid haemorrhage have a three to fivefold increased risk of subarachnoid haemorrhage compared to the general population.

10.3.2 Pattern of inheritance

The inheritance pattern of familial intracranial aneurysms is unknown. The main difficulty in establishing the mode of transmission is that intracranial aneurysms are acquired lesions and often remain asymptomatic. At visual inspection, some pedigrees support autosomal dominant inheritance and others support autosomal recessive or multifactorial transmission; in most, however, the inheritance pattern is unclear (Lozano and Leblanc 1987, Norrgård *et al.* 1987, Bailey 1993, Ronkainen *et al.* 1993, Schievink *et al.* 1994*e*, 1995, Leblanc *et al.* 1995, Bromberg *et al.* 1995*b*, Ronkainen *et al.* 1995*a*). In a segregation analysis of published pedigrees, no single Mendelian model was the overall best fitting. However, several possible patterns of inheritance were identified, and autosomal transmission was the most likely (Schievink *et al.* 1994*e*). This finding suggests that genetic heterogeneity is important in the genetics of intracranial aneurysms (Schievink *et al.* 1994*e*). Genetic heterogeneity had been suspected on the basis of the large number of heritable disorders that have been associated with intracranial aneurysms (Table 9.1).

Although the Saguenay Lac–Saint–Jean region is well known for its large number of consanguineous marriages, De Braekeleer *et al.* (1996) observed that the coefficient of inbreeding was no higher in patients with intracranial aneurysms than in a control population. They also noted a decrease in the frequency of intracranial aneurysms among first-, second-, and third-degree relatives of affected patients. These observations suggest the presence of dominant instead of recessive genes in their reported kinships.

Among families with two affected generations, children suffer SAH at a significantly younger age than the parents (Bailey 1993, Bromberg *et al.* 1995*b*). Although this age difference could be explained by ascertainment bias, disease onset at earlier ages in later generations (genetic anticipation) is increasingly recognized as an expression of unstable deoxyribonucleic acid trinucleotide repeats expanding in subsequent generations. This genetic mechanism has been demonstrated in several dominantly inherited neurodegenerative diseases and may also underlie the inheritance of intracranial aneurysms in some families.

10.3.3 Are familial aneurysms different?

Numerous studies have compared the characteristics of familial intracranial aneurysms with those of nonfamilial (sporadic) aneurysms. These studies have consistently shown that familial aneurysms rupture, on average, about 5 years earlier than sporadic aneurysms (Norrgård *et al.* 1987, Bailey 1993, Schievink *et al.* 1995, Leblanc *et al.* 1995, Ronkainen *et al.* 1995, Bromberg *et al.* 1995*b*). In several populations of siblings, aneurysms more commonly rupture within the same decade of life (Lozano and

Leblanc 1987, Ronkainen *et al.* 1995*a*). Aneurysms of the anterior communicating artery complex are underrepresented in patients with familial aneurysms (Norrgård *et al.* 1987, Bailey 1993, Bromberg *et al.* 1995*b*, Leblanc *et al.* 1995, Schievink *et al.* 1995). Although prospective studies are unavailable, two studies suggest that familial aneurysms rupture at a smaller size than sporadic aneurysms (Lozano and Leblanc 1987, Ronkainen *et al.* 1995*a*). The observed differences are small (1–2 mm) but may be important, particularly for the treatment of small asymptomatic aneurysms. Patients with familial aneurysms also may develop *de novo* aneurysms more often than patients with sporadic aneurysms although the number of observed cases is small (Motuo Fotso *et al.* 1993, Schievink *et al.* 1994*e*, Lebland 1999). An increased proportion of multiple aneurysms (see Fig. 10.3) is also found in patients with familial aneurysms (Norrgård *et al.* 1987, Bailey 1993, Schievink *et al.* 1995, Leblanc *et al.* 1995, Ronkainen *et al.* 1995, Bromberg *et al.* 1995*b*). One hospital-based study suggests that the case-fatality rate of SAH is worse in patients with familial aneurysms (Bromberg *et al.* 1995*c*); however, other studies do not support this observation (Schievink and Schaid 1996, Ronkainen *et al.* 1999). At autopsy patients with familial intracranial aneurysms have had changes in the media of the intra- and extracranial artery that were not present in patients with sporadic aneurysms (Schievink *et al.* 1997*b*). Together, these clinical and pathologic data suggest that familial intracranial aneurysms are different from nonfamilial intracranial aneurysms.

10.3.4 Screening

The benefits of screening for asymptomatic intracranial aneurysms have never been quantified. Several groups, however, have extensive experience with screening for familial intracranial aneurysms using MR angiography. In the absence of any clinical feature or biologic marker that can identify individuals who are most likely to develop intracranial aneurysms, screening for asymptomatic familial intracranial aneurysms may be recommended for first-degree relatives in families with two or more affected members (Schievink *et al.* 1994*e*, Ronkainen *et al.* 1995*b*, 1997, Raaymakers *et al.* 1998, Brown and Soldevilla 1999). With this screening strategy, approximately 10 per cent of individuals are found to have an intracranial aneurysm (Ronkainen *et al.* 1997, Raaymakers *et al.* 1998, Brown and Soldevilla 1999). In approximately a third of these patients, the aneurysms are larger than 5 mm in diameter (Ronkainen *et al.* 1997). Some investigators have recommended screening individuals with only a single family member with an intracranial aneurysm (Bromberg *et al.* 1995*a*,*b*). The absolute lifetime risk for first-degree relatives to suffer an aneurysmal SAH when there is only a single family member with an aneurysm is modest (Schievink *et al.* 1995), however. Furthermore, the yield of such a screening, strategy is fairly low (2–4%) (Ronkainen *et al.* 1998, Raaymakers 1999, The Magnetic Resonance Angiography in Relatives of Patients Study Group 1999). Therefore, screening is seldom recommended for those patients (Schievink 1994*e*, 1997, Ronkainen *et al.* 1995*b*).

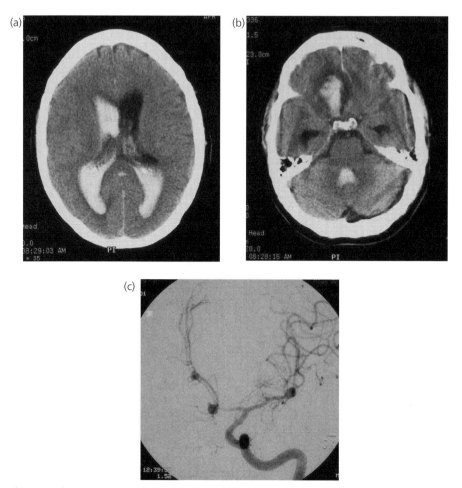

Fig. 10.3 This patient presented with subarachnoid haemorrhage. CT brain imaging on day 1 shows blood in the ventricles (a) and also around the left anterior cerebral artery (b) consistent with a left anterior cerebral artery aneurysm. Intra-arterial angiography (c) confirms a left anterior cerebral artery aneurysm, but also shows asymptomatic left middle cerebral artery and left pericallosal artery aneurysms. Multiple aneurysms are more common in familial cases of aneurysm. (Copyright with Hugh Markus).

There are no guidelines for determining when aneurysm screening should be performed. Several investigators have used sophisticated decision-making analytic models using similar data to determine the optimum age for screening. Widely differing age ranges have been suggested (e.g. Obuchowski *et al.* (1995), <30 years; Leblanc *et al.* (1994), 20–50 years; ter Berg *et al.* (1992), 35–65 years). Ronkainen *et al.* (1996) limit their screening to individuals older than 30 years of age. We have arbitrarily offered screening to those between the ages of 18 and 65 years. To detect *de novo* aneurysms, repeat screening has been suggested at 6-month to 5-year intervals after the initial study (Schievink *et al*. 1991). I currently offer MR angiographic screening to all first-degree relatives between the ages of 18 and 65 years once the familial aggregation of intracranial aneurysms has been established. If MR angiography discloses no aneurysm, screening at 5-year intervals is then recommended. Among patients with affected siblings, screening is offered at 2-year intervals during the decades of life that the siblings were diagnosed with an intracranial aneurysm. Screening should also be considered for children if a family member younger than 18 years has been diagnosed with an intracranial aneurysm. In addition, I recommend screening for persons with a monozygotic (identical) twin who has an intracranial aneurysm.

10.3.5 Evaluation of patients with a familial aneurysm

Patients with an intracranial aneurysm and a family history of intracranial aneurysm or SAH warrant further evaluation. This evaluation primarily consists of obtaining a detailed medical and family history supplemented by a review of the available medical or autopsy records. A review of these records is important because a self-reported family history alone may not prove or refute a diagnosis of intracranial aneurysm or SAH. Consultation by a medical geneticist is often valuable in constructing a pedigree, obtaining records, and evaluating the patient for the presence of heritable disorders that have been associated with intracranial aneurysms. Apart from ADPKD (Schievink *et al*. 1992, Huston *et al*. 1993, Ronkainen *et al*. 1997) and, occasionally, Ehlers–Danlos syndrome type IV (Pope *et al*. 1991, Pollack *et al*. 1997), however, the heritable connective tissue disorders are rarely identified in families with intracranial aneurysms. Familial intracranial aneurysms may be the first manifestation of ADPKD (McConnell *et al*. 1997). Renal ultrasonography is a noninvasive and reliable technique and should therefore be considered to rule out ADPKD. At least one study has reported a low yield of screening for ADPKD in patients with familial intracranial aneurysms (Ronkainen *et al*. 1997). When Ehlers–Danlos syndrome type IV is suspected, collagen type III analyses should be performed on cultured skin fibroblasts to confirm this diagnosis. Finally, adult first-degree relatives should be contacted and advised about the possibilities and uncertainties of invasive and noninvasive screening for asymptomatic intracranial aneurysms.

10.3.6 Intracranial aneurysm gene?

Before the burgeoning capabilities of molecular genetic linkage, several allelic association studies were conducted in patients with intracranial aneurysms using classic markers such as human lymphocyte antigens, red blood cell types, and serum group systems. These studies failed to show any convincing associations (Schievink 1997).

Recent advances in molecular genetics have made linkage studies possible to map the chromosomal locus of a putative intracranial aneurysm gene mutation. One approach is to screen the human genome for intracranial aneurysm genes by testing linkage of a large number of distinct highly polymorphic genetic markers. Such linkage analysis is classically performed in large families with multiple affected members. However, this method (as applied to intracranial aneurysms) is hampered by the genetic heterogeneity, the paucity of well-documented multiple case families, and the uncertainties in designating family members as unaffected if screening does not show an aneurysm.

Another method for studying linkage is to analyze variations in the sharing of marker alleles among affected sibling pairs only. Although this method requires no knowledge of the mode of transmission and only affected family members are studied, very large sample sizes are often required. An alternative approach to locate intracranial aneurysm genes is candidate gene sequence analysis. This analysis involves evaluating the sequence of a gene for a protein plausibly involved in intracranial aneurysm development (e.g., PKD1 or COL3A1, Table 9.1) and determining whether a mutant sequence variation occurs more frequently among affected patients than is predicted by chance. Several laboratories are currently directing their efforts at locating intracranial aneurysm genes using one or more of these approaches.

Polymorphisms of several genes have now been investigated in patients with intracranial aneurysms (Takenaka *et al*. 1998, 1999, Yoon *et al*. 1999, Kokubo *et al*. 2000, Krex *et al*. 2001, Zhang *et al*. 2001). Certain polymorphisms of the angiotensin I-converting enzyme, matrix metalloproteinases, apolipoprotein E, and endoglin genes may be associated with an increased risk for aneurysm development, but these findings need to be confirmed in other groups of aneurysm patients.

Olson *et al*. (1998) performed a sibling-pair linkage analysis in Finnish patients with intracranial aneurysms and identified a susceptibility locus at 19q13.1–13.3 One of the candidate genes in this region is uPAR (urokinase-type plasminogen activator receptor) at 19q13.2. Onda *et al*. (2001) performed a similar analysis in Japanese patients with intracranial aneurysms and identified a locus near the elastin gene at 7q11.

Grond-Ginsbach *et al*. (2002) studied skin biopsies of patients with intracranial aneurysms using electron microscopy and noted abnormal morphology of collagen fibrils and elastic fibers in one-third of patients.

References

Aoyama, T., Francke, U., Gasner, C., *et al*. (1995). Fibrillin abnormalities and prognosis in Marfan syndrome and related disorders. *American Journal of Medical Genetics*, **58**, 169–76.

Bailey, J.C. (1993). Familial subarachnoid haemorrhage. *Ulster Medical Journal*, **62**, 119–26.

Baker, C.J., Fiore, A., Connolly, E.S. Jr, *et al*. (1995). Serum elastase and alpha-1-antitrypsin levels in patients with ruptured and unruptured cerebral aneurysms. *Neurosurgery*, **37**, 56–62.

Belz, M.M., Hughes, R.L., Kaehny, W.D., *et al*. (2001). Familial clustering of ruptured intracranial aneurysms in autosomal dominant polycystic kidney disease. *American Journal of Kidney Diseases*, **38**, 770–6.

Benatar, M.G. (1994). Intracranial fusiform aneurysms in von Recklinghausen's disease: case report and literature review. *Journal of Neurology, Neurosurgery and Psychiatry*, 57, 1279–80.

Brega, K.E., Seltzer, W.K., Munro, L.G., *et al.* (1996). Genotypic variations of type III collagen in patients with cerebral aneurysms. *Surgical Neurology*, 46, 253–7.

Bromberg, J.E.C., Rinkel, G.J.E., Algra, A., *et al.* (1995*a*). Subarachnoid haemorrhage in first and second degree relatives of patients with subarachnoid haemorrhage. *British Medical Journal*, 311, 288–9.

Bromberg, J.E.C., Rinkel, G.J.E., Algra, A., *et al.* (1995*b*). Familial subarachnoid hemorrhage: distinctive features and patterns of inheritance. *Annals of Neurology*, 38, 929–34.

Bromberg, J.E.C., Rinkel, G.J.E., Algra, A., *et al.* (1995*c*). Outcome in familial subarachnoid hemorrhage. *Stroke*, 26, 961–3.

Brown, B.M. and Soldevilla, F. (1999). MR angiography and surgery for unruptured familial intracranial aneurysms in persons with a family history of cerebral aneurysms. *AJR. American Journal of Roentgenology*, 173, 133–8.

Byers, P.H. (1995). Ehlers–Danlos syndrome type IV: a genetic disorder in many guises. *Journal of Investigative Dermatology*, 105, 311–13.

Chambers, W.R., Harper, B.F. Jr, and Simpson, J.R. (1954). Familial incidence of congenital aneurysms of cerebral arteries. *Journal of the American Medical Association*, 155, 358–9.

Chapman, A.B., Rubinstein, D., Hughes, R., *et al.* (1992). Intracranial aneurysms in autosomal dominant polycystic kidney disease. *New England Journal of Medicine*, 327, 916–20.

Chyatte, D., Bruno, G., Desai, S., *et al.* (1999). Inflammation and intracranial aneurysms. *Neurosurgery*, 45, 1137–47.

Cohen, J.R., Sarfati, I., Ratner, L., *et al.* (1990). α_1-Antitrypsin phenotypes in patients with abdominal aortic aneurysms. *Journal of Surgical Research*, 49, 319–21.

Connolly, E.S. Jr, Fiore, A.J., Winfree, C.J., *et al.* (1997). Elastin degradation in the superficial temporal arteries of patients with intracranial aneurysms reflects changes in plasma elastase. *Neurosurgery*, 40, 903–9.

Conway, J.E., Hutchins, G.M., and Tamargo, R.J. (1999). Marfan syndrome is not associated with intracranial aneurysms. *Stroke*, 30, 1632–6.

Corbet, E., Glaisyer, H., Chan, C., *et al.* (1994). Congenital cutis laxa with a dominant inheritance and early onset emphysema. *Thorax*, 49, 836–7.

Cox, D.W. (1994). α_1-Antitrypsin: a guardian of vascular tissue. *Mayo Clinic Proceedings*, 69, 1123–4.

Cox, D.W. (1995). α_1-antitrypsin deficiency. In *The metabolic and molecular bases of inherited disease* (ed. C.R. Scriver, A.L. Beaudet, W.S. Sly, *et al.*), Vol. 3, edn 7, pp. 4125–58. McGraw-Hill, New York.

De Braekeleer, M., Pérusse, L., Cantin, L., *et al.* (1996). A study of inbreeding and kinship in intracranial aneurysms in the Saguenay Lac–Saint–Jean region (Quebec, Canada). *Annals Human Genetics*, 60, 99–104.

Fattori, R., Nienaber, C.A., Descovich, B., *et al.* (1999). Importance of dural ectasia in phenotypic assessment of Marfan's syndrome. *Lancet*, 354, 910–13.

Fick, G.M. and Gabow, P.A. (1994). Natural history of autosomal dominant polycystic kidney disease. *Annual Review Medicine*, 45, 23–9.

Francke, U., Berg, M.A., Tynan, K., *et al.* (1995). A Gly1127Ser mutation in an EGF-like domain of the fibrillin-1 gene is a risk factor for ascending aortic aneurysm and dissection. *American Journal of Human Genetics*, 56, 1287–96.

Gaglio, P.J., Regenstein, F., Slakey, D., *et al.* (2000). Alpha-1 antitrypsin deficiency and splenic artery aneurysm rupture: an association? *American Journal of Gastroenterology*, 95, 1531–4.

Gaist, D., Vaeth, M., Tsiropoulos, I., *et al.* (2000). Risk of subarachnoid haemorrhage in first degree relatives of patients with subarachnoid haemorrhage: follow up study based on national registries in Denmark. *British Medical Journal*, **320**, 141–5.

Godfrey, M. (1993). The Marfan syndrome. In *McKusick's heritable disorders of connective tissue* (ed. P. Beighton), edn 5, pp. 51–135. St. Louis, Mosby.

Graf, C.J. (1965). Spontaneous carotid-cavernous fistula. Ehlers–Danlos syndrome and related conditions. *Archives of Neurology*, **13**, 662–72.

Greene, J.F. Jr, Fitzwater, J.E., and Burgess, J. (1974). Arterial lesions associated with neurofibromatosis. *American Journal of Clinical Pathology*, **62**, 481–7.

Grond-Ginsbach, C., Schnippering, H., Hausser, I., *et al.* (2002). Ultrastructural connective tissue aberrations in patients with intracranial aneurysms. *Stroke*, **33**, 2192–6.

Gutmann, D.H. and Collins, F.S. (1993). The neurofibromatosis type 1 gene and its protein product, neurofibromin. *Neuron*, **10**, 335–43.

Harris, P.C. (1999). Autosomal dominant polycystic kidney disease: clues to pathogenesis. *Human Molecular Genetics*, **8**, 1861–6.

Henkemeyer, M., Rossi, D.J., Holmyard, D.P., *et al.* (1995). Vascular system defects and neuronal apoptosis in mice lacking ras GTPase-activating protein. *Nature*, **377**, 695–701.

Hughes, R., Chapman, A., Rubinstein, D., *et al.* (1996). Recurrent intracranial aneurysms (ICA) in autosomal dominant polycystic kidney disease (ADPKD). *Stroke*, **27**, 178.

Huston, J. III, Torres, V.E., Sullivan, P.P., *et al.* (1993). Value of magnetic resonance angiography for the detection of intracranial aneurysms in autosomal dominant polycystic kidney disease. *Journal of the American Society of Nephrology*, **3**, 1871–7.

Huston, J. III, Torres, V.E., Wiebers, D.O., *et al.* (1996). Follow-up of intracranial aneurysms in autosomal dominant polycystic kidney disease by magnetic resonance angiography. *Journal of the American Society of Nephrology*, **7**, 2135–41.

Iida, H., Naito, T., Hondo, H., *et al.* (1998). Intracranial aneurysms in autosomal dominant polycystic kidney disease detected by MR angiography: screening and treatment. *Nippon Jinzo Gakkai Shi*, **40**, 42–7.

Kimberling, W.J., Fain, P.R., Kenyon, J.B., *et al.* (1988). Linkage heterogeneity of autosomal dominant polycystic kidney disease. *New England Journal of Medicine*, **319**, 913–18.

Kissella, B.M., Sauerbeck, L., Woo, D., *et al.* (2002). Subarachnoid hemorrhage: a preventable disease with a heritable component. *Stroke*, **33**, 1321–6.

Kokubo, Y., Chowdhury, A.H., Date, C., *et al.* (2000). Age-dependent association of apolipoprotein E genotypes with stroke subtypes in a Japanese rural population. *Stroke*, **31**, 1299–306.

Krex, D., Ziegler, A., Schackert, H.K., *et al.* (2001). Lack of association between Endoglin Intron 7 Insertion 7 polymorphism and intracranial aneurysms in a white population: evidence of racial/ethnic differences. *Stroke*, **32**, 2689–94.

Kuivaniemi, H., Prockop, D.J., Wu, Y., *et al.* (1993). Exclusion of mutations in the gene for type III collagen (COL3A1) as a common cause of intracranial aneurysms or cervical artery dissections: results from sequence analysis of the coding sequences of type III collagen from 55 unrelated patients. *Neurology*, **43**, 2652–8.

Leblanc, R., Worsley, K.J., Melanson, D., *et al.* (1994). Angiographic screening and elective surgery of familial cerebral aneurysms: a decision analysis. *Neurosurgery*, **35**, 9–19.

Leblanc, R., Melanson, D., Tampieri, D., *et al.* (1995). Familial cerebral aneurysms: a study of 13 families. *Neurosurgery*, **37**, 633–9.

Lebland, R. (1999). *De novo* formation of familial cerebral aneurysms: case report. *Neurosurgery*, **44**, 871–7.

Liu, X., Wu, H., Byrne, M., *et al.* (1997). Type III collagen is crucial for collagen I fibrillogenesis and for normal cardiovascular development. *Proceedings of the National Academy of Sciences of the USA*, **94**, 1852–6.

Lozano, A.M. and Leblanc, R. (1987). Familial intracranial aneurysms. *Journal of Neurosurgery*, **66**, 522–8.

Majamaa, K., Savolainen, E.-R., and Myllalä V.V. (1992). Synthesis of structurally unstable type III procollagen in patients with cerebral artery aneurysm. *Biochimica et Biophysica Acta*, **138**, 191–6.

McConnell, R.S., Hughes, A.E., Rubinsztein, D.E.C., *et al.* (1997). Gene–environment interactions in familial clustering of cerebral aneurysm formation. *Journal of Neurology, Neurosurgery, and Psychiatry*, **63**, 128.

McConnell, R.S., Rubinsztein, D.C., Fannin, T.F., *et al.* (2001). Autosomal dominant polycystic kidney disease unlinked to the PKD1 and PKD2 loci presenting as familial cerebral aneurysm. *Journal of Medical Genetics*, **38**, 238–40.

Milewicz, D.M., Grossfield, J., Cao, S.-N., *et al.* (1995). A mutation in FBN1 disrupts profibrillin processing and results in isolated skeletal features of the Marfan syndrome. *Journal of Clinical Investigation*, **95**, 2372–8.

Mitchell, M.B., McAnena, O.J., and Rutherford, R.B. (1993). Ruptured mesenteric artery aneurysm in a patient with alpha$_1$-antitrypsin deficiency: etiologic implications. *Journal of Vascular Surgery*, **17**, 420–4.

Mitsui, Y., Nakasaka, Y., Akamatsu, M., *et al.* (2001). Neurofibromatosis type 1 with basilar artery fusiform aneurysm manifesting Wallenberg's syndrome. *Internal Medicine*, **40**, 948–51.

Motuo Fotso, M.J., Brunon, J., Outhel, R., *et al.* (1993). Anéurysmes familiaux, anéurysmes multiples et anéurysmes 'de novo': a propos de deux observations. *Neurochirurgie*, **39**, 225–30.

Nakajima, F., Shibahara, N., Arai, M., *et al.* (2000). Intracranial aneurysms and autosomal dominant polycystic kidney disease: followup study by magnetic resonance angiography. *Journal of Urology*, **164**, 311–13.

Neil-Dwyer, G., Bartlett, J.R., Nicholls, A.C., *et al.* (1983). Collagen deficiency and ruptured cerebral aneurysms. A clinical and biochemical study. *Journal of Neurosurgery*, **59**, 16–20.

Norrgård, Ö., Ångquist, K.-A., Fodstad, H., *et al.* (1987). Intracranial aneurysms and heredity. *Neurosurgery*, **20**, 236–9.

North, K.N., Whiteman, D.A.H., Pepin, M.G., *et al.* (1995). Cerebrovascular complications of Ehlers–Danlos syndrome type IV. *Annals of Neurology*, **38**, 960–4.

Obuchowski, N.A., Modic, M.T., and Magdinec, M. (1995). Current implications for the efficacy of noninvasive screening for occult intracranial aneurysms in patients with a family history of aneurysms. *Journal of Neurosurgery*, **83**, 42–9.

Olson, J., Vongpunsawad, S., Kuivaniemi, H., *et al.* (1998). Genome scan for intracranial aneurysm susceptibility loci using Finnish families. *American Journal of Human Genetics*, **63**, A17.

Olson, J.M., Vongpunsawad, S., Kuivaniemi, H., *et al.* (2002). Search for intracranial aneurysm susceptibility gene(s) using Finnish families. *BMC Medical Genetics*, **3**, 7.

Onda, H., Kasuya, H., Yoneyama, T., *et al.* (2001). Genomewide-linkage and haplotype-association studies map intracranial aneurysm to chromosome 7q11. *American Journal of Human Genetics*, **69**, 804–19.

Østergaard, J.R. and Oxlund, H. (1987). Collagen type III deficiency in patients with rupture of intracranial saccular aneurysms. *Journal of Neurosurgery*, **67**, 690–6.

Pepin, M., Schwarze, U., Superti-Furga, A., *et al.* (2000). Clinical and genetic features of Ehlers–Danlos syndrome type IV, the vascular type. *New England Journal of Medicine*, **342**, 673–80.

Peters, D.J.M. and Breuning, M.H. (2001). Autosomal dominant polycystic kidney disease: modification of disease progression. *Lancet*, **358**, 1439–44.

Poli, P., Peillon, C., Lahda, E., *et al.* (1994). Anévrysmes intracraniens multiples en rapport avec une maladie de Recklinghausen: a propos d'un cas. *Journal of des Maladies Vasculaires*, **19**, 253–5.

Pollack, J.S., Custer, P.L., Hart, W.M., *et al.* (1997). Ocular complications in Ehlers–Danlos syndrome type IV. *Archives of Ophthalmology*, **115**, 416–19.

Pope, F.M., Nicholls, A.C., Narcisi, P., *et al.* (1981). Some patients with cerebral aneurysms are deficient in type III collagen. *Lancet*, **1**, 973–5.

Pope, F.M., Limburg, M., and Schievink, W.I. (1990). Familial cerebral aneurysms and type III collagen deficiency. *Journal of Neurosurgery*, **72**, 156–8.

Pope, F.M., Kendall, B.E., Slapak, G.I., *et al.* (1991). Type III collagen mutations cause fragile cerebral arteries. *British Journal of Neurosurgery*, **5**, 551–74.

Pope, F.M., Narcisi, P., Nicholls, A.C., *et al.* (1996). COL3A1 mutations cause variable clinical phenotypes including acrogeria and vascular rupture. *British Journal of Dermatology*, **135**, 163–81.

Pyeritz, R.E. (1993). The Marfan syndrome. In *Connective tissue and its heritable disorders: molecular, genetic, and medical aspects* (ed. P.M. Royce and B. Steinmann), pp. 437–68. Wiley-Liss, New York.

Pyeritz, R.E., Fishman, E.K., Bernhardt, B.A., *et al.* (1988). Dural ectasia is a common feature of the Marfan syndrome. *American Journal of Human Genetics*, **43**, 726–32.

Raaymakers, T.W. (1999). Aneurysms in relatives of patients with subarachnoid hemorrhage: Frequency and risk factors. MARS Study Group. Magnetic resonance angiography in relatives of patients with subarachnoid hemorrhage. *Neurology*, **53**, 982–8.

Raaymakers, T.W.M., Rinkel, G.J.E., and Ramos, L.M.P. (1998). Initial and follow-up screening for aneurysms in families with familial subarachnoid hemorrhage. *Neurology*, **51**, 1125–30.

Ramirez, F., Gayraud, B., and Pereira, L. (1999). Marfan syndrome: new clues to genotype–phenotype correlations. *Annals of Medicine*, **31**, 202–7.

Reubi, F. (1945). Neurofibromatosis et lésions vasculaires. *Schweizerische Medizinische Wochenschrift*, **75**, 463–5.

Reynolds, D.M., Falk, C.T., Li, A., *et al.* (2000). Identification of a locus for autosomal dominant polycystic liver disease, on chromosome 19p13.2–13.1. *American Journal of Human Genetics*, **67**, 1598–604.

Riccardi, V.M. (1992). *Neurofibromatosis: Phenotype, Natural History and Pathogenesis*. ed 2. Baltimore, Johns Hopkins University.

Ronkainen, A., Hernesniemi, J., and Ryynänen, M. (1993). Familial subarachnoid hemorrhage in east Finland, 1977–1990. *Neurosurgery*, **33**, 787–97.

Ronkainen, Hernesniemi, J., and Tromp, G. (1995*a*). Special features of familial intracranial aneurysms: Report of 215 familial aneurysms. *Neurosurgery*, **37**, 43–7.

Ronkainen, A., Puranen, M.I., Hernesniemi, J.A., *et al.* (1995*b*). Intracranial aneurysms: MR angiographic screening in 400 asymptomatic individuals with increased familial risk. *Radiology*, **195**, 35–40.

Ronkainen, A., Hernesniemi, J., Kuivaniemi, H., *et al.* (1996). Current implications for the efficacy of noninvasive screening for occult intracranial aneurysms in patients with a family history of aneurysms. *Journal of Neurosurgery*, **84**, 534–6.

Ronkainen, A., Hernesniemi, J., Puranen, M., *et al.* (1997). Familial intracranial aneurysms. *Lancet*, **349**, 380–4.

Ronkainen, A., Miettinen, H., Karkola, K., *et al.* (1998). Risk of harboring an unruptured intracranial aneurysm. *Stroke*, **29**, 359–62.

Ronkainen, A., Niskanen, M., Piironen, R., *et al.* (1999). Familial subarachnoid hemorrhage. Outcome study. *Stroke*, **30**, 1099–102.

Rose, B.S. and Pretorius, D.L. (1991). Dissecting basilar artery aneurysm in Marfan syndrome: Case report. *AJNR American Journal of Neuroradiology*, **12**, 503–4.

Ruggieri, P.M., Poulos, N., Masaryk, T.J., *et al.* (1994). Occult intracranial aneurysms in polycystic kidney disease: screening with MR angiography. *Radiology*, **191**, 33–9.

Sakai, L.Y., Keene, D.R., and Engvall, E. (1986). Fibrillin, a new 350-kDa glycoprotein, is a component of extracellular microfibrils. *Journal of Cell Biology*, **103**, 2499–509.

Sakai, N., Nakayama, K., Tanabe, Y., *et al.* (1999). Absence of plasma protease-antiprotease imbalance in the formation of saccular cerebral aneurysms. *Neurosurgery*, **45**, 34–8.

Sasaki, J., Miura, S., Ohishi, H., *et al.* (1995). Neurofibromatosis associated with multiple intracranial vascular lesions: stenosis of the internal carotid artery and peripheral aneurysm of the Huebner's artery; report of a case [Japanese]. *No Shinkei Geka*, **23**, 813–17.

Schievink, W.I. Intracranial aneurysms and Marfan syndrome. *Stroke*, **31** (in press).

Schievink, W.I., Limburg, M., Dreissen, J.J.R., *et al.* (1991). Screening for unruptured familial intracranial aneurysms: Subarachnoid hemorrhage 2 years after angiography negative for aneurysms. *Neurosurgery*, **29**, 434–8.

Schievink, W.I. and Piepgras, D.G. (1991). Cervical vertebral artery aneurysms and arteriovenous fistulae in neurofibromatosis type 1: case reports. *Neurosurgery*, **29**, 760–5.

Schievink, W.I., Torres, V.E., Piepgras, D.G., *et al.* (1992). Saccular intracranial aneurysms in autosomal dominant polycystic kidney disease. *Journal of the American Society of Nephrology*, **3**, 88–95.

Schievink, W.I., Björnsson, J., Parisi, J.E., *et al.* (1994*a*). Arterial fibromuscular dysplasia associated with severe α_1-antitrypsin deficiency. *Mayo Clinic Proceedings*, **69**, 1040–3.

Schievink, W.I., Björnsson, J., and Piepgras, D.G. (1994*b*). Coexistence of fibromuscular dysplasia and cystic medial necrosis in a patient with Marfan's syndrome and bilateral carotid artery dissections. *Stroke*, **25**, 2492–6.

Schievink, W.I., Michels, V.V., and Piepgras, D.G. (1994*c*). Neurovascular manifestations of heritable connective tissue disorders. A review. *Stroke*, **25**, 889–903.

Schievink, W.I., Prakash, U.B.S., Piepgras, D.G., *et al.* (1994*d*). α_1-Antitrypsin deficiency in intracranial aneurysms and cervical artery dissection. *Lancet*, **343**, 452–3.

Schievink, W.I., Schaid, D.J., Rogers, H.M., *et al.* (1994*e*). On the inheritance of intracranial aneurysms. *Stroke*, **25**, 2028–37.

Schievink, W.I., Huston, J. III, Torres, V.E., *et al.* (1995). Intracranial cysts in autosomal dominant polycystic kidney disease. *Journal of Neurosurgery*, **83**, 1004–7.

Schievink, W.I., Schaid, D.J., Michels, V.V., *et al.* (1995). Familial aneurysmal subarachnoid hemorrhage: a community-based study. *Journal of Neurosurgery*, **83**, 426–9.

Schievink, W.I., Katzmann, J.A., and Piepgras, D.G., *et al.* (1996). Alpha-1-antitrypsin phenotypes among patients with intracranial aneurysms. *Journal of Neurosurgery*, **84**, 781–4.

Schievink, W.I. and Schaid, D.J. (1996). The prognosis of familial versus nonfamilial aneurysmal subarachnoid hemorrhage. *Stroke*, **27**, 340–1.

Schievink, W.I. (1997). Genetics of intracranial aneurysms. *Neurosurgery*, **40**, 651–63.

Schievink, W.I. (1997). Intracranial aneurysms. *New England Journal of Medicine*, **336**, 28–40.

Schievink, W.I., Parisi, J.E., Piepgras, D.G., *et al.* (1997*a*). Intracranial aneurysms in Marfan's syndrome: An autopsy study. *Neurosurgery*, **41**, 866–71.

Schievink, W.I., Parisi, J.E., and Piepgras, D.G. (1997*b*). Familial intracranial aneurysms: an autopsy study. *Neurosurgery*, **41**, 1247–52.

Schievink, W.I. and Torres, V.E. (1997). Spinal meningeal diverticula in autosomal dominant polycystic kidney disease. *Lancet*, **349**, 1223–4.

Schievink, W.I., Torres, V.E., Wiebers, D.O., *et al.* (1997*c*). Intracranial arterial dolichoectasia in autosomal dominant polycystic kidney disease. *Journal of the American Society of Nephrology*, **8**, 1298–1303.

Schievink, W.I. (1998). Genetics and aneurysm formation. *Neurosurgery Clinics of North America*, **9**, 485–95.

Schievink, W.I., Katzmann, J.A., and Piepgras, D.G. (1998). Alpha-1-antitrypsin deficiency in spontaneous intracranial arterial dissections. *Cerebrovascular Diseases*, **8**, 42–4.

Schievink, W.I. and Spetzler, R.F. (1998). Screening for intracranial aneurysms in patients with isolated polycystic liver disease. *Journal of Neurosurgery*, **89**, 719–21.

Schievink, W.I., Link, M.J., Piepgras, D.G., *et al.* (2002). Intracranial aneurysms surgery in Ehlers–Danlos syndrome Type IV. *Neurosurgery*, **51**, 607–13.

Schrijver, I., Schievink, W.I., and Godfrey, M. (2002). Spontaneous spinal cerebrospinal fluid leaks and minor skeletal features of Marfan syndrome: a microfibrillopathy. *Journal of Neurosurgery*, **96**, 483–9.

Schwarze, U., Schievink, W.I., Petty, E., *et al.* (2001). Haploinsufficiency for one col3a1 allele of type iii procollagen results in a phenotype similar to the vascular form of Ehlers–Danlos syndrome, Ehlers–Danlos syndrome type iv. *American Journal of Human Genetics*, **69**, 989–1001.

Sekhar, L.N., Bucur, S.D., Bank, W.O., *et al.* (1999). Venous and arterial bypass grafts for difficult tumors, aneurysms, and occlusive vascular lesions: evolution of surgical treatment and improved graft results. *Neurosurgery*, **44**, 1207–24.

Shen, M.H., Harper, P.S., and Upadhyaya, M. (1996). Molecular genetics of neurofibromatosis type 1 (NF1). *Journal of Medical Genetics*, **33**, 2–17.

Sobata, E., Ohkuma, H., and Suzuki, S. (1988). Cerebrovascular disorders associated with von Recklinghausen's neurofibromatosis: a case report. *Neurosurgery*, **22**, 544–9.

St. Jean, P., Hart, B., Webster, M., *et al.* (1996). α_1-antitrypsin deficiency in aneurysmal disease. *Human Heredity*, **46**, 92–7.

Suter W. (1949). Das kongenitale Aneurysma der basalen Hirnarterien und Cystennieren. *Schweizerische Medizinische Wochenschrift*, **79**, 471–6.

Takenaka, K., Yamakawa, H., Sakai, N., *et al.* (1998). Angiotensin I-converting enzyme gene polymorphism in intracranial saccular aneurysm individuals. *Neurological Research*, **20**, 607–11.

Takenaka, K., Sakai, H., Yamakawa, H., *et al.* (1999). Polymorphism of the endoglin gene in patients with intracranial saccular aneurysms. *Journal of Neurosurgery*, **90**, 935–8.

ter Berg, H.W.M., Dippel, D.W.J., Limburg, M., *et al.* (1992). Familial intracranial aneurysms. A review. *Stroke*, **23**, 1024–30.

The Magnetic Resonance Angiography in Relatives of Patients with Subarachnoid Hemorrhage Study Group: Risks and benefits of screening for intracranial aneurysms in first-degree relatives of patients with sporadic subarachnoid hemorrhage. *New England Journal of Medicine*, **341**, 1344–50.

Urashini, R., Ochiai, C., Okuno, S., *et al.* (1995). Cerebral aneurysms associated with von Recklinghausen neurofibromatosis: Report of two cases [Japanese]. *No Shinkei Geka*, **23**, 237–42.

van Dijk, M.A., Chang, P.C., Peters, D.J.M., *et al.* (1995). Intracranial aneurysms in polycystic kidney disease linked to chromosome 4. *Journal of the American Society of Nephrology*, 6, 1670–3.

van den Berg, J.S.P., Pals, G., Arwert, F., *et al.* (1999). Type III collagen deficiency in saccular intracranial aneurysms. Defect in gene regulation? *Stroke*, 30, 1628–31.

Wang, P.S., Longstreth, W.T. Jr, and Koepsell, T.D. (1995). Subarachnoid hemorrhage and family history. A population-based case–control study. *Archives of Neurology*, 52, 202–4.

Yoon, S., Tromp, G., Vongpunsawad, S., *et al.* (1999). Genetic analysis of MMP3, MMP9, and PAI-1 in Finnish patients with abdominal aortic or intracranial aneurysms. *Biochemical and Biophysics Research Communications*, 265, 563–8.

Zhang, B., Dhillon, S., Geary, I., *et al.* (2001). Polymorphisms in matrix metalloproteinase-1, -3, -9, and -12 genes in relation to subarachnoid hemorrhage. *Stroke*, 32, 2198–202.

Zhao, J.Z. and Han, X.D. (1998). Cerebral aneurysm associated with von Recklinghausen's neurofibromatosis: a case report. *Surgical Neurology*, 50, 592–6.

Chapter 11

Familial cerebral arteriovenous malformations

Pierre Labauge

11.1 Introduction

Hereditary cerebral arteriovenous malformations mainly include hereditary haemorrhagic telangectasia (HHT) and familial cavernomas. Both of them belong to the group of capillary malformations. Familial cerebral arteriovenous or venous malformations have not been yet reported.

11.2 Hereditary haemorrhagic telangectasia

Hereditary haemorrhagic telangectasia, also called Osler–Weber–Rendu disease (OMIM # 187300), is an autosomal dominant vascular dysplasia leading to telangectasia and arteriovenous malformations. Disease frequency is close to 2 in 100,000 (Tuente 1964). HHT is highly penetrant. Penetrance is estimated to be almost complete above age of 40 (Porteous *et al.* 1992). Telangectasia may involve many organs including the skin, mucosa, conjunctiva, retina, ears, fingers, gastrointestinal (mostly upper), and kidneys (Fig. 11.1). Cerebral vascular malformations are observed in 6–8 per cent of carriers of the gene and are usually arteriovenous angiomas, arterial aneurysms, venous malformations or indeterminate vascular malformations. In contrast, HHT is never associated with cerebral cavernomas.

11.2.1 Clinical findings

Epistaxes or nose bleeds are the most frequent initial symptom occurring in 90 per cent of symptomatic cases. The mean age of onset is 12 years (Plauchu *et al.* 1989, Aassar *et al.* 1991). The severity of epistaxes is variable; ranging from mild and non-diagnosed to massive, requiring blood transfusion. Pulmonary arteriovenous malformations are one of the most frequent manifestations. The estimated rate is between 4.6 and 23 per cent of the patients with HHT (Vase *et al.* 1985, Plauchu *et al.* 1989). In addition, it was found that 60 per cent of pulmonary arteriovenous fistula are secondary to HHT (Dines *et al.* 1974). Clinical manifestations of these pulmonary malformations include paradoxical embolism with stroke, brain abscess, pulmonary haemorrhage, and heart failure. Angiomas can also occur in the liver in about 8 per cent of the cases, and can result in cirrhosis (Plauchu *et al.* 1989).

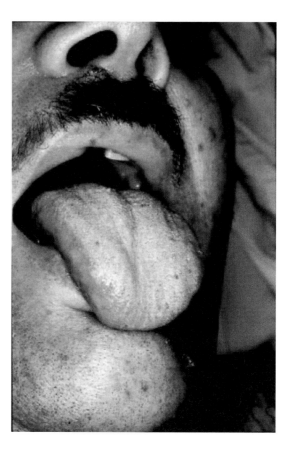

Fig. 11.1 Telangectasia on the tongue of a patient with hereditary haemorrhagic telangectasia (see Plate 3).

Neurological symptoms include migraine, brain abscess, transient ischaemic attacks (TIA), stroke, seizures, and both intracerebral and subarachnoid haemorrhage. Brain abscess, TIA, and ischaemic strokes only occur in patients with pulmonary arteriovenous malformations with right to left shunting. Migraine is frequently observed in HHT patients; 50 per cent of the patients without any cerebral lesions complain of migraine mostly with aura (Steele *et al.* 1993).

11.2.2 Genetic findings

The first gene for HHT (HHT1) was initially mapped to the long arm of the chromosome 9 (9q33–q34.1), between the markers D9S61 and D9S63 (McDonald *et al.* 1994, Shovlin *et al.* 1996). Using positional cloning, the gene was identified in 1994 (McAllister *et al.* 1994). It encodes endoglin, a transforming growth factor-beta (TGFβ) binding protein. Endoglin binds TGFβ isoforms 1 and 3 in combination with the signalling complex of TGFβ receptors types I and II. TGFβ1 plays a role in the migration, proliferation, adhesion and organization of smooth cells recruited by endothelial cells in the early stages of vasculogenesis. It also plays a critical role in angiogenesis. Vascular dysplasia is associated with modifications of TGFβ function. This was the first human disease secondary to a mutation in a member of the TGFβ receptor complex.

A second gene (HHT2) was mapped to chromosone 12q between the markers D12S345 and D12S339 (Heutinck *et al.* 1994, Johnson *et al.* 1995*a*). This gene encodes another TGFβ receptor family member; an activin receptor-like kinase 1 gene (Acvrkl1), which is a member of the serine-threonine kinase receptor family (Johnson *et al.* 1996). Acvrkl1 is expressed in endothelial and vascular smooth muscle cells (Dickson *et al.* 1995). HHT1 and HHT2 highlight the role of receptors for TGFβ family members in vascular differentiation. It is most likely that the effect of the mutations is due to loss of function. A third gene (HHT3) has also been implicated in HHT but has not yet been located or identified (Piantanida *et al.* 1996).

Genotype–phenotype correlations suggest that pulmonary arteriovenous malformations are more frequent in HHT1 than HHT2 and HHT3. HHT2 is also characterized by a later onset and milder clinical course than HHT1.

11.2.3 **Pathogenesis**

The pathogenesis of HHT begins with an early dilatation of post-capillary venules, which progressively enlarge. This enlargement leads to the disappearance of the capillary segments. As the vascular lesion increases in size, the capillary segments disappear. The lesions further evolve resulting in a direct arteriovenous communication. This sequence of events is associated with a perivascular mononuclear cell infiltrate, of which the majority of cells are lymphocytes. Monocytes and macrophages are less common. The recognized manifestations of HHT are secondary to abnormalities in vascular structure.

11.2.4 **Diagnosis**

In spite of the identification of two of the disease-causing genes (endoglin and Acvrkl1), only a clinical diagnosis of HHT can be provided for the majority of individuals. The Scientific Advisory Board of the HHT Foundation International INC (Shovlin *et al.* 2000) have developed consensus clinical diagnostic criteria. The four criteria (epistaxis, telangectasia, visceral lesions, family history) were retained as diagnostic criteria. Diagnosis is likely if at least three criteria are present, possible if only two criteria are present, and unlikely if there are less than two criteria. Capillary microscopy is a useful diagnostic technique, which can be used to identify the typical giant loops seen between the normal capillaries in the nail fold.

11.2.5 **Animal models**

Lee *et al.* (1999) have generated a mice deficient for endoglin (Eng). Eng+/− mice had a normal life expectancy. Eng−/− mice died by embryonic day 1.5 with absence of vascular organization, presence of multiple pockets of red cells on the surface of the yolk sac. The persistence of immature perineural vascular plexus suggests a failure of endothelial remodeling in the Eng$-/-$ embryos. The major vessels (aorta, branchial arteries, and carotid arteries) were atretic. These abnormalities were secondary to poor vascular smooth muscle cell formation. Urness *et al.* (2000) described mice lacking Acvrl1which developed large shunts between arteries and veins. These mice die by mid gestation with severe arteriovenous malformations resulting from fusion of arteries and veins. These results confirm that endoglin and Acvrl1 are essential for angiogenesis, and for the development of distinct arterial and venous vessels.

11.3 **Cerebral cavernous angiomas**

11.3.1 **Introduction**

Cerebral cavernomas, previously called occult vascular malformations, are capillary malformations, mostly located in the central nervous system. They are histologically defined by the occurrence of vascular cavities, without any intervening brain parenchyma, surrounded by endothelial cells and thin connective tissue. They are lacking in elastin, muscular cells, and basal membrane (Fig. 11.2). The occurrence of thrombi of different age, and degrees of calcification, within these cavities suggest that

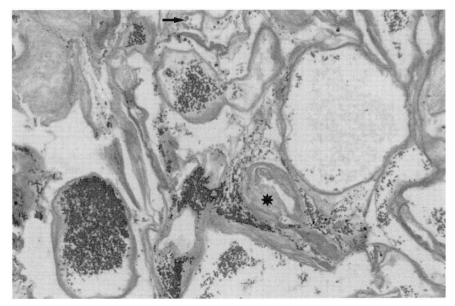

Fig. 11.2 Histological section of a cerebral cavernous angioma. This shows juxtaposition of vascular cavities surrounded by a thin (arrow) or thick (star) endothelial wall. Note the absence of intervening brain parenchyma. (Modified Gomori trichrome stain, magnification × 200.) Courtesy of Professor Françoise Chapon (see Plate 4).

they evolve with time. These malformations are fed by small vessels, without any arteries or veins. Different types of lesions are associated, including venous angiomas, arteriovenous malformations and telangectasias. Such associations support the hypothesis of linkage between different types of vascular malformations. It is becoming recognized that telangectasia and cerebral cavernomas are similar, perhaps identical. Rigamonti *et al.* (1991) proposed that all of these malformations should be referred to as cerebral capillary malformations. In contrast, HHT has never been described with cerebral cavernomas. This has been explained by cerebral cavernomas being related to abnormal development of pre-venule capillaries, and HHT to abnormal development of the post-venule capillaries.

The frequency of cerebral cavernomas is close to 0.5 per cent in the general population (Robinson *et al.* 1991). Eighty per cent of them are supratentorial, 15 per cent are located in the posterior fossa, and 5 per cent are spinal (Otten *et al.* 1989, Aiba *et al.* 1995). Most of them are single (Otten *et al.* 1989). Clinical manifestations consist of cerebral haemorrhage (11–32%), generalized or focal seizures (38–51%), focal signs (12–45%) and headache. However, the clinical penetrance of single lesions seems to be very low. A retrospective study of more than 24,000 autopsies found that only 5 per cent of the individuals with cavernomas found on post-mortem had presented with clinical symptoms (Otten *et al.* 1989). This low penetrance may explain why these lesions were previously under diagnosed.

Magnetic resonance imaging (MRI) is the best tool to diagnose cavernomas. The most typical pattern consist of mixed hyper and hypointense signals, surrounded by a rim of hypointense signal. This decreased signal corresponds to haemosiderin deposits. This pattern is highly specific of cavernomas. Rarely, haemorrhagic metastases can show a similar appearance. A classification into four types can be made on the basis of the MRI patterns (Fig. 11.3) (Zabramski *et al.* 1994). Type 1 describes a hyperintense signal on both T1 and T2 sequences. Type 2 shows a mixture of hyper- and hypointense signals. Type 3 shows hypointense signals on both T1 and T2 sequences. Type 4 shows isointense signal on both T1 and T2 sequences, and hypointense signal on gradient echo (GRE) sequences. Histological correlation has established that type 1 corresponds to acute haemorrhage and type 2 to a mixture of acute and chronic haemorrhage and calcification. The significance of the hypointense signal seen in types 3 and 4 is not clearly understood. It may correspond to cavernomas and telangectasia, but may also represent old haemorrhage.

11.3.2 Familial forms

The first observation of familial forms of cavernomas was reported by Kufs and colleagues in 1928. Further publications reported on a small numbers of families with very heterogeneous degrees of investigation. Only the most recent published families have included MRI examination. In 1995 we initiated a national study in France.

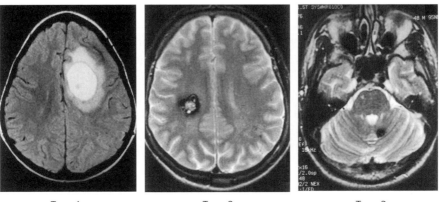

Type 1   Type 2   Type 3

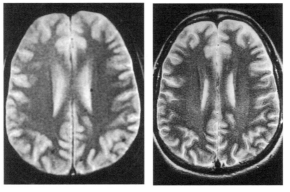

Type 4

Fig. 11.3 Classification of cerebral cavernomas based on MRI patterns. Type 1: hyperintense signal on T2. Type 2: mixed hyperintense and hypointense appearance on T2. Type 3: hypointense signal on T2. Type 4: isointense signal on T2 image (left) and hypointense signal on a GRE sequence (right).

The objectives were to define the clinical features, both neurological and systemic, and the neuroradiological appearances of familial cavernomas (Labauge *et al.* 1998*b*)

Epidemiology

The frequency of familial cavernomas is not well known. Rigamonti *et al.* (1988) estimated that in as many as 54 per cent of patients with cavernomas there was a familial basis. However, sampling bias may influence the results of this study. It was a retrospective study, the patients were non-consecutive, and the families were of Mexican-American descent. We have estimated the prevalence to be approximately 15 per cent (Tournier-Lasserve, unpublished data). A review of the literature has found that most patients with familial cavernomas have multiple lesions. Since these findings, we had prospectively investigated relatives from 22 patients with multiple cavernomas, who appeared to be sporadic cases (i.e. without any known affected relatives). MRI screening of the relatives established a familial condition in 73 per cent (16/22) (Labauge *et al.* 1998*b*).

Clinical findings

The clinical findings of patients with familial cavernomas were defined from a sample of 100 clinically affected patients (Labauge *et al.* 1998*b*). The mean age of onset was 33 years (range 5–74 years). The spectrum of clinical symptoms was: focal and generalized seizures (45%), cerebral haemorrhage (41%), focal signs (11%) and headache (3%). The average age of onset of haemorrhage was lower than the other clinical manifestations (25 versus 38 years, $P < 0.001$) (Rigamonti *et al.* 1988, Labauge *et al.* 1998*b*). These clinical findings are in fact similar to the clinical features of sporadic cavernomas (Del Curling *et al.* 1991, Moriarity *et al.* 1999).

Prognosis of the familial forms

The prognosis of familial cavernomas is not well known. Most patients (78%) will present with only one symptomatic haemorrhage during their lifetime. The remaining patients will present with between 2 and 4 haemorrhagic events. In these the mean time between two events is 37 months (range 3–138 months). The risk of haemorrhagic relapse is 30 per cent at 48 months (Labauge *et al.* 1998*b*).

Follow-up of patients highlighted neuroradiological changes, mostly without any clinical symptoms. The haemorrhagic event rate on MRI was 2.5 per cent per lesion-year, and the size and signal intensity change rate were 1.1 and 1.7 per cent respectively per lesion-year. The observed rate of haemorrhage in familial cavernomas is twice that of sporadic lesions. This rate is increased in brainstem cavernomas and MRI type 1 lesions. In contrast, size, age, and gender do not increase the risk of haemorrhage (Labauge *et al.* 2000, 2001*b*).

The appearance of new lesions is a hallmark of familial cavernomas. The yearly rate is about 0.2 lesions per patient. They are mostly asymptomatic, and seen as hypointense signals on T2 sequences (48%) and are classified as type 3 (Labauge *et al.* 2000, 2001*b*). They usually appear spontaneously, but in rare cases can occur after radiotherapy or gamma-knife treatment (Pozzati *et al.* 1996, Larson *et al.* 1998). The significance of the appearance of new lesions is poorly understood. They could correspond to previously undectable lesions which increase in size by haemorrhage or endothelial proliferation, or may represent true new lesions. Serial MRI with GRE sequences suggests that they are true new lesions (Labauge *et al.* 2001). These findings confirm the dynamic nature of cerebral cavernomas (Detwiler *et al.* 1997).

The long-term prognosis is quite favorable with a preserved independence in 80 per cent of cases. Prognosis mainly depends on whether the brainstem is involved location which is a indicator of poor prognosis, as is also the case for sporadic cases (Del Curling *et al.* 1991, Kondziolka *et al.* 1995, Moriarity *et al.* 1999).

Neuroimaging characteristics

The main neuroimaging feature distinguishing familial from sporadic cavernomas is that lesions are multiple; 83 per cent of familial patients have more than two lesions, with an mean of 7 (range: 1–51) on T2 sequences, of which 80 per cent are supratentorial. Most of them (70%) are seen as hypointense signals (type 3), while 23 per cent show a mixed signal (type 2), and only 7 per cent have a hyperintense signal on both T1 and T2 sequences (type 1). A few patients only have lesions seen as hypointense signals on T1 and T2 sequences (type 3), without any typical cavernomas (type 2).

MRI screening of asymptomatic individuals from affected families, showed that half of them had silent cavernomas. The average number of lesions was 5 (range 1–47) per subject on T2 sequences (Labauge et al. 1998b), which is not statistically different from the symptomatic subjects (Plauchu et al. 1989). These features suggest that clinical penetrance is higher in familial forms than in sporadic cases, and that it is not related to the number of the lesions. The distribution of the lesions is the same in symptomatic and asymptomatic patients, except for the type 1 lesions which are more frequently observed in symptomatic subjects (Labauge et al. 1998a, Brunereau et al. 2000a).

MRI investigation of many families has proved the sensitivity of the GRE sequences. The average number of the lesions detected per subject increased from 5 on T2 sequences, to 16 on GRE sequences ($P < 0.001$). Of the 15 subjects with a single lesion on T2, 5 had multiple lesions on GRE. The sensitivity of GRE also identifies lesions in undiagnosed individuals, since 5 per cent of the subjects with a normal T2 MRI had cavernomas on GRE. Therefore, the risk of misdiagnosing cavernomas in clinically unaffected family members based on T2 sequences is 5 per cent. These results underline the benefit of the routine use of GRE to investigate relatives of patients with familial cavernomas (Labauge et al. 1998b).

Correlation of the lesions number and age

Although cavernomas are classified as vascular malformations, they have to be considered as evolving lesions. The number of the lesions is strongly related to the age of the subjects. While the average number of lesions is five in subjects under 50 years old, it increases to 15 in subjects over 50. This progression is supported by the observation of the appearance of new lesions during a patients lifespan (Brunereau et al. 2000b). Kattapong et al. (1995) have estimated that lesion count increases by one lesion per decade. A three year retrospective study of 40 patients established that new lesions appeared in 28 per cent of them. These were mainly seen as hypointense signals on T1 and T2 sequences and were mainly asymptomatic (Labauge et al. 2000). They usually appear spontaneously, but external factors, such as radiotherapy can promote their occurrence (Larson et al. 1998).

Other locations and associated malformations

Other types of cerebral vascular malformations can be found in patients with familial cavernomas. These include telangectasias, arteriovenous malformations and venous angiomas. The latter, also called developmental venous anomaly (DVA), are most often asymptomatic and diagnosed fortuitously. The risk of evolution and haemorrhage is considered to be very low.

Cavernomas in extraneurological locations are becoming frequently recognized. The histological observation of Wood *et al.* (1957) is a remarkable example. In this report, the autopsy of a patient with multiple cerebral cavernomas, revealed cavernomas in the heart, kidneys, skin, and liver. Histological analysis found that these lesions were of capillary type, similar to cerebral cavernomas.

The most frequently described locations are cutaneous and retinal. Multiple kinds of cutaneous lesions have been described. These include bluish nodules, cherry angiomas, capillary vascular anomalies and eruptive multiple angiokeratomas (Bartolomei *et al.* 1992, Ostlere *et al.* 1996). A distinctive hyperkeratotic cutaneous lesion was reported in 4 French families with cerebral cavernomas (Labauge *et al.* 1999). Cutaneous lesions are congenital, single, mostly located on the lower limbs, and do not evolve. They are subcutaneous venous angioma, with superficial angioma, and covered by a hyperkeratotic reaction. Histological analysis shows abundant dilated capillaries, and blood-filled spaces in the papillary and reticular dermis extending to the hypodermis, with orthokeratosis and hyperkeratosis. Following the criteria established by the International Society for the Study of Vascular Anomalies (Enjolras and Mulliken 1998), they are defined as hyperkeratotic cutaneous capillary venous malformations (HCCVMs). To the best of our knowledge, they have never found without associated cerebral cavernomas.

Cavernomas located in the retina very rare. They are formed by vascular malformations, seen on fundoscopy or fluorescein angiography as capillary lesions, and are unilateral and mostly asymptomatic (Gass 1971, Klein *et al.* 1975, Colvard *et al.* 1978, Goldberg *et al.* 1979, Messmer *et al.* 1983, 1984; Schwartz *et al.* 1984, Pancurak *et al.* 1985, Dobyns *et al.* 1987, Moffat *et al.* 1998). The presence of such lesions in a patient without any past neurological history should be a strong suggestion to the physician to perform brain MRI to determine whether asymptomatic cerebral cavernomas are present (Laberge-Le-Couteulx *et al.* 2002). Recently, other kinds of ocular lesions have been described as choroidal hemangioma (Sarraf *et al.* 2000).

These observations confirm that cavernomas can be seen outside the central nervous system. These systemic cavernomas are also capillary malformations but, unlike cerebral cavernomas, they are stable and not prone to evolution.

11.3.3 Genetic findings

Medical genetics

Analysis of the familial cavernoma pedigrees showed an autosomal dominant inheritance with an equal sex ratio. Half of the obligatory transmitters with cavernomas on MRI are clinically asymptomatic. This finding demonstrtaes that clinical penetrance is incomplete, and close to 50 per cent. Clinical penetrance is higher than in sporadic cavernomas, which is estimated to less than 5 per cent. This difference is attributed to the multiplicity of the lesions in the familial forms. Neuroradiological penetrance is very high, but incomplete. A skipped generation has been found in one family. The age above which neuroradiological penetrance is complete is still unknown.

Analysis of the pedigrees strongly suggests a high degree of clinical and neuroradiological heterogeneity. Anticipation was only found in one report (Siegel *et al.* 1998). MRI screening of relatives of patients with multiple lesions presenting as sporadic cases has shown that 73 per cent of them in fact have a familial form. The absence of familial cavernomas in the remaining 27 per cent index cases can be explained by occurrence of germinal neomutation, somatic mutation, and incomplete neuroradiological penetrance. In these sporadic patients with multiple cavernomas, evolution is similar to that of familial forms, notably with the appearance of new lesions (Labauge *et al.* 2001*a*).

Molecular studies

In 1995, the study of a large Hispano-American family allowed the mapping of a first gene (CCM1) to a 33 centimorgan (cM) interval of the long arm of the chromosome 7 (7q11–q22) (Dubovsky *et al.* 1995). These findings were confirmed by further analysis of five different American families and the interval was reduced to 4 cM between the markers D7S2410 and D7S689 (Günel *et al.* 1995, Johnson *et al.* 1995*b*, Gil-Nagel *et al.* 1996) All of the published Hispano-American families are linked to 7q and share a common haplotype. This founder effect results from a common ancestor (Gûnel *et al.* 1996). In contrast, this haplotype was not shared by either the French families (Laberge-Lecouteulx *et al.* 1999*b*), or a Hispanic families originating from south of Spain (Jung *et al.* 1999). The mapping of CCM1 to chromosome 7q11–q22 was confirmed in the French families (Laberge-Lecouteulx *et al.* 1999*b*). Sixty-five per cent of the French families were consistent with linkage to CCM1. Two other genes, CCM2 and CCM3, have been mapped to the short arm of the chromosome 7 (7p15–p13), and the long arm of chromosome 3 (3q25.2–27) respectively (Craig *et al.* 1998), establishing the genetic heterogeneity of the clinical phenotype. No genotype–phenotype correlation has been established yet.

CCM1/KRIT1 was identified in 1999 (Laberge-LeCouteulx *et al.* 1999*a*, Sahoo *et al.* 1999). Interestingly, the nature of CCM1/KRIT1 mutations appears to be highly stereotyped. To date, all reported CCM-causing KRIT1 mutations are predicted to lead to a premature stop codon (nonsense mutations, nucleotide deletions/insertions with frameshift). No missense mutation has been identified (Cave-Riant *et al.* in press). The only nucleotide substitutions predicted to be missense mutations lead at mRNA level to an abnormal splicing and a premature stop codon. Nonsense mRNA decay (NMD), as a consequence of premature stop codons, has been shown to underlie haploinsufficicency in many disorders. These data suggest that KRIT1 mRNA decay due to the presence of premature stop codons and KRITI haploinsufficicency may be the underlying mechanism of CCM1. These mutations have been found in the families sharing cerebral and non-cerebral cavernomas (Eerola *et al.* 2000). In addition a *de novo* germline mutation has recently been reported (Lucas 2001). The protein KRIT1 which is encoded for by CCM1, contains 736 amino acids, including four ankyrin domains, a FERM domain and a C-terminal portion interacting with Rap1A. The N-terminal region of KRIT 1 contains a NPXY motif required for the interaction of KRIT1 with integrin cytoplasmic domain-associated protein 1 (icap1). KRIT1 interacts with the 200 amino acid isoform of icap (icap1α), but not with the 150 amino acid form resulting from alternating splicing (icap1β) (Zhang *et al.* 2001).

The size of the interval containing CCM2 and CCM3 is unchanged since 1998 and is close to 22 cM. CCM2 and CCM3 are still unidentified.

Acknowledgements

I thank Professor Elisabeth Tournier-Lasserve, Doctor Christian Denier (Lariboisiere Hospital), Professors Laurent Brunereau (CHU de Tours) and Françoise Chapon (CHU de Caen), Doctor Odile Enjolras (Lariboisiere Hospital), and all of the Members of the French Society of Neurosurgery for their help and contribution. I thank David O'Callaghan Ph.D. (INSERM U431) for his critical reading.

References

Aassar, O.S., Friedman, C.M., and White, R.I. (1991). The natural history of epistaxis in hereditary hemorrhagic telangiectasia. *Laryngoscope*, **101**, 977–80.

Aiba, T., Tanaka, R., Koike, T., Kameyama, S., Takeda, N., and Komata, T. (1995). Natural history of intracranial malformations. *Journal of Neurosurgery*, **83**, 56–9.

Bartolomei, F., Lemarquis, P., Alicherif, A., Lepillouer-Prost, A., Sayag, J., and Khalil, R. (1992). Angiomatose cavernomateuse systématisée avec localisations multiples cérébrales et cutanées. *Revue Neurologique*, **148**, 568–70.

Brunereau, L., Labauge, P., Tournier-Lasserve, E., Laberge, S., Lévy, C., Houtteville, J.-P. and the French Society of Neurosurgery. (2000*a*). Familial forms of intracranial cavernous angiomas: MR imaging findings in 51 families. *Radiology*, **214**, 209–16.

Brunereau, L., Laberge, S., Lévy, C., Houtteville J.-P., and Labauge, P. (2000*b*). *De novo* lesions in the familial form of cerebral cavernous angiomas: clinical and MR features in 29 non-Hispanic families. *Surgical Neurology*, **53**, 475–83.

Cave-Riant, F., Denier, C., Labauge, P., *et al.* (2002). Spectrum and expression analysis of KRIT1 mutations in 121 consecutive and unrelated patients with cerebral cavernous malformations. *European Journal of Human Genetics*, **10**, 733–40.

Colvard, D.M., Robertson, D.M., and Trautmann, J.C. (1978). Cavernous hemangioma of the retina. *Annals of Neurology*, **96**, 2042–4.

Craig, H.D., Günel, M., Cepeda, O., *et al.* (1998). Multilocus linkage identifies two new loci for a Mendelian from of stroke, cerebral cavernouas malformation, at 7p15–13 and 3q25.2–27. *Human Molecular Genetics*, **12**, 1851–8.

Del Curling, O.D., Kelly, D., Elster, A.D., *et al.* (1991). An analysis of the natural history of cavernous angiomas. *Journal of Neurosurgery*, **75**, 702–8.

Detwiler, P.L., Porter, R.W., Zabramski, J.M., and Spetzler, R.F. (1997). *De novo* formation of a central nervous system cavernous malformation: implications for predicting risk of hemorrhage. *Journal of Neurosurgery*, 87, 629–32.

Dickson, M.C., Martin, J.S., Cousins, F.M., *et al.* (1995). Defective hematopoiesis and vasculogenesis in transforming growth-factor-beta-1 knock out mice. *Development*, 121, 1845–54.

Dines, D.E., Arms, R.A., Bernatz, P.E., and Gomes, M.R. (1974). Pulmonary arteriovenous fistulas. *Mayo Clinic Proceedings*, 49, 460–5.

Dobyns, W.B., Michels, V.V., Goover, R.V., *et al.* (1987). Familial cavernous malformations of the central nervous system and retina. *Annals of Neurology*, 6, 578–83.

Dubovsky, J., Zabramski, J.M., Kurth, J., *et al.* (1995). A gene responsible for cavernous malformations of the brain maps to chromosome 7. *Human Molecular Genetics*, 4, 453–8.

Eerola, I., Plate, K.H., Spiegel, R., *et al.* (2000). KRIT1 is mutated in hyperkeratotic cutaneous capillary-venous malformation associated with cerebral capillary malformation. *Human Molecular Genetics*, 9, 1351–5.

Enjolras, O. and Mulliken, J.B. (1998). Vascular tumors and vascular malformations (New Issues). *Advances in Dermatology*, 13, 375–423.

Gass, J.D. (1971). Cavernous hemangioma of the retina. A neuro-oculo-cutaneous syndrome. *American Journal of Ophthalmology*, 71, 799–814.

Gil-Nagel, A., Dubovsky, J., Wilcox, K.J., *et al.* (1996). Familial cerebral cavernous angioma: a gene localized to a 15 cM interval on chromosome 7q. *Annals of Neurology*, 39, 807–10.

Goldberg, R.E., Pheasant, T.R., and Shields, J.A. (1979). Cavernous hemangioma of the retina. A four generation pedigree with neurocutaneous manifestations and an example of bilateral retinal involvement. *Annals of Neurology*, 97, 2321–4.

Günel, M., Awad, I.A., Anson, J., and Lifton, R.P. (1995). Mapping a gene causing cerebral cavernous malformation to 7q11.2–q21. *Proceedings of the National Academy of Sciences*, 92, 6620–4.

Günel, M., Awad, I.A., Finberg, K., *et al.* (1996). A founder mutation as a cause of cerebral cavernous malformation in hispanic americans. *New England Journal of Medicine*, 334, 946–51.

Heutinck, P., Haitejema, T., Breedveld, G.J., *et al.* (1994). Linkage of hereditary haemorrhagic telangectasia to chromosome 9q34 and evidence for locus heterogeneity. *Journal of Medical Genetics*, 31, 933–6.

Johnson, D.W., Berg, J.N., Gallione, C.J., *et al.* (1995*a*). A second locus for hereditary haemorrhagic telangectasia maps to chromosome 12. *Genome Research*, 5, 21–8.

Johnson, D.W., Berg, J.N., Baldwin, M.A., *et al.* (1996). Mutations in the activin receptor-like kinase 1 gene in hereditary haemorrhagic telangectasia type 2. *Nature Genetics*, 13, 189–95.

Johnson, E.W., Lyer, L.M., Rich, S.S., *et al.* (1995*b*). Refined localization of the cerebral cavernous malformation gene (*CCM1*) to a 4-cM interval of chromosome 7q contained in a well-defined YAC Contig. *Genome Research*, 5, 368–80.

Jung, H., Labauge, P., Laberge, S., *et al.* (1999). Spanish families with cavernous angiomas do not share the Hispano-American CCM1 haplotype. *Journal of Neurology, Neurosurgery, and Psychiatry*, 67, 551–2.

Kattapong, V.J., Hart, B.L., and Davis, L.E. (1995). Familial cerebral cavernous angiomas: clinical and radiologic studies. *Neurology*, 45, 492–7.

Klein, M., Goldberg, M.F., and Cotlier, E. (1975). Cavernous hemangioma of the retina. Report of four cases. *Annals of Ophthalmology*, 9, 1213–21.

Kondziolka, D., Lunsford, L.D., and Kestle, J.R.W. (1995).The natural history of cerebral cavernous malformations. *Journal of Neurosurgery*, 83, 820–4.

Labauge, P., Laberge, S., Brunereau, L., *et al.* (1998*a*). Clinical and genetic study of 57 French familial cavernomas pedigrees. *Neurology*, **50**, A441.

Labauge, P., Laberge, S., Brunereau, L., Lévy, C., Tournier-Lasserve, E and the Société Française de Neurochirurgie. (1998*b*). Hereditary cerebral cavernous angiomas: clinical and genetic features in 57 French families. *Lancet*, **352**, 1892–7.

Labauge, P., Enjolras, O., Bonerandi, J.J., *et al.* (1999). An association between autosomal dominant cerebral cavernomas and a distinctive hyperkeratotic cutaneous vascular malformation in 4 families. *Annals of Neurology*, **45**, 250–4.

Labauge, P., Brunereau, L., Laberge, S., and Lévy, C., and Houtteville, J.P. (2000). Natural history of familial cavernomas: a retrospective clinical and MRI study of 40 patients. *Neuroradiology*, **42**, 327–32.

Labauge, P., Brunereau, L., Coubes, P., *et al.* (2001*a*). Appearance of new lesions in two non familial cerebral cavernomas patients. *European Neurology*, **45**, 83–8.

Labauge, P., Brunereau, L., Laberge, S., and Houtteville, J.P. (2001*b*). A prospective follow-up of 33 asymptomatic patients with familial cerebral cavernomas. *Neurology*, **57**, 1825–8.

Laberge-Le Couteulx, S., Jung, H.H., Labauge, P., *et al.* (1999*a*). Truncating mutations in *KRIT1*, a protein interacting with rap1A, cause hereditary cavernous angiomas. *Nature Genetics*, **23**, 189–93.

Laberge-Le Couteulx, S., Labauge, P., Marechal, E., Maciazek, J., and Tournier-Lasserve, E. (1999*b*). Genetic heterogeneity and absence of founder effect in a series of 36 French cerebral cavernous angiomas families. *European Journal of Human Genetics*, **7**, 499–504.

Laberge-Le Couteulx, S., Brezin, A., Fontaine, B., Tournier-Lasserve, E., and Labauge, P. (2002). KRIT I/CCM1 truncating mutation in a patient with cerebral and retinal cavernous angiomas. *Archives of Ophthalmology*, **120**, 217–18.

Larson, J.J., Ball, W.S., Bove K.E., Crone, K.R., and Tew, J.M. (1998). Formation of intracerebral cavernous malformations after radiation treatment for central nervous system neoplasia in children. *Journal of Neurosurgery*, **88**, 51–6.

Lee, D.Y., Sorensen, L.K., Brooke, B.S., *et al.* (1999). Defective angiogenesis in mice lacking endoglin. *Science*, **284**, 1534–7.

Lucas, M., Costa, A.F., Montori, M., *et al.* (2001). Germline mutations in the CCM1 gene, encoding Krit1, cause cerebral cavernous malformations. *Annals of Neurology*, **49**, 529–32.

McAllister, K.A., Grogg, K.M., Johnson, D.W., *et al.* (1994). Endoglin, a TGF-beta binding protein of endothelial cells, is the gene for hereditary haemorrhagic telangectasia type I. *Nature Genetics*, **8**, 345–51.

McDonald, M.T., Papenberg, K.A., Ghosh, S., *et al.* (1994). A disease locus for hereditary haemorrhagic telangectasia maps to 9q33–34. *Nature Genetics*, **6**, 197–204.

Messmer, E., Laqua, H., Wessing, A., Spitznas, M., and Weidle, E. (1983). Nine cases of cavernous hemangioma of the retina. *American Journal of Ophthalmology*, **95**, 383–90.

Messmer, E., Font, R.L., Laqua, H., Höpping, W., and Naumann, G.O.H. (1984). Cavernous hemangioma of the retina. Immunohistochemical and ultrastructural observations. *Archives of Ophthalmology*, **102**, 413–18.

Moffat, K.P., Lee, M.S., and Ghosh, M. (1988). Retinal cavernous hemangioma. *Canadian Journal of Ophthalmology*, **23**, 133–5.

Moriarity, J.L., Wetzel, M., Clatterbuck, R.E., *et al.* (1999). The natural history of cavernous malformations: a prospective study of 68 patients. *Neurosurgery*, **44**, 1166–73.

Ostlere, L., Hart, Y., and Misch, K.J. (1996). Cutaneous and cerebral haemangiomas associated with eruptive angiokeratomas. *British Journal of Dermatology*, **135**, 98–101.

Otten, P., Pizzolato, G.P., Rilliet, B., and Berney, J. (1989). A propos de 131 cas d'angiomes caverneux (cavernomes) du SN.C, repérés par l'analyse rétrospective de 24 535 autopsies. *Neurochirurgie*, 35, 82–3.

Pancurak, J., Goldberg, M.F., Frenkel, M., and Crowell, R.M. (1985). Cavernous hemangioma of the retina. Genetic and central nervous system involvement. *Retina*, 5, 215–20.

Piantanida, M., Buscarini, E., Dellavecchia, C., *et al.* (1996). Hereditary haemorrhagic telangectasia with extensive liver involvement is not caused by either HHT1 or HHT2. *Journal of Medical Genetics*, 33, 441–3.

Plauchu, H., de Chadarevian, J.P., Bideau, A., and Robert, J.M. (1989). Age-related clinical profile of hereditary hemorrhagic telangectasia in an epidemiologically recruited population. *American Journal of Medical Genetics*, 32, 291–7.

Porteous, M.E.M., Burns, J., and Proctor, S.J. (1992). Hereditary haemorrhagic telangectasias: a clinical analysis. *Journal of Medical Genetics*, 29, 527–30.

Pozzati, E., Acciari, N., Tognetti, F., Marliani, F., and Giangaspero, F. (1996). Growth, subsequent bleeding and de novo appearance of cerebral angiomas. *Neurosurgery*, 4, 662–70.

Rigamonti, D., Johnson, P.C., Spetzler, R.F., Hadley, M.N., and Drayer, B.P. (1991). Cavernous malformations and capillary telangectasia: a spectrum within a single pathological entity. *Neurosurgery*, 8, 60–4.

Rigamonti, D., Hadley, M.N., Drayer, B.P., *et al.* (1988). Cerebral cavernous malformations. Incidence and familial occurrence. *New England Journal of Medicine*, 319, 343–7.

Robinson, J.R., Awad, I.A., and Little, J.R. (1991). Natural history of the cavernous angioma. *Journal of Neurosurgery*, 75, 709–14.

Russel, D.S. and Rubenstein, L.J. (1989). *Pathology of tumors of the nervous system*. 5th edn. Williams and Wilkins, Baltimore, MD, pp. 730–6.

Sahoo, T., Johnson, E.W., Thomas, J.W., *et al.* (1999). Mutations in the gene encoding *KRIT1*, a Krev-1/rap1a binding protein cause cerebral cavernous malformations (CCM1). *Human Molecular Genetics*, 8, 2325–33.

Sarraf, D., Payne, A.M., Kitchen, N.D., *et al.* (2000). Familial cavernous hemangioma. An expanding ocular spectrum. *Archives of Ophthalmology*, 118, 969–73.

Schwartz, A.C., Weaver, G., Bloomfield, R., and Tyler, M.E. (1984). Cavernous hemangioma of the retina, cutaneous angiomas and intracranial vascular lesion by computed tomography and nuclear magnetic resonance imaging. *American Journal of Ophthalmology*, 98, 483–7.

Shovlin, C.L., Hughes, J.M.B., Tuddenhal. E.G.D., *et al.* (1996). A gene for hereditary haemorrhagic telangectasia maps to chormosome 9q3. *Nature Genetics*, 6, 205–9.

Shovlin, C.L., Guttmacher, A.E., Buscarini, E., *et al.* (2000). Diagnostic criteria for hereditary hemorrhagic telangiectasia (Rendu–Osler–Weber syndrome). *American Journal of Medical Genetics*, 6, 66–7.

Siegel, A.M., Andermann, E., Badhwar, A., *et al.* (1998). Anticipation in familial cavernous angioma: a study of 52 families from International Familial Cavernous Angioma Study. *Lancet*, 352, 1676–7.

Steele, J.S., Nath, P.U., Burn, J., and Porteous, M.E.M. (1993). An association between migrainous aura and hereditary telangectasia. *Headache*, 33, 145–8.

Tuente, W. (1964). Klinik und Genetik der Oslerschen Kranheit. *Z. Menschl. Vererb. Konstitutionsl*, 37, 221–50.

Urness, L.D., Sorensen, L.K., and Li, D.Y. (2000). Arteriovenous malformations in mice lacking activin receptor-like kinase-1. *Nature Genetics*, 26, 328–31.

Vase, P., Holm, M., and Arendrup, H. (1985). Pulmonary arteriovenous fistulas in hereditary haemorrhagic telangectasia. *Acta Medica Scandinavica*, **218**, 105–9.

Wood, M.W., White, R.J., and Kernohan, K.W. (1957). Cavernous hemangiomatosis involving the brain, spinal cord, heart, skin and kidney. Report of a case. *Staff Meetings of the Mayo Clinic*, **32**, 249–54.

Zabramski, J.M., Washer, T.M., Spetzler, R.F., *et al.* (1994). The natural history of familial cavernous malformations. Results of an ongoing study. *Journal of Neurosurgery*, **80**, 422–32.

Zhang, J., Clatterbruck, R.E., Rigamonti, D., *et al.* (2001). Interaction between krit1 and icap1a infers perturbation of integrin b1-mediated angiogenesis in the pathogenesis of cerebral cavernous malformation. *Human Molecular Genetics*, **10**, 2953–60.

Chapter 12

The genetics of paediatric stroke

Fenella Kirkham and Mara Prengler

12.1 Introduction

Unlike in adults atherosclerosis is a relatively uncommon cause of stroke in childhood, while Mendelian conditions, and some chromosomal abnormalities, causing stroke are much more common. There is a long list of inherited conditions which predispose to cerebrovascular disease and stroke in childhood (Natowicz and Kelley 1987, Pavlakis *et al.* 2000), but our understanding of the precise mechanisms has been limited until recently. Several conditions with cerebral vascular manifestations are now being intensively studied. A classification of monogenic disorders leading to childhood stroke is given in Table 12.1; this is by aetiological mechanism, although a number of causes can result in stroke by more than one mechanism. Many of these affect children and young adults in a similar fashion and are dealt with in detail in chapters on monogenic ischaemic stroke (Chapter 6), and haemorrhagic stroke (Chapters 9–11). Here cross-references are made to the appropriate chapters in Table 12.1.

There are several single gene disorders with a highly significant predisposition to stroke, such as sickle cell disease (SCD), homocystinuria, Menkes' disease and Neurofibromatosis (Roach and Riela 1995, Pavlakis *et al.* 2000). These conditions provide an opportunity to investigate gene–gene and gene–environment interactions, as the reasons why some but not all of these patients develop stroke is not well understood. In addition, the mechanisms that trigger cerebrovascular disease in children, in whom atherosclerosis is minimal, may lead to insights into the initiation of endothelial damage in general. As for adult stroke, genes controlling intermediate risk factors, such as hypertension and hyperhomocysteinaemia, may be important in children. This chapter will look at the available data on risk factors for stroke in children which may have a genetic basis. SCD, a recessively inherited condition which is the commonest cause of childhood stroke world-wide, will be considered in more detail as an example of the complex issues involved.

12.2 Phenotype of childhood stroke

Except for children with SCD, in whom the incidence is similar to that for elderly adults in the general population (Earley *et al.* 1998), stroke is relatively rare in children and there are few large well-documented series. The incidence of childhood stroke is

Table 12.1a Monogenic causes of arterial ischaemic childhood stroke

Category	Aetiological mechanism	Examples	Section number or external reference
Arterial ischaemia	Cardioembolic	Cardiomyopathies: primary/secondary	Natowicz and Kelley 1987
		Familial atrial myxoma	
		Familial dysrhythmias	
	Thrombotic/thromboembolic	Haemaglobinopathies	Section 12.3
		Sickle cell disease	
		Haemaglobin SC disease	
		Metabolic	
		Homocysteinuria	Section 12.8.2
		Dyslipoproteinaemias	Section 12.8.4
		Prohrombotic	Section 12.8.3
		Protein C or S deficiency	
		ATIII deficiency	
		APC resistance	
	Vascular anomalies associated with ischaemic stroke	Moya–Moya disease and syndrome	Sections 6.3.1 and 12.6
		Fibromuscular displasia	
		Kohlmeier–Degos disease	
		Familial arterial dissection	Section 12.5
	Others	Fabry's disease	Section 6.4.1
		Neurofibromatosis Type 1 (NK1)	Section 6.3.5
		Inherited immunodeficiency syndromes	Section 12.8.5
		Pseudoxanthoma elasticum	Section 6.3.4
		Menke's disease	

Table 12.1b Other monogenic causes of childhood stroke

Category	Aetiological mechanism	Examples	Section number
Haemorrhagic	Vascular malformations	Hereditary haemorrhagic telangectasia	Section 11.2
		Familial arteriovenous malformations	
		Familial cavernomas	Section 11.3
	Aneurysms	Familial aneurysms	Section 10.3
Venous thrombosis	Prothrombotic disorders	Protein C or S deficiency	Section 12.7
		ATIII deficiency	
		APC resistance	
		Prothrombin 20210 mutation	
		Hyperhomocysteinaemia	
Mitochrondial		Melas	Section 6.7
Chromosomal Abnormalities		Down syndrome	
		Williams syndrome	

at least 2.5 per 100,000 (Broderick *et al*. 1993). There is a wide variety of clinical presentations, including seizures secondary to venous sinus thrombosis and acute hemiparesis, often related to arterial stoke but sometimes in the context of metabolic stroke, for example, secondary to mitochondrial disease (Pavlakis *et al*. 2000). Around half of childhood strokes are ischaemic (Broderick *et al*. 1993). Approximately half the children with a first-ever arterial ischaemic stroke have a known predisposing cause, such as SCD or congenital cardiac anomaly (Ganesan *et al*. 2002). For the remainder, the stroke is, at least initially, unexplained.

Of the 212 children presenting with arterial ischaemic stroke to Great Ormond Street Hospital (London, UK) from 1978 to 2002, 44 had underlying conditions with Mendelian inheritance: 38 with SCD, 1 with sickle cell trait, 1 with neurofibromatosis type 1, 1 with cystinuria and 3 with genetic causes of immumodeficiency. In addition, 4 had chromosomal abnormalities (3 with Down syndrome and 1 with Williams syndrome). Three had parents with stroke (2 children with cryptogenic stroke whose parent had had an arterial stroke and 1 with HIV infection whose parent had had a sinovenous thrombosis) and there was a pair of siblings with stroke and cerebrovascular disease in the context of SCD, a condition in which family history of stroke is relatively common (Driscoll *et al*. 1997). A positive family history of stroke in other relatives was elicited for a further 35 patients. Haemorrhagic stroke and venous sinus thrombosis are also seen in childhood and may occur in the context of illnesses with Mendelian inheritance (Al-Jarallah *et al*. 2000, de Veber and Andrew 2001), but there are few data available on family history. Stroke also occurs in the neonatal period, in around 1 in 4000 births, and is an important cause of hemiplegic cerebral palsy (Lynch and Nelson 2001).

Although there is no epidemiologically based data, studies from large teaching hospitals have reported that children with arterial stroke have an early recurrence risk for stroke of 10–25 per cent (Riikonen and Santavouri 1994, Abram *et al*. 1996, Ganesan *et al*. 1998, Sträter *et al*. 2002). About 80 per cent of children with arterial stroke have abnormal conventional or magnetic angiography studies (Shirane *et al*. 1992, Ganesan *et al*. 2002). Typical abnormalities include stenosis or occlusion of the distal internal carotid or middle cerebral arteries, internal carotid or vertebral dissection, Moya–Moya syndrome (Ganesan *et al*. 1997, Husson *et al*. 2002), and occasionally rarer patterns such as cerebral vasculitis (Lanthier *et al*. 2002). Relatively few children presenting with stroke have congenital cerebral arteriographic anomalies which do not change over time. Longitudinal studies show that 25–50 per cent of abnormal arteriograms become completely normal at follow-up (Chabrier *et al*.1998, Prengler *et al*. 2000), while others may develop progressive cerebrovascular disease (e.g. Moya–Moya syndrome) (Prengler *et al*. 2000).

12.3 Sickle cell disease

The best studied population is that with SCD, where the majority of children with stroke have large vessel disease (Stockman *et al*. 1972) with intimal hyperplasia

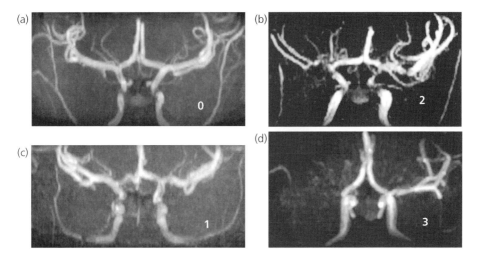

Fig. 12.1 MRA children with SCD (Kirkham *et al.* 2001). (a) Normal (grade 0); (b) mild (grade 1) turbulence; (c) moderate (grade 2) turbulence; (d) severe (grade 3) turbulence.

pathologically (Rothman *et al.* 1986). Twenty-five per cent of patients have had a stroke by the age of 45; ischaemic stroke predominates in childhood while the majority of adults have spontaneous intracerebral or subarachnoid hamorrhage (Ohene-Frempong *et al.* 1998). Cerebrovascular disease may now be diagnosed non-invasively in asymptomatic patients using transcranial Doppler ultrasound to detect very high velocities in the internal carotid/middle cerebral artery as an indicator of critical stenosis (Adams *et al.* 1997). At some stage during follow-up, around 7–8 per cent have velocities $>200 \, \text{cm s}^{-1}$, which predicts a 40 per cent risk of stroke over the next 3 years. Turbulence may also be recognized and graded on MRA (Kirkham *et al.* 2001*a*) (Fig. 12.1). There are, however, well-documented patients with SCD and apparent stroke who do not have arteriographic abnormalities and may have other risk factors, such as recent chest crisis or poor cardiac function (Wood 1978, Ganesan *et al.* 2002). Venous sinus thrombosis has also been documented (Pavlakis *et al.* 1989). The genetic and environmental basis of these stroke syndromes is likely to be different. In addition, there is a little evidence that the vascular disease may improve or deteriorate under poorly understood genetic or environmental influences and this may determine the clinical presentation, for example, with ischaemic or haemorrhagic stroke.

In this population, in contrast to most children with strokes who do not have SCD, silent infarction, possibly related to small vessel disease, occurs in up to 25 per cent (Kinney *et al.* 1999, Saunders *et al.* 2001) (Fig. 12.2) and may progress silently (Pegelow *et al.* 2002) or predict clinical stroke (Miller *et al.* 2001) as well as being associated with cognitive difficulties (Armstrong *et al.* 1996, Watkins *et al.* 1998). Clinical transient

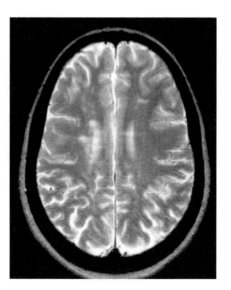

Fig. 12.2 'Silent' cerebral infarction in the deep white matter in a child with SCD.

ischaemic attacks also predict stroke, with a relative risk of 56 (95% CIs 12–285) (Ohene-Frempong *et al.* 1998) and seizures also appear to be a marker for cerebrovascular disease and silent infarction in this population (Kinney *et al.* 1999). For patients with homozygous sickle cell disease, 10–16 per cent have seizures at some stage, compared with around 1 per cent for the general population, while for those with haemoglobin SC disease, the figure is around 7 per cent. Seizures herald the onset of stroke in around 20 per cent of patients. This very complex recessively inherited disease illustrates the need for a very careful description of the phenotype when attempting to look for genes for stroke and other neurological complications. The genetic predisposition to large and small vessel disease, silent and clinical infarction, seizures and cognitive deterioration could be very different or could be linked in some way to environmental exposure, for example, to infection, poor nutrition (Osuntokun 1979) or hypoxaemia (Kirkham *et al.* 2001*b*).

The cellular characteristic of the typical 'sickle-shaped' red blood cells was first described at the beginning of the twentieth century (Herrick 1910). Pauling *et al.* (1949) described the abnormal haemoglobin (Hb) SS molecule and described this as a 'molecular disease'. In SCD, an abnormal beta globin gene codes the substitution of the amino acid valine for glutamic acid (Ingram 1957) which is normally present at the sixth position from the amino terminus of the beta globin chain (β6 Glut→Val). The resulting Hb S is unstable and has an increased propensity to polymerise under certain physical conditions. Historically, the sickle gene has conferred a selective advantage by virtue of a relative resistance to falciparum malaria in heterozygotes with sickle cell trait, which otherwise does not appear to be associated with disease

(Serjeant 1997), although there are few data looking at the effect on stroke risk in elderly adults. However, homozygotes (with both Hb genes coding for Hb S, HbSS) have a
serious life-threatening disease, sickle cell anaemia. There are two other common
genotypes included under the term SCD: Hb SC disease and sickle cell-beta thalassaemia, where one Hb gene codes for Hb S and the other codes for another abnormality of the beta globin chain (either Hb C (HbSC) or β-thalassaemia (HbSβthal).

Sickle cell disease is found mainly in Equatorial Africa, where 10–30 per cent of
individuals have sickle cell trait. However the sickle cell gene has different haplotypes.
The African haplotypes are Senegal, Benin and Bantu. The Benin haplotype is also
found in different foci in Mediterranean countries, such as Italy, Sicily, Greece, Spain,
Portugal, Israel and North Africa, and as far as Western Arabia (Serjeant 1997). The
Asian haplotype is an independent mutation of the HbSS gene, presenting a different
structure from the African haplotype, and it is found in Eastern Saudi Arabia and India
(Serjeant 1997). On the other hand, the origins of SCD in the New World come from
the Atlantic slave trade of millions of West Africans to North America, the Caribbean
and Brazil between 1450 and 1870, and because of this the frequency of SCD is now
high in the Americas. One in 600 African Americans has sickle cell anaemia, and 8 per
cent are heterozygous carriers of the sickle cell trait (Steinberg 1999). There are more
than 10,000 patients with SCD in the UK, it is the commonest inherited condition in
inner cities, and the population is increasing. In the Caribbean, the frequency of the
major genotypes of sickle cell disease at birth in Jamaica are 1 in 300 for homozygous
SCD, 1 in 500 for sickle/C disease, 1 in 3000 for sickle/β^+ thalassaemia, and 1 in 7000
for sickle cell/β° thalassaemia (Serjeant 1997). In North America, the three African Hb
S-linked haplotypes, Benin, Bantu, and Senegal vary in frequency, with, for example,
a higher proportion of the Senegal haplotype in the Deep South.

The risk factors for complications, including stroke, in SCD remain poorly understood (Weatherall 1995). There is a familial predisposition to stroke but the number of
familial cases are small (Driscoll et al. 1997). Predisposition for stroke is related in part
to HbS gene genotype. Stroke is commoner in homozygous sickle cell anaemia (HbSS)
and S/β^0-thalassaemia whereas Hb SCD and S/β^+-thalassaemia typically have a milder
course (Serjeant 1997). Powars and her colleagues provided evidence that a low fetal
Hb, below 8 per cent, was a risk factor for stroke, but subsequent studies have
confirmed this. However, patients from Saudi Arabia, who have a high Hb F level, have
a low incidence of complications, including stroke and silent infarction (Adekile et al.
2002). In African-Americans, there is a high incidence of individuals with only
three α-globin genes and α-thalassaemia. Alpha thalassaemia is protective for stroke
probably because Hb is higher and the percentage of Hb S is lower (Pavlakis et al. 1989,
Serjeant 1997, Sarnaik and Ballas 2001). A haplotype of the HbS gene, Senegal B^S
globin gene, is considered a risk factor for silent infarcts (Kinney et al. 1999), but Powars
and colleagues found lower rates of overt stroke with this haplotype (Powars 1990). The
Bantu haplotype may be related to severe disease (Powars et al. 1990) but in another

study, those with the Central African Republic haplotypes were at higher risk (Sarnaik and Ballas 2001).

12.4 Childhood stroke associated with inherited cardiac disease

In contrast to studies in young adults, previously undiagnosed cardiac disease such as patent foramen ovale appears to be uncommon (Ganesan *et al.* 2002). In fact, certain forms of congenital heart abnormality, particularly those of the arch and aortic valve, are associated with primary cerebrovascular disease (Schievink *et al.* 1996, Lutterman *et al.* 1998) (e.g. Moya–Moya syndrome, dissection and aneurysm) rather than cardiac embolus or venous sinus thrombosis. Abnormalities of vascular embryogenesis at the time of neural crest development and inherited connective tissue disease may be associated with cerebrovascular, as well as cardiovascular, disease.

12.5 Childhood stroke associated with arterial dissection

Dissection of the extracranial and intracranial vasculature is certainly an important cause of stroke in children but may have been missed in the past (Ganesan *et al.* 1999). In the Great Ormond Street series, 14/212 children with stroke in an arterial distribution had radiological evidence for dissection (Ganesan *et al.* 2002), and the figure was 20 per cent in a recent French study in which all of 59 consecutive children had conventional arteriography in the acute phase (Chabrier *et al.* 2000). Arterial dissections in association with congenitally bicuspid aortic valve may be secondary to a familial abnormality in the development of neural crest tissue (Schievinck and Mokri 1995). It is likely that there is an underlying connective tissue disorder in many cases of vascular dissection, particularly those occurring spontaneously. Ultrasonographic abnormalities may be demonstrated (Brandt *et al.* 1998) and a minority have abnormalities of type III collagen with or without typical Ehlers–Danlos type IV syndrome (van den Berg *et al.* 1998). The adult polycystic kidney and α-1 antitrypsin genes may be responsible for a significant proportion of spontaneous arterial dissection (Schievinck *et al.* 1994*a,b*) as well as aneurysm formation. However, α-1 antitrypsin was normal in the 8 patients with arterial dissection in the GOSH series in whom it was measured and hereditary connective tissue disorders with a unique phenotype appear to be as common (Schievinck *et al.* 1998).

12.6 Moya–Moya disease and syndrome

Primary Moya–Moya disease is relatively common in Asia, particularly in Japan, and sporadic primary cases are also relatively common in this population (Table 12.2). In the USA and Europe, however, most cases are of Moya–Moya syndrome secondary

Table 12.2 Causes of Moya–Moya disease and syndrome

Primary Moya–Moya disease
Secondary Moya–Moya syndrome
Mendelian disorders
Neurofibromatosis
Marfan's syndrome
Noonan syndrome
Sickle cell disease
Hereditrary spherocytosis
Alagile syndrome
Hereditary prothrombotic dosorders
Bicuspid aortic valve/coarctation of aorta
Tuberose sclerosis complex
Pseudoxanthoma elasticum
Chromosomal disorders
Down syndrome
Williams syndrome

to other conditions with Mendelian inheritance, such as Neurofibromatosis (Tomsick *et al*. 1976), Marfan's syndrome (Terada *et al*. 1999), Noonan syndrome (Ganesan and Kirkham 1997b), hereditary spherocytosis (Tokunaga *et al*. 2001) and SCD (Dobson *et al*. 2002) or chromosomal disorders such as Down (Dai *et al*. 2000) and Williams syndromes. Moya–Moya has also been documented in the Alagille syndrome (Woolfenden *et al*. 1999, Connor *et al*. 2002), a syndrome which usually presents with liver disease secondary to paucity of the bile ducts, which is usually caused by mutations in the Jagged-1 gene (about half of which are inherited) which is responsible for signalling during embryonic development (Piccoli and Spinner 2001). Bicuspid aortic valve and coarctation of the aorta are also associated with Moya–Moya (Lutterman *et al*. 1998, Christiaens *et al*. 2000). Environmental triggers, such as irradiation for optic glioma in Neurofibromatosis (Grill *et al*. 1999) and the severity of anaemia in spherocytosis, may also be important and there is also evidence for a role of prothrombotic disorders (Bonduel *et al*. 2001). The relative importance of genetic and environmental factors remains controversial and although the radiological appearances are similar, there may be important differences in pathology.

In primary Moya–Moya disease, there is a systemic vasculopathy in addition to the occlusion of the circle of Willis, which is characterized by eccentric thickening of the intima and probably involves excessive amounts of elastin and collagen. There is considerable evidence that primary Moya–Moya disease has a genetic basis, probably polygenic. Approximately 10 per cent of primary cases are familial and 80 per cent of monozygotic twins are concordant (Ganesan *et al*. 1997, Kaneko *et al*. 1998). Familial Moya–Moya disease in the Japanese appears to be linked to markers on chromosome 3p (Ikeda *et al*. 1999) and a Greek family has also been reported (Zaferiou *et al*. 2002);

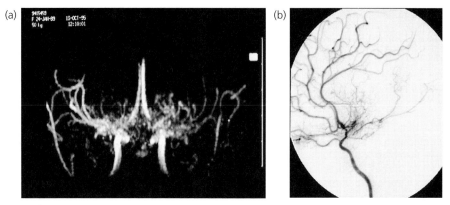

Fig. 12.3 MRA (a) and conventional carotid arteriography (b) demonstrating the Moya–Moya (puff-of-smoke) appearance of collaterals in a child with distal internal carotid stenosis.

interestingly the genes for Marfan disease and von Hippel–Lindau disease also map to 3p. Williams' syndrome, which is associated with cerebrovascular as well as cardio-vascular disease, results from a mutation on chromosome 7q in a region which includes the elastin gene. Interestingly, in familial Moya–Moya, there is now evidence for involvement of a second gene on chromosome 17q25, close to the gene for Neurofibromatosis type 1 (Yamauchi *et al.* 2000). There may be a third locus on chromosome 6 close to the HLA genes (Inoue *et al.* 2000). Typical radiological appearances of Moya–Moya are shown in Fig. 12.3.

12.7 Childhood cerebral venous thrombosis

This presents in neonates, usually as seizures, and in older children, with similar non-specific symptoms as in adults (de Veber and Andrew 2001). The diagnosis may be missed unless an MR venogram is performed but infarcts in a parieto-occipital distribution would be suggestive. Genetic causes of thrombophilia, including Factor V Leiden, prothrombin 20210, polymorphisms of the plasminogen activator inhibitor-1 (Baumeister *et al.* 2000) and the thermolabile variant of the methylene tetrahydrofolate reductase gene (Hiller *et al.* 1998, Kosch *et al.* 2001) are probably risk factors, together with environmental triggers such as systemic illness or infection, dehydration and iron deficiency anaemia.

12.8 Intermediate risk factors for childhood stroke

12.8.1 Hypertension

Hypertension is one of the most important risk factors for stroke in young adults (You *et al.* 1997), as well as in the elderly, but has largely been ignored in the paediatric literature. In a recent series, 54 per cent of children with cryptogenic and 46 per cent of those with symptomatic stroke had a systolic BP >90th percentile and there was a significant association with cerebral arterial abnormalities (Ganesan *et al.* 2002). Blood pressure is relatively lower in patients with SCD in comparison to controls. However, in SCD an associated relative hypertension is associated with increased risk of CVD (Rodgers *et al.* 1993) and ischaemic stroke (Ohene-Frempong *et al.* 1998). The A3 and A4 alleles of the GT-repeat polymorphism of the angiotensinogen gene appear to be associated with a fourfold risk of clinical stroke in SCD, perhaps because of an effect on blood pressure (Tang *et al.* 2001).

12.8.2 Hyperhomocysteinaemia and homocystinuria

Classical homocystinuria (deficiency of cystathionine β-synthase) has long been recognized as an important cause of arterial vascular disease and infarction and may present with stroke in infancy, childhood and adolescence (Lu *et al.* 1996, Cardo *et al.* 1999*a*). There is considerable evidence that it is high levels of homocysteine which predispose to vessel abnormalities (Perry *et al.* 1995). Reduction in the activity of the 5,10-methylene tetrahydrofolate reductase gene results in reduction of 5-methyl tetrahydrofolate for the conversion of homocysteine to methionine and therefore in hyperhomocysteinemia. Whereas the large number of mutations of cystathionine β-synthase are all relatively rare, there is a common thermolabile variant of the methylene tetrahydrofolate reductase gene, for which about 60 per cent of Caucasians are heterozygous and 5–15 per cent homozygous. In adults, stroke risk is linked to homocysteine and folate levels, but there is no clear association with thermolabile methylene tetrahydrofolate reductase status, perhaps because of the confounding effect of acquired risk factors in this age group or simply because studies have been underpowered (Markus *et al.* 1997, Kelly *et al.* 2002, Madonna *et al.* 2002). Hyperhomocysteinaemia appears to be a risk factor for childhood (van Beynum *et al.* 1999, Cardo *et al.* 1999*b*) and neonatal (Hogeveen *et al.* 2002) stroke. Homozygosity for the thermolabile methylene tetrahydrofolate reductase polymorphism appears to be a risk factor for primary (Nowak-Göttl *et al.* 1999, Cardo *et al.* 2000, Prengler *et al.* 2001) and for recurrent (Prengler *et al.* 2001) non-sickle stroke in childhood in Northern Europe, but not in Turkey (Akar *et al.* 2001*a*). There is no evidence for an effect of any of the other common genes influencing homocysteime metabolism in the Turkish population (Akar *et al.* 2001*a*), but there are few data from other populations to date.

Apart from genetic predisposition, homocysteine levels are also influenced by intake of folate, vitamin B12 and vitamin B6. For example, homocysteine levels appear to be higher in patients with SCD who have stroked than in those who have not, and are inversely related to red cell folate (Houston *et al.* 1997), despite the relatively low prevalence of the thermolabile methylene tetrahydrofolate reductase mutation in AfroCaribbeans (Andrade *et al.* 1998). Homocysteine levels were higher in adults with arterial dissection than in controls in one series, but the MTHFR polymorphism was not associated (Pezzini *et al.* 2002). Vitamin supplementation, which carries no known risks, appears to reduce homocysteine levels (Jacques *et al.* 1999).

12.8.3 Disorders of coagulation

Recognized disorders of coagulation occur acutely in up to 38 per cent of children with childhood stroke (de Veber *et al.* 1998), but up to half resolve within 3 months of the ictus and the prevalence of known inherited coagulopathies is around 10 per cent in previously well patients (Ganesan *et al.* 1998). Williams *et al.* (1997) quoted a higher figure of 25 per cent, but this series included a high proportion of children with SCD, in which prothrombotic abnormalities are known to be common, but are not necessarily associated with stroke and cerebrovascular disease (Liesner *et al.* 1998).

Factor V Leiden, which is common in Caucasian populations and is the commonest cause of activated protein C resistance, is an important risk factor for venous thrombosis in adults. The mutation has been linked to neonatal (Thorarensen *et al.* 1999, Lynch *et al.* 2001) and childhood stroke (Ganesan *et al.* 1996, Zenz *et al.* 1997; Kenet *et al.* 2000, Nowak-Göttl *et al.* 1999). Factor V Leiden is rare in Afro-Caribbeans and at present, there is little evidence for a link with stroke for this or any other genetically determined prothrombotic disorder in patients with SCD (Kahn *et al.* 1997, Andrade *et al.* 1998, Liesner *et al.* 1998).

Other candidate genes, such as the prothrombin 20210 mutation, appear to be risk factors for cerebral venous thrombosis, and at the present time there is no evidence for an association with arterial stroke in this age group (Zenz *et al.* 1997, Gaustadnes *et al.* 1998). Data from the Great Ormond Street database are similar, with only 2/116 of the arterial stroke patients heterozygous for the prothrombin 20210 gene (Ganesan *et al.* 2002) and no difference from controls. A significant proportion of children with stroke have multiple prothrombotic disorders (de Veber *et al.* 1998, Deda *et al.* 2002) and there is evidence for interaction, for example, between the factor V Leiden mutation and hyperhomocysteinaemia (Mandel *et al.* 1996, Szolnoki *et al.* 2000). Factor V Leiden does seem to be associated with large infarcts in adults (Szolnoki *et al.* 2001) and with poor prognosis in neonatal stroke (Mercuri *et al.* 2001). Interestingly, the only child in our series who had a recurrent stroke after arteriography was also the only one who was heterozygous for the factor V Leiden and the prothrombin 20210 gene mutations and homozygous for the thermolabile methylene tetrahydrofolate reductase gene.

There are few data on the role of other polymorphisms, for example, the ACE D polymorphism (Szolnoki *et al.* 2000, 2001) or the apolipoprotein E genotype (Weir *et al.* 2001) in childhood stroke, although they might be associated with specific subtypes of different prognostic significance. One child with a stroke has been reported to be homozygous for the 99 Leu to Phe mutation affecting the heparin binding site for antithrombin (Kuhle *et al.* 2001). The plasminogen activator inhibitor-1 promoter polymorphism 4G/5G, which is associated with decreased fibrinolytic activity, does not appear to play a role in arterial stroke (Nowak-Göttl *et al.* 2001, Akar *et al.* 2001*b*) and there appears to be no association with polymorphisms of the platelet collagen receptor $\acute{\alpha}2\beta1$ (Akar *et al.* 2001*c*).

12.8.4 Lipid abnormalities

In a recent series of childhood stroke, nine per cent of those in whom random cholesterol was measured had high levels, while 31 per cent had high triglyceride levels and 22 per cent had high lipoprotein (a) (Ganesan *et al.* 2002), a risk factor for atherosclerosis in adults. In another series, apolipoprotein abnormalities were seen more commonly in association with childhood stroke (Abram *et al.* 1996). Although the genes controlling lipoprotein (a) levels in children have not yet been elucidated, levels do appear to be increased in a significant proportion of patients with arterial stroke in a Caucasian population in Germany (Nowak-Göttl *et al.* 1999), and are a risk factor for recurrent stroke (Sträter *et al.* 2002).

12.8.5 Infection, inflammation, and immune deficiency

At least a third of cases of childhood stroke occur in the context of infection (Riikonen *et al.* 1994, Ganesan *et al.* 2002). Frank immunodeficiency, either inherited or acquired also appears to be an occasional association (Ganesan *et al.* 2002). Recently, several children with otherwise cryptogenic stroke following chickenpox have been documented and a causative link has been proposed (Ganesan and Kirkham 1997*a*, Sébire *et al.* 1999, Askalan *et al.* 2001). Typically, there is infarction within the basal ganglia associated with stenosis of the middle cerebral artery close to the lenticulostriate vessels arteriographically, but Moya–Moya syndrome has also been described (Ganesan and Kirkham 1997*a*). There may be direct invasion of the vessel wall but there are cases of histologically documented arteritis without viral invasion and it is likely that several mechanisms, including thrombosis and the immune response, are involved.

In SCD, high leukocyte count is a risk factor for stroke (Balkaran *et al.* 1992, Miller *et al.* 2000) and cerebrovascular episodes are often precipitated by infections. This group of patients is also relatively immunodeficient, in part secondary to splenic autoinfarction or surgical removal of the spleen. Work has started on the question of whether genetic modulators of the immune response are important in the development of cerebrovascular disease and stroke. For example, sickle cells which are coated in immunoglobulin adhere more firmly to endothelium, but there is no evidence for an association between stroke and polymorphisms of the low affinity immunoglobulin receptors (Taylor *et al.* 2002*a*).

The host inflammatory response may also play a role in, for example, determining levels of intermediary cytokines, which may have harmful effects on the endothelium, although work on the genetic basis of these complex pathways and their relationship to cerebrovascular disease is at an early stage. Interestingly, in a pilot study, there was a trend suggesting that the TNF-$\acute{\alpha}$ (-308) A allele was linked to stroke in SCD

(Hoppe *et al.* 2001). The TNF locus is in linkage dysequilibrium with human leukocyte (HLA) antigens. In recent years, evidence for HLA-susceptibility for stroke was found in the class I HLA-B and class II DRB loci in children with and without SCD (Mintz *et al.* 1992, Aoyagi *et al.* 1995, Inoue *et al.* 1997, Styles *et al.* 2000). However, there does not appear to be an association between *Varicella*-associated crytogenic stroke and HLA type (Kluger *et al.* 2001) and the relative importance of HLA type in the determination of stroke risk in childhood remains very controversial.

12.8.6 Vascular adhesion

Adhesion of red and white cells and of platelets appears to be an important mechanism of endothelial damage in SCD and may play a role in stroke of other aetiologies such as Moya–Moya (Soriano *et al.* 2002). It is clear that sickle erythrocytes adhere more avidly to vascular endothelial cells than normal erythrocytes (Hebbel 1997). In addition, neutrophil and platelet adhesion to the vascular endothelium and activation have been found in adults and children with SCD (Setty and Stuart 1996, Solovey *et al.* 1997, Wun *et al.* 1997, Fadlon *et al.* 1998, Inwald *et al.* 2000). Hypoxia increases adhesion to the endothelial of sickle red cells (Setty and Stuart 1996), neutrophils and monocytes (Inwald *et al.* 2000).

There is evidence that different molecular mechanisms are involved in the adhesion of red and white cells and platelets to the vascular endothelium in SCD and in stroke in general. These mechanisms include adhesive ligands (e.g. von Willebrand factor) and molecules on the RBCs and endothelial cell surfaces (e.g. vascular cell adhesion molecule, VCAM-1, intercellular adhesion molecule Type 1, ICAM-1 and E-selectin) (Setty and Stuart 1996). VCAM-1 is of particular interest in SCD, as this cellular adhesion molecule appears to co-ordinate the inflammatory response by recruiting leukocytes and mice depleted of it have a high leukocyte count. As high white cell count predicts stroke in children with SCD, the possibility that there are variations in the VCAM-1 gene accounting for stroke susceptibility is currently under investigation. Interestingly, there is a high density of single nucleotide polymorphisms in the VCAM-1 gene in the Afro-Caribbean population and one of these variant alleles, G1238C, has been shown to be associated with protection from stroke in the Jamaican population, in comparison with the wild allele (Taylor *et al.* 2002*b*). This work will need repeating in a larger population with neuroimaging of cases and controls but suggests that resequencing of genes in a susceptible population will yield polymorphisms which can then be studied using a variety of methodologies. For SCD, there is also considerable interest in looking at polymorphisms which may influence susceptibility to malaria, such as CD-36 (Taylor *et al.* 2000).

12.8.7 Nitric oxide

Nitric oxide (NO) may play an important role in determining whether or not the endothelium is damaged (Prengler *et al.* 2002). NO is one of the most potent vasodilators and a regulator of the normal vasculature tone, cell adhesion and thrombosis. There is a delicate balance between hypoxia driven vasoconstriction and NO driven vasodilatation in hypoxic conditions. Thus, NO biosynthesis may also be a key factor in the pathogenesis of vascular occlusion and stroke in SCD. Abnormal NO metabolism has recently been demonstrated in sickle mice (Kaul *et al.* 2000). NO has been shown to decrease sickle erythrocyte adherence to vascular endothelial cells (Space *et al.* 2000) and in a rat model of disease, sickle erythrocytes decrease cerebral blood flow after inhibition of NO synthase (French *et al.* 1997). In stroke in adults, genetic studies have looked at common polymorphisms in endothelial NO synthase (eNOS), such as Glu–Asp[298], which may be processed abnormally in the cell, resulting in a cleaved protein that may be defective. There are few data in children (Akar *et al.* 2000) and the evidence in adults is conflicting (MacLeod *et al.* 1999, Elbaz *et al.* 2000), perhaps reflecting different distributions of stroke syndromes between populations, but this approach might be worthwhile in SCD, as failure to produce NO might result in increased vasoconstriction, increased sickle erythrocyte–endothelial adhesion and hence an increased probability of vascular occlusion.

12.9 Summary and future directions

Although conditions with a clear genetic basis are commonly associated with childhood stroke, we are a long way from understanding the mechanisms. A very clear description of the phenotype will be important, as for example the genetic basis of cerebrovascular disease with the angiographic appearances of Moya–Moya may be very different from that associated with venous sinus thrombosis, even if the underlying SCD is the same. The relative importance of intermediate factors, such as prothrombotic disorders, abnormalities of homocysteine metabolism and factors affecting endothelial function may be very different in different populations. To date, most studies have used a candidate gene approach and a case control design, which has limitations (Gambaro *et al.* 2000) but international collaboration might allow more sophisticated approaches. It is likely that stroke in childhood occurs secondary to interactions between several genes and the environment and teasing out the relative importance of each component will be complex. The hope is that an understanding of the genetic basis of childhood stroke will lead to better management of this important group of patients.

References

Abram, H., Knepper, E., Warty, V.S., and Painter, M.J. (1996). Natural history, prognosis and lipid abnormalities of idiopathic ischemic childhood stroke. *Journal of Child Neurology*, 11, 276–82.

Adams, R.J., McKie, V.C., Carl, E.M., *et al.* (1997). Long-term stroke risk in children with sickle cell disease screened with transcranial Doppler. *Annals of Neurology*, 42, 699–704.

Adekile, A.D., Yacoub, F., Gupta, R., *et al.* (2002). Silent brain infarcts are rare in Kuwaiti children with sickle cell disease and high Hb F. *American Journal of Hematology*, 70, 228–31.

Akar, N., Akar, E., Deda, G., and Sipahi, T. (2000). No association between Glu/Asp polymorphism of NOS3 gene and ischemic stroke. *Neurology*, **55**, 460–1.

Akar, N., Akar, E., Ozel, D., Deda, G., and Sipahi, T. (2001*a*). Common mutations at the homocysteine metabolism pathway and pediatric stroke. *Thrombosis Research*, **102**, 115–20.

Akar, N., Duman, T., Akar, E., Deda, G., and Sipahi, T. (2001*b*). The alpha2 Gene alleles of the platelet collagen receptor integrin alpha2 beta1 in Turkish children with cerebral infarct. *Thrombosis Research*, **102**, 121–3.

Akar, N., Akar, E., Yilmaz, E., and Deda, G. (2001*c*). Plasminogen activator inhibitor-1 4G/5G polymorphism in Turkish children with cerebral infarct and effect on factor V 1691 A mutation. *Journal of Child Neurology*, **16**, 294–5.

Al-Jarallah, A., Al-Rifai, M.T., Riela, A.R., and Roach, E.S. (2000). Nontraumatic brain hemorrhage in children: etiology and presentation. *Journal of Child Neurology*, **15**, 284–9.

Andrade, F.L., Annichino-Bizzacchi, J.M., Saad, S.T., Costa, F.F., and Arruda, V.R. (1998). Prothrombin mutant, factor V Leiden, and thermolabile variant of methylenetetrahydrofolate reductase among patients with sickle cell disease in Brazil. *American Journal of Hematology*, **59**, 46–50.

Aoyagi, M., Ogami, K., Matsushima, Y., Shikata, M., Yamamoto, M., and Yamamoto, K. (1995). Human leukocyte antigen in patients with moyamoya disease. *Stroke*, **26**, 415–17.

Armstrong, F.D., Thompson, R.J., Wang, W., *et al.* (1996). Cognitive functioning and brain magnetic resonance imaging in children with sickle cell disease. *Pediatrics*, **97**, 864–70.

Askalan, R., Laughlin, S., Mayank, S., Chan, A., MacGregor, D., Andrew, M., Curtis, R., Meaney, B., and de Veber, G. (2001). Chickenpox and stroke in childhood: a study of frequency and causation. *Stroke*, **32**, 1257–62.

Balkaran, B., Char, G., Morris, J.S., Thomas, P.W., Serjeant, B.E., and Serjeant, G.R. (1992). Stroke in a cohort of patients with homozygous sickle cell disease. *Journal of Pediatrics*, **120**, 360–6.

Baumeister, F.A., Auberger, K., and Schneider, K. (2000). Thrombosis of the deep cerebral veins with excessive bilateral infarction in a premature infant with the thrombogenic 4G/4G genotype of the plasminogen activator inhibitor-1. *European Journal Pediatrics*, **159**, 239–42.

Bonduel, M., Hepner, M., Sciuccati, G., Torres, A.F., Tenembaum, S., and de Veber, G. (2001). Prothrombotic disorders in children with Moyamoya Syndrome. *Stroke*, **32**, 1786–92.

Brandt, T., Hausser, I., Orberk, E., Grau, A., Hartschuh, W., Anton-Lamprecht, I., and Hacke, W. (1998). Ultrastructural connective tissue abnormalities in patients with spontaneous cervicocerebral artery dissections. *Annals of Neurology*, **44**, 281–5.

Broderick, J., Talbot, G.T., Prenger, E., Leach, A., and Brott, T. (1993). Stroke in children within a major metropolitan area: the surprising importance of intracerebral hemorrhage. *Journal of Child Neurology*, **8**, 250–5.

Cardo, E., Campistol, J., Vilaseca, A., Caritg, J., Ruiz, S., Kirkham, F., and Blom, H.J. (1999*a*). Stroke in infancy in a child with homocystinuria. *Developmental Medicine and Child Neurology*, **41**, 132–5.

Cardo, E., Vilaseca, M.A., Campistol, J., Artuch, R., Colome, C., and Pineda, M. (1999*b*). Evaluation of hyperhomocysteinemia in children with stroke. *European Journal of Paediatric Neurology*, **3**, 113–17.

Cardo, E., Monrós, E., Colomé, C., Artuch, R., Campistol, J., Pineda, M., and Vilaseca, M.A. (2000). 677C→T polymorphism of the 5,10-methylenetetrahydrofolate reductase gene, mild hyperhomocysteinemia, and vitamin status in children with stroke. *Journal of Child Neurology*, **15**, 295–8.

Chabrier, S., Rodesch, G., Lasjaunias, P., Tardieu, M., Landrieu, P., and Sébire, G. (1998). Transient cerebral arteriopathy: a disorder recognized by serial angiograms in children with stroke. *Journal of Child Neurology*, **13**, 27–32.

Chabrier, S., Husson, B., Lasjaunias, P., Landrieu, P., and Tardieu, M. (2000). Stroke in childhood: outcome and risk of recurrence according to the mechanism, in a series of 59 patients. *Journal of Child Neurology*, **15**, 290–4.

Christiaens, F.J., Van den Broeck, L.K., Christophe, C., and Dan, B. (2000). Moyamoya disease (moyamoya syndrome) and coarctation of the aorta. *Neuropediatrics*, **31**, 47–8.

Connor, S.E., Hewes, D., Ball, C., and Jarosz, J.M. (2002). Alagille syndrome associated with angiographic moyamoya. *Child's Nervous System*, **18**, 186–90.

Dai, A.I., Shaikh, Z.A., and Cohen, M.E. (2000). Early-onset Moyamoya syndrome in a patient with Down syndrome: case report and review of the literature. *Journal of Child Neurology*, **15**, 696–9.

Deda, G., Icagasioglu, D., Caksen, H., and Akar, N. (2002). Combined genetic defects in a child with ischemic stroke: case report. *Journal of Child Neurology*, **17**, 533–4.

de Veber, G. and Andrew, M. (2001). Canadian Pediatric Ischemic Stroke Study Group. Cerebral sinovenous thrombosis in children. *New England Journal of Medicine*, **345**, 417–23.

de Veber, G., Monagle, P., Chan, A., *et al.* (1998). Prothrombotic disorders in infants and children with cerebral thromboembolism. *Archives of Neurology*, **55**, 1539–43.

Dobson, S.R., Holden, K.R., Nietert, P.J., Cure, J.K., Laver, J.H., Disco, D., and Abboud, M.R. (2002). Moyamoya syndrome in childhood sickle cell disease: a predictive factor for recurrent cerebrovascular events. *Blood*, **99**, 3144–50.

Driscoll, M., Hurlet, A., Berman, B., Files, B., and Byrne, J. (1997). Stroke in sib-pairs with sickle cell disease. *Blood*, **90**, 264a (abstract).

Earley, C.J., Kittner, S.J., Feeser, B.R., *et al.* (1998). Stroke in children and sickle-cell disease. *Neurology*, **51**, 169–76.

Elbaz, A., Poirier, O., Moulin, T., Chedru, F., Cambien, F., and Amarenco, P. (2000). Association between the Glu298Asp polymorphism in the endothelial constitutive nitric oxide synthase gene and brain infarction. The GENIC Investigators. *Stroke*, **31**, 1634–9.

Fadlon, E., Vordermeier, S., Pearson, T.C., Mire-Sluis, A.R., Dumonde, D.C., Phillips, J., Fishlock, K., and Brown, K.A. (1998). Blood polymorphonuclear leukocytes from the majority of sickle cell patients in the crisis phase of the disease show enhanced adhesion to vascular endothelium and increased expression of CD64. *Blood*, **91**, 266–74.

French, J.A., Kenny, D., Scott, J.P., Hoffmann, R.G., Wood, J.D., Hudetz, A.G., and Hillery, C.A. (1997). Mechanisms of stroke in sickle cell disease: sickle erythrocytes decrease cerebral blood flow in rats after nitric oxide synthase inhibition. *Blood*, **89**, 4591–9.

Gambaro, G., Anglani, F., and D'Angelo, A. (2000). Association studies of genetic polymorphisms and complex disease. *Lancet*, **355**, 308–11.

Ganesan, V., Kelsey, H., Cookson, J., Osborn, A., and Kirkham, F.J. (1996). Activated protein C resistance in childhood stroke. *Lancet*, **347**, 260 (letter).

Ganesan, V. and Kirkham, F.J. (1997a). Mechanisms of ischaemic stroke after chickenpox. *Archives of Disease in Childhood*, **76**, 522–5.

Ganesan, V. and Kirkham, F.J. (1997b). Noonan syndrome and moyamoya. *Pediatric Neurology*, **16**, 256–8.

Ganesan, V. and Kirkham, F.J. (1998). Recurrence after ischaemic stroke in childhood. *Developmental Medicine and Child Neurology*, Suppl 79, 7 (abstract).

Ganesan, V., Isaacs, E., and Kirkham, F.J. (1997). Variable presentation of cerebrovascular disease in monovular twins. *Developmental Medicine and Child Neurology*, **39**, 628–31.

Gaustadnes, M., Rudiger, N., and Ingerslev, J. (1998). The 20210 A allele of the prothrombin gene is not a risk factor for juvenile stroke in the Danish population. *Blood Coagulation & Fibrinolysis*, **9**, 663–4.

Ganesan, V., Savvy, L., Chong, W.K., and Kirkham, F.J. (1999). Conventional cerebral angiography in the investigation of children with ischaemic stroke. *Pediatric Neurology*, **20**, 38–42.

Ganesan, V., McShane, M.A., Liesner, R., Cookson, J., Hann, I., and Kirkham, F.J. (1998). Inherited prothrombotic states and ischaemic stroke in childhood. *Journal of Neurology Neurosurgery Psychiatry*, **65**, 508–11.

Ganesan, V., Prengler, M., McShane, M.A., Wade, A., and Kirkham, F.J. (2003). Investigation of risk factors in children with arterial ischemic stroke. *Annals of Neurology*, **53**, 167–73.

Grill, J., Couanet, D., Cappelli, C., Habrand, J.L., Rodriguez, D., Sainte-Rose, C., and Kalifa, C. (1999). Radiation-induced cerebral vasculopathy in children with neurofibromatosis and optic pathway glioma. *Annals of Neurology*, **45**, 393–6.

Hebbel, R.P. (1997). Adhesive interactions of sickle erythrocytes with endothelium. *Journal of Clinical Investigation*, **100**, S83–6.

Herrick, J.B. (1910). Peculiar elongated and sickle-shaped red corpuscles in a case of severe anemia. *Archives of Internal Medicine*, **6**, 517–54.

Hiller, C.E.M., Collins, P.W., Bowen, D.J., Bowley, S., and Wiles, C.M. (1998). Inherited prothrombotic risk factors and cerebral venous thrombosis. *Quarterly Journal of Medicine*, **91**, 677–80.

Hoppe, C., Cheng, S., Grow, M., Silbergleit, A., Klitz, W., Trachtenberg, E., Erlich, H., Vichinsky, E., and Styles, L. (2001). A novel multilocus genotyping assay to identify genetic predictors of stroke in sickle cell anaemia. *British Journal of Haematology*, **114**, 718–20.

Houston, P.E., Rana, S., Sekhsaria, S., Perlin, E., Kim, K.S., and Castro, O.L. (1997). Homocysteine in sickle cell disease: relationship to stroke. *American Journal of Medicine*, **103**, 192–6.

Husson, B., Rodesch, G., Lasjaunias, P., Tardieu, M., and Sebire, G. (2002). Magnetic resonance angiography in childhood arterial brain infarcts: a comparative study with contrast angiography. *Stroke*, **33**, 1280–5.

Ikeda, H., Sasaki, T., Yoshimoto, T., Fukui, M., and Arinami, T. (1999). Mapping of a familial moyamoya disease gene to chromosome 3p24.2–p26. *American Journal of Human Genetics*, **64**, 533–7.

Ingram, V.M. (1957). Gene mutation in human hemoglobin: the chemical difference between normal and sickle cell hemoglobin. *Nature*, **180**, 326–9.

Inoue, T.K., Ikezaki, K., Sasazuki, T., Ono, T., Kamikawaji, N., Matsushima, T., and Fukui, M. (1997). DNA typing of HLA in the patients with moyamoya disease. *Japanese Journal of Human Genetics*, **42**, 507–15.

Inoue, T.K., Ikezaki, K., Sasazuki, T., Matsushima, T., and Fukui, M. (2000). Linkage analysis of moyamoya disease on chromosome 6. *Journal of Child Neurology*, **15**, 179–82.

Inwald, D.P., Kirkham, F.J., Peters, M.J., *et al.* (2000). Platelet and leukocyte activation in childhood sickle cell disease: association with nocturnal hypoxaemia and disease severity. *British Journal of Haematology*, **111**, 474–81.

Jacques, P.F., Selhub, J., Bostom, A.G., Wilson, P.W., and Rosenberg, I.H. (1999). The effect of folic acid fortification on plasma folate and total homocysteine concentrations. *New England Journal of Medicine*, **340**, 1449–54.

Kahn, M.J., Scher, C., Rozans, M., Michaels, R.K., Leissinger, C., and Krause, J. (1997). Factor V Leiden is not responsible for stroke in patients with sickling disorders and is uncommon in African Americans with sickle cell disease. *American Journal of Hematology*, **54**, 12–15.

Kaneko, Y., Imamoto, N., Mannoji, H., and Fukui, M. (1998). Familial occurrence of moyamoya disease in the mother and four daughters including identical twins. *Neurologia Medico-Chirurgica* (Tokyo), **38**, 349–54.

Kaul, D.K., Liu, X.D., Fabry, M.E., and Nagel, R.L. (2000). Impaired nitric oxide-mediated vasodilation in transgenic sickle mouse. American Journal of Physiology. *Heart and Circulatory Physiology*, **278**, H1799–806.

Kelly, P.J., Rosand, J., Kistler, J.P., Shih, V.E., Silveira, S., Plomaritoglou, A., and Furie, K.L. (2002). Homocysteine, MTHFR 677C→T polymorphism, and risk of ischemic stroke: results of a metaanalysis. *Neurology*, **59**, 529–36.

Kenet, G., Sadetzki, S., Murad, H., Martinowitz, U., Rosenberg, N., Gitel, S., Rechavi, G., and Inbal, A. (2000). Factor V Leiden and antiphospholipid antibodies are significant risk factors for ischemic stroke in children. *Stroke*, **31**, 1283–8.

Kinney, T.R., Sleeper, L.A., and Wang, W.C. (1999). Silent cerebral infarcts in sickle cell anemia: a risk factor analysis. *Pediatrics*, **103**, 640–5.

Kirkham, F.J., Calamante, F., Bynevelt, M., Gadian, D.G., Cox, T.C., Evans, J.P.M., and Connelly, A. (2001a). Perfusion MR abnormalities in patients with Sickle cell Disease: relation to symptoms, infarction and cerebrovascular disease. *Annals of Neurology*, **49**, 477–85.

Kirkham, F.J., Hewes, D.K.M., Hargrave, D., Wade, A., Lane, R., Liesner R., and Evans, J. (2001b). Nocturnal hypoxaemia predicts CNS events in sickle cell disease. *Lancet*, **357**, 1656–9.

Kluger, G., Hubmann, M., Vogler, L., and Berz, K. (2001). Lack of association between childhood stroke after varicella and human leukocyte antigen (HLA)-B51. *European Journal of Paediatric Neurology*, **5**, 259–60.

Kosch, A., Junker, R., Baumgarten, A., Schobess, R., Kurnik, K., Heller, C., Straeter, R., and Nowak-Gottl, U. (2001). Venous sinus thrombosis: first multivariate analysis of inherited prothrombotic conditions and underlying triggering factors in a cohort of caucasian children. (Abstract): *Blood*, **98** (Suppl 16), 51a no. 206.

Kuhle, S., Lane, D.A., Jochmanns, K., Male, C., Quehenberger, P., Lechner, K., and Pabinger, I. (2001). Homozygous antithrombin deficiency type II (99 Leu to Phe mutation) and childhood thromboembolism. *Thrombosis and Haemostasis*, **86**, 1007–11.

Lanthier, S. (2002). Primary angiitis of the central nervous system in children: 10 cases proven by biopsy. *Journal of Rheumatology*, **29**, 1575–6.

Liesner, R., Mackie, I., Cookson, J., McDonald, S., Chitolie, A., Donohoe, S., Evans, J., Hann, I., and Machin, S. (1998). Prothrombotic changes in children with sickle cell disease: relationships to cerebrovascular disease and transfusion. *British Journal of Haematology*, **103**, 1037–44.

Lu, C.-Y., Hou, J.-W., Wang, P.-J., Chiu, H.H., and Wang, T.R. (1996). Homocystinuria presenting as fatal common carotid artery occlusion. *Pediatric Neurology*, **15**, 159–62.

Lutterman, J., Scott, M., Nass, R., and Geva, T. (1998). Moyamoya syndrome associated with congenital heart disease. *Pediatrics*, **101**, 57–60.

Lynch, J.K. and Nelson, K.B. (2001). Epidemiology of perinatal stroke. *Current Opinion in Pediatrics*, **13**, 499–505.

Lynch, J.K., Nelson, K.B., Curry, C.J., and Grether, J.K. (2001). Cerebrovascular disorders in children with the factor V Leiden mutation. *Journal of Child Neurology*, **16**, 735–44.

MacLeod, M.J., Dahiyat, M.T., Cumming, A., Meiklejohn, D., Shaw, D., and St Clair, D. (1999). No association between Glu/Asp polymorphism of NOS3 gene and ischemic stroke. *Neurology*, **53**, 418–20.

Madonna, P., de Stefano, V., Coppola, A., Cirillo, F., Cerbone, A.M., Orefice, G., and Di Minno, G. (2002). Hyperhomocysteinemia and other inherited prothrombotic conditions in young adults with a history of ischemic stroke. *Stroke*, **33**, 51–6.

Mandel, H., Brenner, B., Berant, M., Rosenberg, N., Lanir, N., Jakobs, C., Fowler, B., and Seligsohn, U. (1996). Coexistence of hereditary homocystinuria and factor V Leiden—effect on thrombosis. *New England Journal of Medicine*, **334**, 763–8.

Markus, H.S., Nadira, A., Swaminathan, R., Sankaralingam, A., Molloy, J., and Powell, J. (1997). A common polymorphism in the methylenetetrahydrofolate reductase gene, homocysteine, and ischaemic cerebrovascular disease. *Stroke*, **28**, 1739–43.

Mercuri, E., Cowan, F., Gupte, G., Manning, R., Laffan, M., Rutherford, M., Edwards, A.D., Dubowitz, L., and Roberts, I. (2001). Prothrombotic disorders and abnormal neurodevelopmental outcome in infants with neonatal cerebral infarction. *Pediatrics*, **107**, 1400–4.

Miller, S.T., Sleeper, L.A., Pegelow, C.H., *et al.* (2000). Prediction of adverse outcomes in children with sickle cell disease. *New England Journal of Medicine*, **342**, 83–9.

Miller, S.T., Macklin, E.A., Pegelow, C.H., *et al.* (2001). The Cooperative Study of Sickle Cell Disease. Silent infarction as a risk factor for overt stroke in children with sickle cell anemia: a report from the Cooperative Study of Sickle Cell Disease. *Journal of Pediatrics*, **139**, 385–90.

Mintz, M., Epstein, L.G., and Koenigsberger, M.R. (1992). Idiopathic childhood stroke is associated with human leukocyte antigen (HLA)-B51. *Annals of Neurology*, **31**, 675–7.

Natowicz, M. and Kelley, R.I. (1987). Mendelian etiologies of stroke. *Annals of Neurology*, **22**, 175–92.

Nowak-Göttl, U., Sträter, R., Heinecke, A., Koch, H.G., Schuierer, G., and von Eckardstein, A. (1999). Lipoprotein (a) and genetic polymorphisms of clotting factor, V., prothrombin and methylenetetrahydrofolate reductase are risk factors of ischaemic stroke in childhood. *Blood*, **94**, 3678–82.

Nowak-Göttl, U., Strater, R., Kosch, A., *et al.* (2001). The plasminogen activator inhibitor (PAI)-1 promoter 4G/4G genotype is not associated with ischemic stroke in a population of German children. Childhood Stroke Study Group. *European Journal of Haematology*, **66**, 57–62.

Ohene-Frempong, K., Weiner, S.J., Sleeper, L.A., *et al.* (1998). Cerebrovascular accidents in sickle cell disease: rates and risk factors. *Blood*, **91**, 288–94.

Osuntokun, B.O. (1979). Undernutrition and infectious disorders as risk factors for stroke (with special reference to Africans). *Advances in Neurology*, **25**, 161–74.

Pauling, L., Italo, H.A., Singer, S.J., *et al.* (1949). Sickle cell anemia: a molecular disease. *Science*, **110**, 543–6.

Pavlakis, S.G., Prohovnik, I., Piomelli, S., and DeVivo, D.C. (1989). Neurological complications of Sickle Cell Disease. *Advances in Pediatrics*, **36**, 247–76.

Pavlakis, S.G., Kingsley, P.B., and Bialer, M.G. (2000). Stroke in children: genetic and metabolic issues. *Journal of Child Neurology*, **15**, 308–15.

Pegelow, C.H., Macklin, E.A., Moser F.G., *et al.* (2002). Longitudinal changes in brain magnetic resonance imaging findings in children with sickle cell disease. *Blood*, **99**, 3014–8.

Perry, I.J., Refsum, H., Morris, R.W., Ebrahim, S.B., Ueland, P.M., and Shaper, A.G. (1995). Prospective study of serum total homocysteine concentration and risk of stroke in middle-aged British men. *Lancet*, **346**, 1395–8.

Pezzini, A., Magoni, M., Corda, L., Pini, L., Medicina, D., Crispino, M., Pavia, M., Padovani, A., and Grassi, V. (2002). Alpha-1-antitrypsin deficiency-associated cervical artery dissection: report of three cases. *European Neurology*, **47**, 201–4.

Piccoli, D.A. and Spinner, N.B. (2001). Alagille syndrome and the Jagged1 gene. *Seminars in Liver Disease*, **21**, 525–34.

Powars, D.R., Chan, L., and Schroeder, W.A. (1990). Beta-S-gene-cluster haplotypes in sickle cell disease: clinical implications. *The American Journal of Pediatric hematology/oncology*, 12, 367–74.

Prengler, M., Cox, T.C., Klein, N., Evans, J.P.M., Bynevelt, M., Chong, W.K., and Kirkham, F.J. (2000). Progressive cerebrovascular disease in childhood stroke: associations and effect on recurrence risk. *Developmental Medicine and Child Neurology*, 42 (Suppl 85), 47.

Prengler, M., Sturt, N., Krywawych, S., Surtees, R., and Kirkham, F. (2001). The homozygous thermolabile variant of the methylenetetrahydrofolate reductase gene: a risk factor for recurrent stroke in childhood. *Developmental Medicine and Child Neurology*, 43, 220–5.

Prengler, M., Pavlakis, S.G., Prohovnik, I., and Adams, R.J. (2002). Sickle cell disease: the neurological complications. *Annals Neurology*, 51, 543–52.

Riikonen, R. and Santavuori, P. (1994). Hereditary and acquired risk factors for childhood stroke. *Neuropediatrics*, 25, 227–33.

Roach, E.S. and Riela, A.R. (1995). *Pediatric cerebrovascular disorders*, 2nd edn. Futura, Armonk, New York.

Rodgers, G.P., Walker, E.C., and Podgor, M.J. (1993). Is 'relative' hypertension a risk factor for vaso-occlusive complications in sickle cell disease? *The American Journal of the Medical Sciences*, 305, 150–6.

Rothman, S.M., Fulling, K.H., and Nelson, J.S. (1986). Sickle cell anemia and central nervous system infarction: a neuropathological study. *Annals of Neurology*, 20, 684–90.

Sarnaik, S.A. and Balla, S.K. (2001). Molecular characteristics of pediatric patients with sickle cell anemia and stroke. *American Journal of Hematology*, 67, 179–82.

Saunders, D.E., Bynevelt, M., Hewes, D.K.M., Cox, T.C., Chong, W.K., Evans, J.P., and Kirkham, F.J. (2001). MRI in children with sickle cell disease without overt stroke. *Developmental Medicine and Child Neurology*, 43 (Suppl 90), 27.

Schievink, W.I. and Mokri, B. (1995). Familial aorto-cervicocephalic arterial dissections and congenitally bicuspid aortic valve. *Stroke*, 26, 1935–40.

Schievink, W.I., Michels, V.V., and Piepgras, D.G. (1994a). Neurovascular manifestations of heritable connective tissue disorders. A review. *Stroke*, 25, 889–903.

Schievink, W.I., Mokri, B., and Piepgras, D.G. (1994b). Spontaneous dissections of the cervicocephalic arteries in childhood and adolescence. *Neurology*, 44, 1607–12.

Schievink, W.I., Mokri, B., Piepgras, D.G., and Gittenberger-de Groot, A.C. (1996). Intracranial aneurysms and cervicocephalic arterial dissections associated with congenital heart disease. *Neurosurgery*, 39, 685–90.

Schievink, W.I., Wijdicks, E.F., Michels, V.V., Vockley, J., and Godfrey, M. (1998). Heritable connective tissue disorders in cervical artery dissections: a prospective study. *Neurology*, 50, 1166–9.

Serjeant, G.R. (1997). Sickle-cell disease. *Lancet*, 350, 725–30.

Sébire, G., Meyer, L., and Chabrier, S. (1999). Varicella as a risk factor for cerebral infarction in childhood: a case-control study. *Annals of Neurology*, 45, 679–80.

Setty, B.N. and Stuart, M.J. (1996). Vascular cell adhesion molecule-1 is involved in mediating hypoxia-induced sickle red blood cell adherence to endothelium: potential role in sickle cell disease. *Blood*, 88, 2311–20.

Shirane, R., Sato, S., and Yoshimoto, T. (1992). Angiographic findings of ischaemic stroke in children. *Child's Nervous System*, 8, 432–6.

Solovey, A., Lin, Y., Browne, P., Choong, S., Wayner, E., and Hebbel, R.P. (1997). Circulating activated endothelial cells in sickle cell anemia. *New England Journal of Medicine*, 337, 1584–90.

Space, S.L., Lane, P.A., Pickett, C.K., and Weil, J.V. (2000). Nitric oxide attenuates normal and sickle red blood cell adherence to pulmonary endothelium. *American Journal of Hematology*, 63, 200–4.

Sträter, R., Becker, S., von Eckardstein, A., Gutsche, S., Junker, R., Kurnik, K., Schobess, R., and Nowak-Göttl, U. (2002). Prospective evaluation of risk factors for recurrent stroke during childhood—results of the 5-year follow-up. *Lancet*, **360**, 1540–5.

Steinberg, M.H. (1999). Management of sickle cell disease. *New England Journal of Medicine*, **340**, 1021–30.

Stockman, J.A., Nigro, M.A., Mishkin, M.M., and Oski, F. (1972). Occlusion of the large cerebral vessels in sickle cell anemia. *New England Journal of Medicine*, **287**, 846–9.

Styles, L.A., Hoppe, C., Klitz, W., Vichinsky, E., Lubin, B., and Trachtenberg, E. (2000). Evidence for HLA-related susceptibility for stroke in children with sickle cell disease. *Blood*, **95**, 3562–7.

Szolnoki, Z., Somogyvari, F., Szabo, M., and Fodor, L. (2000). A clustering of unfavourable common genetic mutations in stroke cases. *Acta Neurologica Scandinavia*, **102**, 124–8.

Szolnoki, Z., Somogyvari, F., Szolics, M., Szabo, M., and Fodor, L. (2001). Common genetic mutations as possible aetiological factors in stroke. *European Neurology*, **45**, 119–20.

Tang, D.C., Prauner, R., Liu, W., Kim, K.H., Hirsch, R.P., Driscoll, M.C., and Rodgers, G.P. (2001). Polymorphisms within the angiotensinogen gene (GT-repeat) and the risk of stroke in pediatric patients with sickle cell disease: a case-control study. *American Journal of Hematology*, **68**, 164–9.

Taylor, J.G., Tang, D., Leitman, S., Heller, S., Serjeant, G.R., Rodgers, G.P., and Chanock, S.P. (2000). Identification of single nucleotide polymorphisms (SNPS) in cell adhesion molecules for a pilot study of stroke and sickle cell disease. *Blood*, **96**, 486a (Suppl 1, abstract).

Taylor, J.G., Tang, D., Foster, C.B., Serjeant, G.R., Rodgers, G.P., and Chanock, S.J. (2002a). Patterns of low affinity immunoglobulin receptor polymorphisms in stroke and sickle cell disease. *American Journal of Hematology*, **69**, 109–14.

Taylor, J.G., Tang, D.C., Savage, S., Leitman, S.F., Heller, S.I., Serjeant, G.R., Rodgers, G.P., and Chanock, S.J. (2002b). Variants in the VCAM1 gene and risk for symptomatic stroke in sickle cell disease. *Blood*. Prepublished DOI 10.1182/blood-2001-12-0306.

Terada, T., Yokote, H., Tsuura, M., Nakai, K., Ohshima, A., and Itakura, T. (1999). Marfan syndrome associated with moyamoya phenomenon and aortic dissection. *Acta Neurochirurgica* (Wien), **141**, 663–5.

Thorarensen, O., Ryan, S., Hunter, J., and Younkin, D.P. (1997). Factor V Leiden mutation: an unrecognized cause of hemiplegic cerebral palsy, neonatal stroke, and placental thrombosis. *Annals of Neurology*, **42**, 372–5.

Tomsick, T.A., Luskin, R.R., Chambers, A.A., and Benton, C. (1976). Neurofibromatosis and intracranial arterial occlusive disease. *Neuroradiology*, **11**, 229–34.

Tokunaga, Y., Ohga, S., Suita, S., Matsushima, T., and Hara, T. (2001). Moyamoya syndrome with spherocytosis: effect of splenectomy on strokes. *Pediatric Neurology*, **25**, 75–7.

van Beynum, I.M., Smeitink, J.A., den Heijer. M., *et al.* (1999). Hyperhomocysteinemia: a risk factor for ischemic stroke in children. *Circulation*, **99**, 2070–2.

van den Berg, J.S., Limburg, M., Kappelle, L.J., Poele Pothoff, M.T., and Blom, H.J. (1998). The role of type III collagen in spontaneous cervical arterial dissections. *Annals of Neurology*, **43**, 494–8.

Watkins, K.E., Hewes, D.K.M., Connelly, A., Kendall, B.E., Kingsley, D.P.E., Evans, J.P.M., Gadian, D.G., Vargha-Khadem, F., and Kirkham, F.J. (1998). Cognitive deficits associated with frontal lobe infarction in children with sickle cell disease. *Developmental Medicine and Child Neurology*, **40**, 536–43.

Weatherall, D.J. (1995). The molecular basis of phenotypic diversity in genetic disease. *Annals of New York Academy Science*, **758**, 245–60.

Weir, C.J., McCarron, M.O., Muir, K.W., Dyker, A.G., Bone, I., Lees, K.R., and Nicoll, J.A. (2001). Apolipoprotein E genotype, coagulation, and survival following acute stroke. *Neurology*, 57, 1097–100.

Williams, L.S., Garg, B.P., Cohen, M., Fleck, J.D., and Biller, J. (1997). Subtypes of ischemic stroke in children and young adults. *Neurology*, 49, 1541–5.

Wood, D.H. (1978). Cerebrovascular complications of sickle cell anemia. *Stroke*, 9, 73–5.

Woolfenden, A.R., Albers, G.W., Steinberg, G.K., Hahn, J.S., Johnston, D.C., and Farrell, K. (1999). Moyamoya syndrome in children with Alagille syndrome: additional evidence of a vasculopathy. *Pediatrics*, 103, 505–8.

Wun, T., Paglieroni, T., Tablin, F., Welborn, J., Nelson, K., and Cheung, A. (1997). Platelet activation and platelet–erythrocyte aggregates in patients with sickle cell anemia. *The Journal of Laboratory and Clinical Medicine*, 129, 507–16.

Yamauchi, T., Tada, M., Houkin, K., Tanaka, T., Nakamura, Y., Kuroda, S., Abe, H., Inoue, T., Ikezaki, K., Matsushima, T., and Fukui, M. (2000). Linkage of Familial Moyamoya Disease (Spontaneous Occlusion of the Circle of Willis) to Chromosome 17q25. *Stroke*, 31, 930–5.

You, R.X., McNeil, J.J., O'Malley, H.M., Davis, S.M., Thrift, A.G., and Donnan, G.A. (1997). Risk factors for stroke due to cerebral infarction in young adults. *Stroke*, 28, 1913–18.

Zafeiriou, D.I., Ikeda, H., Anastasiou, A., Vargiami, E., Vougiouklis, N., Katzos, G., Gombakis, N., Matsushima, Y., and Kirkham, F.J. (2003). Familial moyamoya disease in a Greek family: further evidence for linkage to chromosome 3P24.2–P26. *Brain Development* (in press).

Zenz, W., Bodo, Z., Plotho, J., *et al.* (1997). Factor V Leiden and prothrombin gene G 20210 A variant in children with ischemic stroke. *Thrombosis and Haemostasis*, 80, 763–6.

Chapter 13

Investigating a patient with stroke for genetic causes

Hugh S. Markus

13.1 Introduction

Most cases of stroke have a multi-factorial pathogenesis. In such cases, although a genetic predisposition may be a risk factor in individual patients, identifying the underlying genetic basis is usually impossible, and is clinically not relevant. In contrast in a minority of stroke patients, abnormalities in a single gene are primarily responsible for the stroke. In this group, identifying the underlying genetic abnormality is not only often realistic, but may also have important implications for both clinical management, and genetic testing of other family members. In many cases, particularly when stroke is only one part of a systemic monogenic disorder, diagnosis is not difficult. However, in other cases it can be difficult not only to determine whether stroke in a young individual has a monogenic basis, but also to identify the underlying genetic predisposition. This chapter will address two issues. First, how can one determine whether stroke in an individual patient is due to a monogenic disorder? Second, what is the most practical way to determine the underlying gene defect or diagnosis? Some patients present with a dementia, but have evidence of cerebral ischaemia, and a separate section covers this presentation. An important consideration when dealing with single-gene disorders causing stroke is genetic counselling. This issue is covered at the end of the chapter.

13.2 Is the stroke due to a monogenic disorder?

In many patients with stroke secondary to monogenic disorders, this is only one manifestation of a systemic disease. For example, most patients with sickle cell disease (SCD), in whom stroke is an important complication, have already presented with other manifestations of the disease such as painful crises. A patient presenting with subarachnoid haemorrhage due to a ruptured berry aneurysm, as a complication of polycystic kidney disease, may have already presented with renal disease. In such cases diagnosis is not a problem. Similarly, many patients come from a family with an already diagnosed single-gene disorder. However, in patients without these features diagnosis is more difficult.

A number of clues should alert one to the possibility of an underlying single-gene defect. These include: a family history of stroke, other cardiovascular disease or dementia; a young age of onset (less than 50 years); an atypical or more complex presentation which fits best with one of the monogenic stroke disorders (e.g., late onset complex migraine followed by lacunar stroke as occurs in CADASIL); or other

Table 13.1 Monogenic causes of ischaemic stroke

Mechanism	Examples	Notes	Gene

Cardioembolic	Cardiomyopathies
	  Primary
	  Secondary
	Familial dysrhythmias
			Various

Small vessel disease	CADASIL
	Fabry's disease
		X linked
		Also large vessel
		  disease, and
		  cardioembolism
			Notch 3
			α-galactosidase A

Premature atherosclerosis	Dyslipidaemias		Various
	Homocysteinuria/ Hyperhomocysteinaemia	Also prothrombotic	Cystathione β synthase MTHFR
Prothrombotic states	Protein S and C deficiency Antithrombin III deficiency APC resistance		Protein S and C genes Antithrombin III gene Ledien factor V mutation

	Familial anticardiolipin
	  syndrome
	Familial Sneddon's
	  syndrome
			Unknown
			
			Unknown

Haemoglobinopathies	Sickle cell disease	Sludging during crises Vasculopathy Moya–Moya in adults	Globin genes
Mitochondrial disorders	MELAS		Mitochondrial mutations
Arterial dissection	Ehlers–Danlos syndrome Fibromuscular dysplasia Marfan syndrome		Procollagen gene Unknown Fibrillin
Chanelopathies	Familial hemiplegic migraine		Calcium channel gene
Others	Neurofibromatosis	Vaso-occlusive disease	Neurofibronin

	Pseudoxanthoma
	  elasticum
	Moya–Moya
		Vaso-occlusive
		  disease
			Unknown
			
			Unknown

specific abnormalities on clinical assessment consistent with a particular monogenic disorder.

A key step in identifying the underlying disorder is accurate phenotyping, or stroke subtyping. The major single-gene disorders causing ischaemic stroke and cerebral haemorrhage are shown in Tables 13.1 and 13.2. It can be seen that the majority of these result in specific stroke subtypes. For example, CADASIL, which is perhaps the most common monogenic condition causing ischaemic stroke, results in small vessel disease but does not result in large vessel disease or cardioembolic stroke. The connective tissue disorders, such as Ehlers–Danlos syndrome, cause ischaemic stroke primarily through carotid and vertebral artery dissection rather than through small vessel disease, or atherosclerosis. There are some exceptions to this rule. For example, SCD can cause ischaemic stroke either by sludging and thrombosis during crises, or via a vasculopathy particularly affecting the large intracerebral vessels. It can also cause cerebral haemorrhage due to a secondary Moya–Moya syndrome particularly in adults. Nevertheless, even in such cases defining the underlying cause of stroke will aid in making the diagnosis.

Therefore, in all cases the first step should be to subtype stroke according to a simple pathophysiological classification, as shown in Table 13.1 for cerebral ischaemia and Table 13.2 for cerebral haemorrhage. This involves a careful history and examination,

Table 13.2 Monogenic causes of cerebral haemorrhage

Mechanism	Examples	Gene
Aneurysms	Primary familial SAH	Unknown
	Secondary	
	Polycystic kidney disease	Polycystin 1 and 2
	Marfan syndrome	Fibrillin
	Ehlers–Danlos type IV	Type III procollagen gene
	Fibromuscular dysplasia	Unknown
Amyloid angiopathy	Dutch type	Amyloid precursor protein
	Italian type	Amyloid precursor protein
	Flemish type	Amyloid precursor protein
	Icelandic type	Cystatin
Arteriovenous malformations	Hereditary haemorrhagic telangectasia (HHT)	HHT1, HHT2, HHT3
	Cerebral cavernous angiomas	CCM1, CCM2, CCM3
Bleeding disorders	Haemophilia A and B	Factor VIII and IX
	Other Factor deficiencies	Various
	Fibrinogen deficiency	Fibrinogen
Moya–Moya	Idiopathic	Unknown
	Secondary	
	Sickle cell disease	Globin gene
	Prothrombotic disorders	Various

brain imaging preferably with magnetic resonance imaging (MRI) rather than computed tomography, imaging of the extra and intracerebral vessels with ultrasound and/or magnetic resonance angiography, electocardiography and echocardiography. In individual cases further specific investigations will be required. For example, in suspected carotid dissection the optimal first line investigation is cross-sectional MRI imaging through the internal carotid artery throughout its course from the bifurcation to the skull base. Similarly in patients suspected of having amyloid angiopathy gradient echo MRI is particularly useful as it shows evidence of old cerebral haemorrhage. This initial subtyping may lead directly onto further more invasive investigations, such as intra-arterial angiography in a case of suspected Moya–Moya syndrome.

13.3 Family history

Taking an accurate family history is crucial in diagnosing single-gene disorders causing stroke. Frequently, this is poorly performed and on more detailed testing a patient for whom a family history of 'nil relevant' has been recorded in the notes, turns out to have a highly significant family history. It is best to adopt a systematic approach and work stepwise through the patient's father, mother, individual sibs, and then more distant relatives. For each family member, I would recommend asking specifically whether that member is alive, if they are dead at what age they died and of what disease, if they are alive what age they are, and whether they have ever suffered stroke. One should ask whether specific members have suffered from other cardiovascular disease including sudden death and myocardial infarction, and whether they suffered from dementia which may well have had a vascular basis. Its is also important to ask about other neurological disease which can sometimes be confused with stroke. For example, particularly before its existence was more widely appreciated, cases of CADASIL were diagnosed as multiple sclerosis due to a similar age of onset and some similarities in the MRI appearances. Therefore, a patient who gives a family history of multiple sclerosis may in fact have a family history of CADASIL. A family history of other potentially related diseases may also be important. This is often easiest to ask for once the stroke subtype has been determined. For example, in a patient with carotid dissection one might ask about a family history of joint hypermobility or skin abnormalities. Similarly in a patient with suspected CADASIL a family history of complex migraine, depression or other psychiatric disease, or encephalopathy may be highly relevant.

It can often be helpful to get confirmation of specific details of the family history either from other family members or from the patient's family doctor. This is particularly important in individuals who have cognitive impairment or speech disorder secondary to their stroke. Interviewing a patient with their spouse, sibling, or child is frequently useful. Sometimes a patient may not know full details of their family history when first questioned and in these cases they can often perform useful research by asking other family members. It may be helpful to identify one informant within a

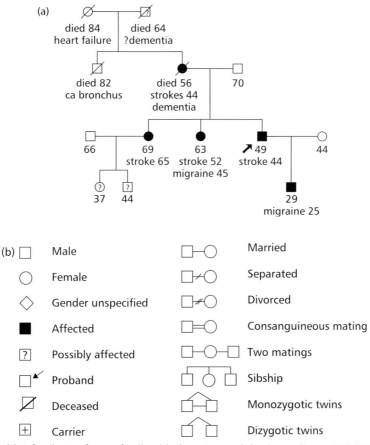

Fig. 13.1 (a) A family tree from a family with the autosomal dominant disease CADASIL, created using a standard software package. Standard symbols, illustrated in (b), are used to indicate the status of individuals. Additional information, such as the presence of cardinal symptoms and their age of onset, can be added under each individual.

family who is prepared to compile an accurate family history from other relatives. It is also important to record any consanguinous relationships.

The family history can be clearly represented with a family tree using standard symbols (see Fig. 13.1). There are a number of commercially available software packages that will create a family tree as in Fig. 13.1(a).

13.4 Clues to the diagnosis of monogenic ischaemic stroke on history, examination, and investigation

A number of clinical systemic features, or particular appearances on brain imaging or other investigations are particularly useful in identifying certain specific single-gene disorders causing ischaemic stroke. Some of these are summarized in Table 13.3.

Table 13.3 Clues to diagnosis of monogenic ischaemic stroke

Examples	History	Examination	Imaging/useful tests

Cardiomyopathies
  Primary
  Secondary
			Echocardiography

Familial dysrhythmias			Electrocardiography

CADASIL	Migraine with
	  aura
	Depression
			MRI: pattern of
			  involvement
			Skin biopsy

Fabry's disease	Episodic painful
	  crises
	Anhydrosis
		Skin and mucosal
		  angiokeratoma
		Corneal dystrophy
		Proteinuria
		Cardiac disease	

Dyslipidaemias		Xanthalasma Atherosclerosis elsewhere	Serum lipids

Homocysteinuria	Venous
	  thrombosis
		Atherosclerosis
		  elsewhere
		Ectopic/dislocated lens
		Skeletal deformities
		Mental retardation
			Urinary homocysteine
			Serum homocysteine

Hyperhomocysteinaemia	Venous
	  thrombosis
		Atherosclerosis
		  elsewhere
			Serum homocysteine

Protein S and C deficiency	Venous thrombosis		Protein C and S levels
Antithrombin III deficiency	Venous thrombosis		Antithrombin III assay
APC resistance	Venous thrombosis		APC assay
Familial anticardiolipin syndrome	Spontaneous miscarriages Venous thrombosis		Anticardiolipin antibody
Familial Sneddon's syndrome		Livedo reticularis	Anticardiolipin antibody
Sickle cell disease	Painful crises	Anaemia	Haemoglobin electrophoresis

MELAS	Migraine
	Seizures
	External
	  opthalmoplegia
	Sensorineural
	  deafness
	Dementia
		Myopathy	MRI; rapidly resolving
			  lesions
			Muscle biopsy
			CSF lactate

(continued)

Table 13.3 (continued)

Examples	History	Examination	Imaging/useful tests
Ehlers–Danlos syndrome IV	Easy bruising	Thin translucent skin Facial appearance (see Section 9.2.2)	Skin biopsy
Fibromuscular dysplasia	Hypertension	Hypertension	Angiography
Marfan syndrome		Marfanoid habitus Ectopia lentis	
Familial hemiplegic migraine	Hemiplegic migraine Migraine coma		
Neurofibromatosis		Cafe au lait spots Neurofibromas Axillary freckling	
Pseudoxanthoma elasticum		Skin papules Retinal mottling and angioid streaks	
Moya–Moya			CT/MRI Watershed infarcts New vessels on angiography

Full details of the single-gene disorders which can cause ischaemic stroke, presented according to a pathophysiological classification, are covered in Chapter 6, and only certain clinical features particularly useful in diagnosis are discussed below.

13.4.1 CADASIL

Although firm data on the prevalence of different single-gene disorders causing stroke is not available, it is now apparent that CADASIL is much more frequent that was previously thought, and is perhaps the most common single-gene disorder causing ischaemic stroke. There are a number of useful pointers to the disease on history (Desmond *et al.* 1999, and Section 6.2.1). About 60 per cent of patients have migraine. This usually begins in the 20s or 30s, and in the great majority of cases is complex migraine with aura that may be visual, somatosensory, or confusional. Depression prior to the onset of stroke occurs in a significant number of individuals. Strokes, when they occur are always due to small vessel disease and tend to be classical lacunar syndromes such as pure motor stroke or sensorimotor stroke. A recently recognized presentation of CADASIL is with a sub-acute encephalopathy which resolves over 1–2 weeks (Schon *et al.* 2003). This usually follows a typical complex migraine attack,

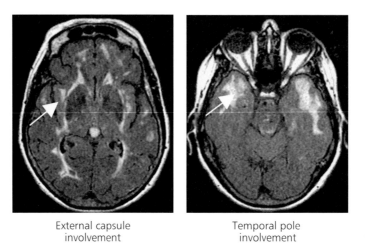

External capsule
involvement

Temporal pole
involvement

Fig. 13.2 Useful diagnostic MRI feature in CADASIL. Involvement of the external capsule and anterior temporal lobe are shown.

and is often accompanied by epilepsy, extensor plantars, and cortical signs. It is frequently misdiagnosed as encephalitis.

The MRI scan appearance is crucial in making a diagnosis of CADASIL. T2-weighted or FLAIR sequences show a combination of leukoaraiosis, both in the periventricular region and centrum semiovale, and small focal lacunar infarcts. Although this alone does not help one distinguish the disease from sporadic lacunar stroke with leukoaraiosis, which is most common in hypertensive patients, there are a number of relatively specific MRI features. The most useful is involvement of the anterior temporal poles (Auer *et al.* 2001, O'Sullivan *et al.* 2001), which occurs early in CADASIL and has a sensitivity and specificity of about 90 per cent in diagnosing the disease (Markus *et al.* 2002). Involvement of the external capsule is also common, occurring in 90 per cent or more of symptomatic patients, although it is less specific (Markus *et al.* 2002). Typical examples of these appearances are shown in Fig. 13.2. In contrast to sporadic lacunar stroke in which involvement of the corpus callosum is rare, it can frequently occur in CADASIL, and this sometimes leads to misdiagnosis as multiple sclerosis.

With a consistent clinical history and MRI appearance one can often be relatively sure of the diagnosis of CADASIL. However, skin biopsy to look for granular osmiophilic material is often useful at this stage, as it is positive in 50 per cent or more of individuals and is 100 per cent specific for CADASIL (Ebke *et al.* 1997, Markus *et al.* 2002). These deposits (see Fig. 6.2) are only visible on electron microscopy and light microscopic appearances are not diagnostic. The underlying genetic defect can be found by screening the notch 3 gene for mutations which are highly stereotyped and all result in disruption of a odd number (usually a single) cysteine residue (Joutel *et al.* 1997). In practice screening the whole gene is very time consuming and therefore most laboratories would start by screening exon 4 in which about 70 per cent of mutations occur (Joutel *et al.* 1997), and then progressing to exons 3, 5, and 6. Screening these four exons has been shown to identify 90 per cent of cases in a British population study (Markus *et al.* 2002).

13.4.2 Mitochondrial disease

Mitochondrial disease is often raised as a possibility in a young patient with ischaemic stroke (see Section 6.7). While it is a rare cause, it can be difficult to diagnose in many cases. Although stroke can occur as part of a variety of mitochondrial disease syndromes, the classical presentation is as part of the picture of MELAS with migraine, seizures, external ophthalmoplegia, sensorineural deafness, and progression to dementia. The neurological deficits seen may evolve in the setting of a febrile illness with vomiting and seizures, and may be transient or permanent (Ciafaloni *et al.* 1992). Because MELAS is due to mutations in mitochondrial DNA the disease is maternally transmitted, although there is not always an obvious family history. There are a number of clues on neuroimaging which may aid in the diagnosis. One typical pattern is for there to be moderate sized 'infarcts' involving both the cortex and subcortex and particularly affecting the occipital and posterior parietal regions. A characteristic feature of these 'infarcts' is that they do not always obey arterial territories, and may show striking resolution on follow-up imaging. A typical case is shown in Fig. 13.3 and 13.4. This rapid resolution is highly characteristic of MELAS. At the time of infarction magnetic resonance spectroscopy can show the presence of a bifid lactate peak within the infarct although this is not specific as it frequently occurs in acute infarcts due to other causes. Cerebrospinal fluid examination may show elevated lactate in the CSF compared with the plasma.

Muscle biopsy typically shows ragged red fibres, but is not always positive, and its interpretation can be complicated by the phenomena of heteroplasmy. This is where there is a variation in the expression of mutated mitochondrial DNA within different tissues. Therefore a large biopsy is often more useful in excluding the disease than a small muscle biopsy. A number of mutations have been reported to cause MELAS and other mitochondrial disorders. The most common mutations causing MELAS are in the *tRNA^{leucine}*(UUR) gene; an A3243G mutation in about 75 per cent, and T3271C in about 10 per cent (Ciafaloni *et al.* 1992). Occasional other mutations have been reported, and in about 10 per cent of cases no mutation can be found. Most laboratories test routinely for the two commonest mutations. Patients with typical MELAS mutations and stroke, but without ragged red fibres, have been described, and stroke can be part of overlap syndromes between MELAS and other mitochondrial disorders including MERRF (myoclonus epilepsy and ragged red fibres) and the Kearns–Sayre syndrome.

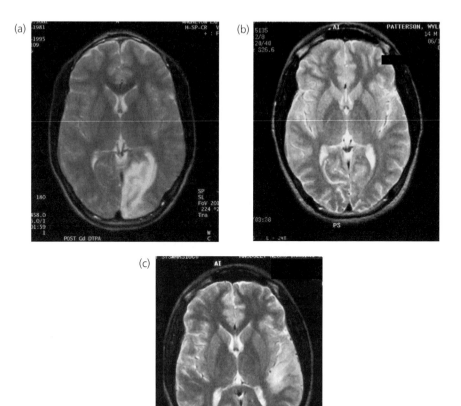

Fig. 13.3 MELAS. One typical neuroradiological pattern seen in MELAS is of 'large infarcts' particularly in the occipito-parietal regions and posterior temporal regions. These may not obey arterial boundaries. A typical example is shown in this series from a boy who was 13 years old at presentation (a). He presented with a right homonymous hemianopia, and a left occipital high signal lesion was seen on the T2-weighted MRI. A characteristic feature of these 'infarcts' is that marked resolution may occur on repeat imaging as can be seen on this repeat scan (b) performed a few months later. The next year he presented with complex partial seizures and a repeat MRI showed another 'infarct' in the left temporal lobe (c).

13.4.3 Disease with associated skin features

A number of skin abnormalities may point to particular systemic diseases causing stroke. Although stroke is not a major feature of dyslipidaemias, these patients may have evidence of cholesterol depositions such as xanthalasma as well as evidence of atherosclerosis elsewhere. Neurofibromatosis is a rare cause of stroke particularly in younger individuals, and

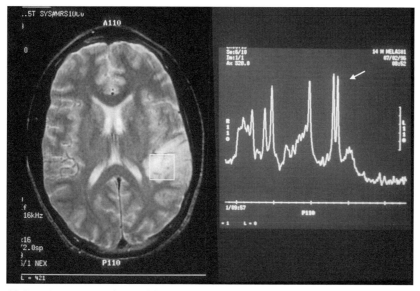

Fig. 13.4 MELAS. Lactate detected by magnetic resonance spectroscopy in a patient with MELAS. This is same patient shown in Fig. 13.3. Proton spectroscopy was carried out at the time of his presentation with seizures and a left temporal lobe lesion. A voxel was placed over the lesion, shown on the left image. The spectra shows a prominent bifid peak at the resonance of lactate.

stroke occurs due to a vasculopathy (see Section 6.3.5). Patients may show café au lait spots as well as cutaneous neurofibromas. Fabry's disease (see Section 6.4.1) is an X linked recessive disorder due to α-galactosidase A deficiency. Progressive accumulation of ceramidetrihexoside within the intima and media of blood vessels results in luminal narrowing, and complications such as stroke and myocardial ischaemia. Stroke most commonly occurs from the third decade onwards and may be secondary to small vessel disease, large vessel disease, or due to the associated cardiac disease with secondary embolism. The presence of angiokeratoma as well as painful acroparaesthesiae and proteinuria may point to the disease. The cerebral vasculopathy is best visualized on T2-weighted MRI which initially demonstrates periventricular hyperintensities and lacunar infarcts indicative of small vessel disease, and subsequently progresses with age to affect the larger vessels leading to symptomatic infarcts which appear in the cortical grey matter. Skin abnormalities in patients with carotid dissection may indicate an underlying connective tissue disorder (see below).

13.4.4 **Prothrombotic disorders**

A number of prothrombotic disorders have been associated with stroke including protein C and S deficiency, antithrombin III deficiency, and activated protein C (APC) resistance. These disorders are much more important risk factors for venous thrombosis including cerebral venous thrombosis. Most studies have suggested they are not important for middle age and elderly stroke (see Section 8.4.1) but may be important in certain families with younger onset stroke (see Section 12.8.3). A clue to their diagnosis is a family history, or past history, of venous thrombosis. In view of their major association with venous as opposed to arterial thrombosis, in stroke patients with one of these disorders it is always worth excluding a patent foramen ovale on echocardiography. In such a patient stroke could be due to venous thrombosis with paradoxical embolism. These diagnoses can be made on blood prothrombotic testing but the results of this have to be interpreted with caution. Proving a causal association in an individual patient is complicated by the fact that reduced levels of protein C and S may occur transiently after stroke. Low levels can also been seen in other diseases including liver disease, disseminated intravascular coagulation and renal disease, or in patients on warfarin therapy. Therefore it may be necessary to confirm an underlying gene defect by serial sampling of levels and screening other family members. APC resistance is usually due to a single underlying mutation, the Leiden factor V mutation. However, even if one detects the heterozygous state one needs to be cautious before attributing it as the cause of stroke. It occurs in about 5 per cent of normal individuals and therefore could be an innocent bystander.

13.4.5 Anticardiolipin syndrome and Sneddon's syndrome

Familial anticardiolipin and lupus anticoagulant syndromes (Mackie *et al.* 1987) are rare causes of stroke. Clues to the diagnosis include a past history of recurrent spontaneous miscarriage or infertility, and venous thrombosis. Strokes may be large vessel disease, or small vessel disease, and amaurosis fugax can occur. The anticardiolipin antibody is detected on a blood sample and is usually markedly elevated, but should be repeated as non-specific elevations of this antibody have been reported in patients with sporadic ischaemic stroke. Sneddon's syndrome is a related disease in which anticardiolipin antibodies are often found, although they are not invariably present. The typical blotchy rash of livedo reticularis is characteristic of Sneddon's syndrome and other features include TIAs, strokes, and dementia. The vast majority of cases of both anticardiolipin syndrome and Sneddon's syndrome are sporadic. The very rare familial cases can only be identified by family history and testing other family members. Familial Sneddon's syndrome appears to have an autosomal dominant inheritance (Berciano 1988).

13.4.6 Homocysteinuria and hyperhomocysteinaemia

Homocysteineuria presents with a classical phenotype including skeletal deformities with a marfanoid habitus, mental retardation, ectopia lentis, and thromboembolic events. Such cases will present to paediatric neurologists and diagnosis is often not difficult, and can be made by the detection of homocysteine in the urine (see Section 6.4.2).

However, homocysteine may still be the cause of stroke in adults presenting without these other clinical features. It is now easy to test for homocysteine levels in the serum. Moderate elevations (>15 mmol/l) are common in patients with sporadic stroke, but greater elevations (>25 mmol/l) suggest that it could be a major factor in stroke pathogenesis. Homocysteine can also be reduced secondary to folic acid or B vitamin deficiency. Samples are best measured fasting, although a random level is useful if levels are markedly elevated. In patients with severe hyperhomocysteinaemia or homocysteineuria, the most common underlying genetic defect is in the cystathione beta-synthase gene. There are a number of relatively common mutations. Lesser degrees of homocysteinaemia are often caused by mutations in the methylene tetrahydrafolate reductase gene (MTHFR) There is a single common mutation (C677T) which underlies this abnormality, and genotyping for this mutation is available in many laboratories. Most individuals are heterozygous for this mutation but occasional individuals with markedly elevated homocysteine are homozygous.

13.4.7 Carotid and vertebral artery dissection

About half of cases of carotid and vertebral dissection occur secondary to trauma, and in most of these cases there appears to be no pre-existing abnormality. The remainder occur spontaneously, or after minimal trauma. In the majority of these cases there is no obvious underlying familial condition, although recent studies, which have performed skin biopsies in spontaneous dissections, have suggested that underlying abnormalities of connective tissue may be relatively common (Brandt *et al.* 2001). However, in a few families there is a clear underlying monogenic disorder responsible for the dissection. Responsible diseases include Ehlers–Danlos syndrome type IV and fibromuscular dysplasia. A diagnosis of Ehlers–Danlos syndrome is suggested by easy bruising, translucent skin with visible veins, characteristic facial features, and rupture of arteries, uterus, or intestines, skin laxity and joint hypermobility (Section 6.3.2). Fibromuscular dysplasia may have a genetic basis although the underlying gene remains unknown. The typical beading appearance can be seen on angiography. In most patients with spontaneous carotid or vertebral dissection recurrence is rare, and the disease remains a unilateral disorder. However, in patients who have recurrent or bilateral dissection, one should always look particularly hard for an underlying connective tissue disorder.

13.5 Clues to the diagnosis of monogenic haemorrhagic stroke on history, examination, and investigation

A similar approach, with accurate determination of the stroke subtype, is equally crucial for patients with cerebral haemorrhage. In many cases, it is possible to determine the underlying pathophysiological mechanisms leading to cerebral haemorrhage, and this is frequently easier than in patients with cerebral ischaemia. The initial brain imaging appearances are very useful. The presence of subarachnoid blood, or detection of subarachnoid blood on lumbar puncture, will usually lead to angiography to look for a cerebral aneurysm. Patients with underlying familial disorders frequently have multiple aneurysms, as well as a family history of cerebral haemorrhage or sudden death, and this is covered in detail in Chapter 10.

13.5.1 Clues from neuroimaging appearances

In patients with parenchymal haemorrhage, the pattern may give clues to the underlying disorder. Lobar haemorrhage, particularly if recurrent, alerts one to a possible diagnosis of amyloid angiopathy. In such a case the next investigation is gradient echo MRI. On this sequence, haemosiderin deposition is seen as signal loss. In patients with amyloid angiopathy it will frequently show evidence of old asymptomatic haemorrhage. The presence of multiple haemorrhages on these sequences is one of the Boston criteria for diagnosis of amyloid angiopathy (see Section 9.3.3). Angiography for subarachnoid haemorrhage will also pick up most cases of cerebral haemorrhage secondary to Moya–Moya disease. Although secondary haemorrhage may be seen on CT imaging, arteriovenous malformations can only be well seen on MRI. This is especially true for cavernous angiomas, which are poorly seen on CT unless there is associated calcification, but can be well seen on MRI. In addition to the angioma, a surrounding area of signal loss due to haemosiderin deposition can be identified (Fig. 13.5).

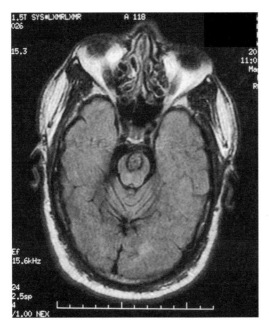

Fig. 13.5 A brainstem cavernous angioma showing a surrounding rim of low signal, secondary to haemosiderin deposition from previous bleeding.

13.5.2 Associated systemic disease

A number of systemic features may be useful in diagnosis in patients with cerebral haemorrhage. Some of these are listed in Table 13.4. Familial cerebral aneurysms may either be primary without obvious systemic disease, or secondary to systemic disease. For example, patients may have a family, or past, history of polycystic kidney disease and hypertension. Imaging of the kidneys will show the typical cysts. Polycystic kidney disease is associated with berry aneurysms. Fibromuscular dysplasia is also associated with berry aneurysms and this will usually be detected on angiography, when typical beading of the arteries is seen. Marfan syndrome has been most associated with aortic

Table 13.4 Clues to diagnosis of monogenic cerebral haemorrhage

Examples	History	Examination	Imaging/tests
Subarachnoid haemorrhage			Angiography
Primary familial SAH			
Secondary			
Polycystic kidney disease		Polycystic kidneys Hypertension	Renal ultrasound
Marfan syndrome		Marfanoid habitus Ectopic/dislocated lens	
Ehlers–Danlos type IV	Easy bruising	Thin translucent skin Facial appearance (see Section 9.2.2)	Skin biopsy
Fibromuscular dysplasia			Angiography
Amyloid angiopathy			Gradient echo MRI
Dutch type		Dementia	
Italian type		Dementia	
Flemish type		Dementia	
Icelandic type		Dementia (less common)	
AVMs			
Hereditary haemorrhagic telangectasia (HHT)	Nose bleeds	Cutaneous telangectasia	
Cerebral cavernous angiomas		Cutaneous angiomas	Gradient echo MRI
Bleedings disorders			
Haemophilia A and B	Systemic bleeding	Arthritis	
Other Factor deficiencies	Systemic bleeding		
Fibrinogen deficiency	Systemic bleeding		
Moya–Moya			Watershed infarcts Angiography
Idiopathic			
Secondary			
Sickle cell disease	Painful crises	Anaemia	Haemoglobin electrophoresis

aneurysms, and giant aneurysms sometimes affecting the internal carotid artery. The association with berry aneurysms is much weaker. Clues to this diagnosis include a Marfanoid habitus, dislocated lens, high arched palate, and aortic regurgitation. Ehlers–Danlos type IV has also been associated with fusiform internal carotid artery aneurysms and carotid-cavernous fistulae, but not particularly with berry aneurysms. Coarctation of the aorta has been associated with an increased occurrence of berry aneurysms, although part of this may result from the associated hypertension. This diagnosis should be raised by the associated severe hypertension.

13.5.3 Amyloid angiopathy

Dementia or a family history of dementia can be an important clue to the diagnosis of amyloid angiopathy (Section 9.9.3). Dementia is more common with the angiopathies associated with mutations in the amyloid precursor protein (Dutch type, Italian type, Flemish type) than with amyloid angiopathy associated with cystatin mutations (Icelandic type). The location of the cerebral haemorrhages and the appearances on gradient echo MRI (described above) are crucial in diagnosis. The diagnosis can be proven on brain biopsy on which amyloid deposits, which show birefringence on Congo red staining, can be seen.

13.5.4 Hereditary haemorrhagic telangectasia

Hereditary haemorrhagic telangectasia (Osler–Weber–Rendu) disease is a systemic disease leading to both telangectasia and cerebral arteriovenous malformation (see Section 11.2). Therefore the presence of telangectasia, which can affect many organs including the skin, mucosa, conjunctiva, retina, ears, fingers, gastrointenstinal tract particularly the upper tract, and kidneys, is an important clue to diagnosis. Nose bleeds or epistaxis is the most frequent initial symptom occurring in 90 per cent of cases and is an important clue to diagnosis. Pulmonary arteriovenous malformations are also frequent, and clinical manifestations of these which may point to the diagnosis include paradoxical embolism with stroke, brain abscess, pulmonary haemorrhage, and heart failure. Migraine is also frequently observed in hereditary haemorrhagic telangectasia.

13.5.5 Cerebral cavernomas

In contrast to hereditary haemorrhagic telangectasia, which is a systemic disease, cerebral cavernomas are capillary malformations which are mostly located in the central nervous system (see Section 11.3). These are best diagnosed on MRI (Fig. 13.4), and an important clue to a familial basis is the presence of multiple cavernous angiomas. For example, in one study of 22 patients with multiple cavernomas who appeared to be sporadic cases (i.e. without any known affected relatives) MRI screening of the relatives established a familial basis in 73 per cent (Labauge et al. 1998). Despite the fact that the disease is primarily in the brain, systemic manifestations may occur which can be an important clue to diagnosis. The most commonly described locations are cutaneous. These include blueish nodules, cherry angiomas, capillary vascular anomalies, and eruptive multiple angiokeratomas. These cutaneous lesions are mostly located on the lower limbs, are often single, and do not evolve.

13.5.6 Familial bleeding disorders

Patients with cerebral haemorrhage secondary to coagulation disorders such as haemophilia usually have the diagnosis already established. Typical features include recurrent episodes of pain and swelling in weight bearing joints due to haemarthrosis, and haematuria in the absence of any genitourinary pathology. Delayed bleeding hours or days after injury involving any organ is a classical feature.

13.5.7 Moya–Moya syndrome

Moya–Moya syndrome often presents in the late teens or early adulthood with subarachnoid haemorrhage. Occlusion of the basal intracerebral vessels early in life is followed by new vessel formation. These friable new vessels may bleed. A typical appearance on angiography with a 'puff of smoke' is seen. This syndrome occurs on an idiopathic basis particularly in the Far East but is also seen in Caucasians. It can be familial (Sections 6.3.1 and 12.6). It can also occur secondary to other conditions causing basal intracerebral vessel occlusion. These include SCD and in such patients the diagnosis is usually apparent, and there may have been previous ischaemic events earlier in life. Although the occlusive vessel disease can be seen on intracerebral magnetic resonance angiography, the typical new vessel formation is often only seen on intra-arterial angiography. A typical angiographic appearance is shown in Fig. 13.6. A clue to diagnosis from brain imaging is the presence of watershed infarcts. These are in the territories most distal to the origin of the supplying arteries, which are therefore the areas with lowest perfusion pressure. These include traditional watershed regions in the frontal cortex between the anterior and middle cerebral artery territories, and in the posterior parietal cortex between middle and posterior cerebral artery territories. They also include the internal watershed regions as illustrated in Fig. 13.6(a).

13.6 Other useful pointers to an underlying single-gene disorder

Despite the clues from history, examination and imaging findings, it can frequently be difficult to decide which patients with stroke are worth screening for monogenic disorders, and which monogenic disorders to screen for. In practice the phenotype often points one to particular monogenic disorders. For example, in a 45-year-old man with recurrent lacunar stroke, late onset complex migraine, a family history of stroke, and

(a)

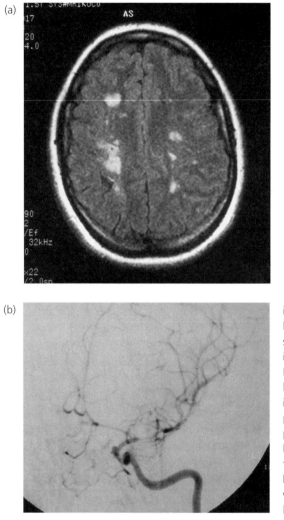

(b)

Fig. 13.6 Moya–Moya syndrome. This patient had extensive vasculopathy of the basal intracerebral vessels including bilateral middle cerebral artery stenosis. She presented with ischaemic stroke in her late teens. Her FLAIR MRI scan (a) shows bilateral areas of ischaemia in the internal watershed region. This pattern is commonly seen in the presence of large vessel haemodynamic ischaemia, as in this case. Angiography (b) shows a left middle cerebral artery stenosis with new vessel formation, the hallmark of Moya–Moya.

typical MRI features of CADASIL, one would go straight for confirmatory tests for CADASIL. However, in patients with isolated stroke without systemic signs or other diagnostic findings, whether or not to screen for monogenic disorders can be a difficult decision. There is no firm guidance from good population based studies. Nevertheless, as a general rule in patients with ischaemic stroke it is only worth screening if there is a strong family history of stroke or vascular dementia, or the patient has unexplained stroke at a young age (less than 50 years). In such cases it is only worth screening for the monogenic disorders likely to cause that particular stroke subtype, for example, notch 3 mutations in patients with small vessel disease. In a recent study in which over 200 patients with a phenotype of lacunar stroke with or without leukoaraiosis were screened for notch 3 mutations, a mutation was found in only one individual who was a man of age 38 years (Dong *et al.* 2003). The overall mutation carrier frequency was 0.05 per cent (95% CI 0.0–2.0); for individuals with lacunar stroke and leukoaraiosis with first stroke at ≤ 65 years it was 2.0 per cent (95% CI 0.4–10.9), and 11.1 per cent (95% CI 2.5–44.5) for disease onset ≤ 50 years. It is important to remember when evaluating family history, that a family history of stroke at any age is seen in about a third of an unselected group of patients with 'mulitfactorial' ischaemic stroke, while a family history of young stroke at age less than 65 years is seen in about 13 per cent (Hassan *et al.* 2002). Therefore, the presence of a family history does not necessarily imply a monogenic cause.

13.7 Investigating a patient with vascular dementia for genetic causes

Vascular dementia, like stroke, is a heterogeneous syndrome. Dementia can occur due to a single-strategic infarct in a location such as the thalamus, due to multiple infarcts involving both the cortex and subcortex, and probably most commonly due to diffuse ischaemic damage to subcortical structures. The most common cause of this latter type of dementia is small vessel disease in hypertensive patients. Such patients typically present with problems with executive and attentional function.

All of the monogenic stroke disorders considered above can potentially cause dementia. However a number are more likely to present with dementia, and this may help in diagnosis. In addition, some disorders characteristically present with dementia in the absence of clinical stroke-like events, but with neuroimaging appearances consistent with ischaemia. Investigating such patients for a monogenic disorder requires a similar approach to that outlined for ischaemic stroke and cerebral haemorrhage above. It is particularly useful to categorize patients according to their neuroimaging appearances, and type of cognitive deficit, in deciding on a differential diagnosis.

An important category of patients are those with white matter abnormalities on T2-weighted or FLAIR MRI. Important genetic causes of this presentation include the ischaemic small vessel arteriopathies particularly CADASIL, and the amyloid angiopathies.

CADASIL is dealt with in detail in Section 6.2.1, and useful pointers to diagnosis are mentioned in the section on ischaemic stroke above. Patients with CADASIL frequently suffer a subcortical dementia in the later stage of the disease. However lesser degrees of cognitive impairment may occur early in the disease prior to the onset of dementia, and executive and attentional function are affected early. For example, in one study in eight asymptomatic non-demented patients, abnormalities were found in all individuals with the Wisconsin Card Sorting Test, and in five out of eight individuals with the Trail Making Test. The deficits appeared in some of these individuals without a history of major vascular events (Taillia *et al.* 1998). In one study of 64 CADASIL patients, a significant inverse correlation was found between total lesion volume and mini mental score examination. There appeared to be a possible threshold effect on lesion volume on this score (Dichgans *et al.* 1999). As well as these minor degrees of cognitive impairment, occasional CADASIL patients can present with an advanced dementia without stroke-like episodes.

CADASIL accounts for the vast majority of monogenic small vessel cerebral arteriopathies. Familial young-adult onset arteriosclerotic leukoencephalopathy with alopecia and lumbago without arterial hypertension is a rare cause of ischaemic stroke and dementia which has been reported only in Japanese families (Section 6.2.2). Seventeen cases have been reviewed by Fukutake and Hirayama (1995). There was a male predominance with a ratio of 7.5–1, and the age of onset was usually 25–30 years. Approximately half of the patients suffered ischaemic strokes which appeared usually to be lacunar syndromes, and all developed a progressive subcortical dementia with pseudo-bulbar palsy and pyramidal signs. Acute lumbago and diffuse baldness were frequent accompanying features. Neuroimaging showed a combination of small white matter infarcts and leukoaraiosis, and autopsy demonstrated arteriosclerosis of the small penetrating arteries in the white matter, basal ganglia, brainstem, and spinal cord.

The autosomal dominant amyloid angiopathies are covered in detail in Section 3.3 . In addition to recurrent cerebral haemorrhage, these diseases can cause dementia. In patients with hereditary cerebral haemorrhage with amyloidosis Dutch type, dementia can develop after the first cerebral haemorrhage, but sometimes it is the first or only symptom of the disease. The neuropsychological profile here differs from that seen in CADASIL with more prominent 'cortical' signs, and prominent features include constructional apraxia, agnosia and agraphia, and difficulties with calculation and language (Haan *et al.* 1990). The progression of dementia can be in a step-wise fashion related to the strokes, but in occasional patients a progressive cognitive decline has been documented in the absence of strokes. Neuroimaging shows cerebral haemorrhage and/or evidence of white matter ischaemia seen as high signal on T2-weighted MRI. Gradient echo MRI is particularly useful in showing evidence of old haemorrhages consistent with the disease (see Section 3.3). Hereditary cerebral haemorrhage with amyloidosis Icelandic type, usually causes intracerebral haemorrhage at an earlier age with an onset of between 20 and 30 years. However one family has been reported with late onset dementia, with some family members having intracerebral haemorrhage and others not (Greenberg *et al.* 1993).

A further type of amyloid angiopathy which presents predominantly with dementia and other neurological features, rather than stroke-like episodes, is familial British dementia with amyloid angiopathy. The prominent features of this disease are a dementia, spastic paraparesis, and progressive cerebellar ataxia, although occasionally haemorrhage and stroke-like episodes can occur (Plant *et al.* 1990). Unlike the Dutch and Icelandic hereditary amyloid angiopathies, the disorder is a primary dementia with severe hippocampal pathology unrelated to the vascular involvement. MRI shows multiple white matter lesions, high signal on T2-weighted scans and hypodense on T1-weighted scans. These are distributed throughout the cerebral white matter but particularly prominent and confluent around the anterior and posterior horns of the lateral ventricles in advanced cases. A recent overview has described the clinical and neuropsychological features (Mead *et al.* 2000). Progressive memory loss is almost universal. When subjects with early disease were studied the most consistent cognitive impairment was in delayed memory recall tasks. The amyloid has been shown to result from the 4 kDa insoluble protein called ABRi. This protein is the abnormal product of a gene, the BRI gene on chromosome 13. In familial British dementia there is a point mutation in a stop-codon resulting in a longer than normal 277 residue precursor protein (Vidal *et al.* 1999).

Another extremely rare disease which can cause haemorrhagic strokes and dementia has been described in a family of Spanish descent (Iglesias *et al.* 2000). Patients presented with dementia and/or intracerebral haemorrhage between the ages of 58 and 81. On neuroimaging there was a patchy leukoencephalopathy with prominent periventricular leukoaraiosis, striking bilateral cortical occipital calcifications, and external carotid artery dysplasia. Skin biopsy showed previously unreported changes in the basal laminar of capillaries visible on electron microscopy. These included a multi-layered appearance and round shaped micro-calcification. The underlying genetic abnormality remains uncertain.

Other disorders in which dementia may be a prominent feature include Sneddon's syndrome, and MELAS. In the latter dementia is a frequent feature but follows the typical stroke-like episodes described earlier in the chapter. Dementia can also be a feature of SCD arising either from multiple strokes, strategic infarcts, or possibly from more diffuse damage. A slowly progressive encephalopathy, which may be due to small vessel disease in a manner similar to that seen in other small vessel disease arteriopathies, has been reported in patients with SCD (Pavlakis *et al.* 1989).

13.8 Genetic counselling

A diagnosis of a monogenic cause of stroke has major implications both for the patient and other family members. These include a combination of complex emotional, psychological and social issues. Therefore, it is vital that the patient or asymptomatic relative is carefully counselled before genetic testing is performed. This is best performed in a structured environment such as a Clinical Genetics Clinic, or a specialized Stroke Genetics Clinic. It can be provided by a number of different health professionals but those providing counselling require detailed knowledge of the clinical features and prognosis of the condition itself, detailed knowledge of its genetics, and an appreciation of the psychological and social implications of a diagnosis.

It should be remembered that tests which are not obviously 'genetic tests' could in fact give a genetic diagnosis. For example in a patient with a family history of CADASIL, if an MRI scan is performed and this shows typical neuroimaging appearances, then one can be almost 100 per cent sure that that individual has the mutation. Therefore, before performing such tests a similar level of counselling should be provided to that given before carrying out DNA mutation analysis.

There are a number of components to successful genetic counselling which can be summarized under different headings:

1. *Information collection.* This involves reviewing the clinical history of the individual being counselled including the presence of any symptoms suggestive of monogenic stroke, reviewing the family pedigree and constructing this if necessary, and understanding the social and psychological background of the individual.

2. *Explanation.* This phase involves explaining the process of genetic diagnosis. It involves giving detailed information about the disease and its prognosis. This is greatly aided by having appropriate information sheets. A typical information sheet for CADASIL that is used in our Department is shown in Fig. 13.7. The methods used to obtain a genetic diagnosis are reviewed. These will differ for different monogenic stroke disorders and also different family members. For example in a family with CADASIL in whom a specific mutation has been previously found, it is relatively easy to test for other family members. However in a family in whom a mutation has not been found and a diagnosis has been made on neuroimaging and skin biopsy appearances, other family members who would like genetic testing will have to have this on the basis of MRI scans and skin biopsies. Neither test is 100 per cent sensitive and therefore the sensitivity in an individual of a particular age being studied will need to be discussed.

   The potential pros and cons of genetic testing can then be reviewed. At this stage it is helpful for the individual to consider what implications a positive diagnosis might have, both psychologically and socially. This session offers an ideal opportunity to answer the many other questions that subjects usually have. It is important to point out however that whether or not they have genetic testing is entirely up to them and there is no right or wrong decision.

3. *Contemplation.* Once the individual has all the information necessary to make their decision, it is important to leave time for them to consider the options and come up with a definite decision. In some patients with symptomatic disease in whom finding the cause is important for therapeutic reasons, it is sometimes appropriate to progress rapidly on to genetic testing. However, in asymptomatic family members it is generally advisable to leave a period of weeks from the initial counselling until genetic tests are performed. We usually leave a period of at least four weeks.

4. *Diagnostic testing.* An appointment is made for the individual to return to clinic. If they wish to proceed with genetic testing the appropriate tests can now be performed. This is a good opportunity to ensure that the patient has a complete understanding of both the implications of testing, and the sensitivity and specificity of the test.

5. *The results of genetic testing.* If genetic testing is performed a further appointment is made for the patient to re-attend to receive the results. If the results show a positive

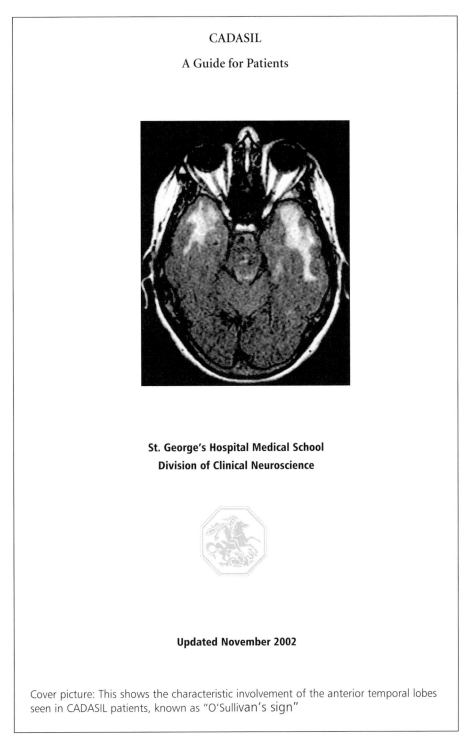

CADASIL

A Guide for Patients

St. George's Hospital Medical School
Division of Clinical Neuroscience

Updated November 2002

Cover picture: This shows the characteristic involvement of the anterior temporal lobes seen in CADASIL patients, known as "O'Sullivan's sign"

Fig. 13.7 (continued)

What is CADASIL?

CADASIL is an abbreviation for a long name describing a rare hereditary form of stroke (cerebral autosomal dominant arteriopathy with subcortical infarcts and leucoencephalopathy). The disease usually presents with multiple small strokes but migraine is also a prominent feature. There's been a lot of interest in the disease recently because the underlying genetic abnormality was recently demonstrated.

What does genetic mean?

In many diseases genetic factors are important. This means that part, or all of the risk, is passed down from one's parents. Certain diseases are caused by an abnormality in one single gene and CADASIL is one of these diseases. Genes produces proteins which are necessary for normal functioning of the body. Everybody has two copies of each gene, one passed down from their mother, and one from their father. In CADASIL, an abnormality in only one of these two copies results in the disease. We refer to this as autosomal dominant inheritance. A consequence of this is that if you have CADASIL, you have one normal copy and one abnormal copy of the gene. If you have a child, he or she will receive one copy of the gene from you, and one from your partner. Therefore there is a 50/50 chance that any child of yours will have the CADASIL gene and will be at risk of developing CADASIL.

What causes CADASIL?

We now know that CADASIL results from an abnormality in one very small part of the notch 3 gene. We think that the protein produced by the notch 3 gene, is responsible for communication between cells within the body, although much work is still required on this subject. As yet, we don't know why the abnormalities in the notch 3 gene in individuals with CADASIL, result in the disease. It is likely that it will take a number of years to fully understand the process.

Although we don't fully understand the process, we do know that patients with CADASIL suffer from progressive damage within small blood vessels. This is likely to lead to both reduced blood flow and an inability of the blood vessels to regulate blood flow. Although abnormalities in blood vessels can be found throughout the body, they appear to be most severe in the brain, and only produce problems noticed by the person with CADASIL within the brain. We believe that the abnormalities within the brain result in reduced blood flow to certain parts of the brain.

What are the features of the disease?

Most people with the disease will suffer from strokes. These most commonly first occur in the 30s to 50s although we are discovering that the disease can be very variable and in some people no problems may occur until their 60s. There are a few individuals identified with CADASIL who remain well in their 70s; our oldest patient remains well at 82 years of age. The strokes are what we refer to as lacunar strokes (literally meaning a small lake or hole in the brain). Because they are small, they tend to be fairly mild and individuals often recover well. The most common type of stroke is weakness affecting one side of the body. If recurrent strokes occur, this can lead to persistent disability which is most usually arm or leg weakness, or slurring of the speech.

Fig. 13.7 (continued)

Migraine is another common feature of the disease. This most commonly starts in the 20s but the onset is variable. Usually this is what we call "complex" migraine. This means that in addition to the headache there are short-lived neurological symptoms, most commonly, some disturbance of vision or numbness down one side of the body or speech disturbance.

Individuals with CADASIL can suffer from anxiety or depression. Not surprisingly, depression is very frequent after any stroke and usually improves with time and treatment if necessary. However, occasionally, depression may occur before any other symptoms of CADASIL. Rarely, seizures epilepsy) occurs as part of CADASIL. Over time, as the disease progresses, memory problems may occur and if these become severe, they are likely to occur in the 50s or 60s. An unusual feature is of the onset of a confusion and reduced consciousness over a period of hours or days, sometimes with fever and seizures; this often follows a migraine attack. It recovers completely over 1 to 2 weeks.

Investigations in an individual suspected of having CADASIL

1. Brain scan

A magnetic resonance scan (MR) is usually performed and shows characteristic appearances with abnormalities in the deeper parts of the brain or white matter. Involvement of certain brain areas including a region called the anterior temporal lobe appears to be a useful guide to the diagnosis. This is a safe scan that involves no radiation but some people find it rather claustrophobic. This scan may be repeated to determine whether the disease is progressing.

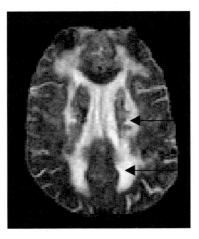

2. Skin biopsy

CADASIL results in characteristic changes in the blood vessels. For obvious reasons it is difficult to look at the blood vessels within the brain. However, even though CADASIL

Fig. 13.7 (continued)

itself only produces symptoms within the brain, abnormalities within the blood vessels can frequently be seen elsewhere in the body. The easiest way to look for these is in the skin. A very small skin biopsy is easily performed under local anaesthetic. It is important this is processed in a special way allowing it to be looked at under high magnification using an electron microscope. Under this magnification, in patients with CADASIL, one can frequently see abnormal collections of material called GOM (granular osmiophilic material) as shown by the arrows in the figure. If these GOM are present we can be almost certain that the individual does have CADASIL. However, the skin biopsy can be normal. It appears that GOM can be detected on skin biopsy in about half of CADASIL patients, but further studies are required to determine the exact figure.

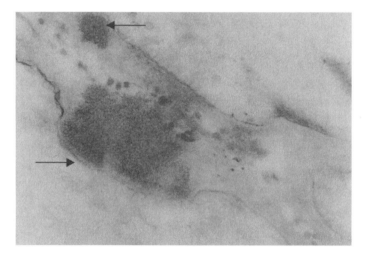

3. Genetic testing

If we can detect an abnormality on genetic testing, we can be 100% sure that someone has CADASIL. In CADASIL the abnormalities that occur are all within one gene which is called the notch 3 gene. However, this gene is made up of many thousands of building blocks (base pairs). In CADASIL, there is an abnormality in only one of these. It can be a very time-consuming process, excluding an abnormality in the whole gene. For this reason routine genetic testing of the whole gene, is not offered in CADASIL. Luckily, most of the abnormalities tend to occur in certain parts of the gene (referred to as exons 3 and 4) and by screening just this part of the gene it's possible to diagnose about 60–70% of cases of CADASIL. A few laboratories world wide offer this screening process. In Britain about 75% of mutations occur in exon4, and about 20% in exons 3,5 and 6 combined. If one member of a family has CADASIL, any other member of the same family that also has CADASIL, will have exactly the same underlying genetic abnormality. If we know where the abnormality is, as in such cases, we can much more easily determine whether it's present. Therefore, once we've found the underlying abnormality within a particular family, it's relatively easy to determine whether other family members are affected.

Fig. 13.7 (continued)

Is there any treatment for CADASIL?

There is no specific treatment for CADASIL available at the moment. In the long run, we hope that now that we know the underlying genetic abnormality, we will be able to discover exactly how this results in the blood vessel damage, and therefore design drugs to prevent this damage. However, this is likely to be a number of years away. Aspirin has been shown to reduce the risk of recurrent stroke by about a third, and most doctors would recommend that patients with CADASIL take a small dose of aspirin per day (75–300mg/day). Occasionally we also use other drugs to reduce blood clotting, such as dipyridamole (persantin) and clopidogrel (plavix). We feel that it's important to prevent any other damage to the blood vessels. For this reason, it is important not to smoke, and that blood pressure and cholesterol are checked, and treated if abnormal. It is also advisable not to take the combined oral contraceptive pill, and recent studies suggest that it is probably best to avoid hormone replacement therapy.

If required during attacks of migraine, standard migraine painkillers can be taken. These include drugs such as migraleve. . If attacks are more frequent (more than once every month or two) it may be worth trying drugs which reduce the frequency of attacks migraine, rather than just wait for an attack and treat it. This include drugs such as the beta-blocker propanolol.

It is important to look for, and treat when necessary, depression in patients with CADASIL. This can be treated with standard anti-depressant drugs and can often respond very well.

Should other members of the family be tested for the disease?

For the reasons explained above, if one member of a family has CADASIL there is a 50/50 chance that other members of the family will also be at risk of the disease. It is possible to look for this in two ways. Firstly, if the underlying genetic abnormality is known, it is relatively simple to look for it in other family members. This will allow us to be 100% sure whether or not an individual carries the CADASIL gene, and is at risk from the disease. Secondly it is possible to carry out magnetic resonance scanning in other family members. This can frequently pick up the characteristic changes of the disease in the 20s before symptoms occur.

Before testing family members for CADASIL, it is very important that a careful discussion of the pros and cons is carried out. This is usually performed by a genetic counsellor. The knowledge that a healthy person is likely to develop CADASIL can obviously be very distressing, and it is possible that it could influence a number of factors including things such as life insurance. Therefore we would normally only test other family members if they were absolutely certain that this is what they wanted to be done. It would be extremely unusual for us to test children.

A potential advantage of being tested for the disease is that it is possible to determine whether one's children are at risk of the disease. For example, if one of your parents has CADASIL you have a 50/50 chance of having the abnormal gene. If you have the abnormal gene, any children you have, also have a 50/50 chance of having the abnormal gene. However, if the abnormal gene has not been passed to you, your children are at no risk. Furthermore, if tests do show that you have the abnormal gene, it is now possible to determine whether the baby has a genetic abnormality fairly early in the pregnancy.

Fig. 13.7 (continued)

If you wished, if the abnormality was present, you could then have a termination. Clearly there are important ethical issues, and individual people have different views on how they would like to address these. If you are keen on having such genetic testing during pregnancy, it is very important that you discuss this well before you plan to become pregnant.

St. George's Hospital Medical School and CADASIL

In the Department of Clinical Neuroscience at St George's we have a particular interest in CADASIL . We have both a research programme in the disease and run a clinical service for patients with CADASIL.

a) Clinical Service
At St George's Hospital we have a specialised CADASIL clinic at which we see patient suspected of having CADASIL or family members who wish to have genetic screening. This is usually held in the first Tuesday (afternoon) of the month. We have facilities to perform skin biopsies in the clinic. We are always happy to see referrals there; if you wish to be seen please ask your GP or hospital consultant to refer you to Professor Markus, Department of Neurology, St George's Hospital, Blackshaw Road, Tooting, London SW17.
The Medical Genetics department at St George's performs notch 3 mutation analysis for CADASIL. Samples can be sent via your local genetics department directly to Medical Genetics (c/o Rohan Taylor), St George's Hospital.

b) Research
We have carried out a British CADASIL prevalence study to find out how common CADASIL is in Great Britain. This was funded by a grant from the National Health Service Research & Development. We have already identified over 50 families with CADASIL in Great Britain. By continuing to study more patients with CADASIL, we are hoping to answer many of the unresolved issues. These include things such as why the disease can come on at different ages in different people, and why different people can suffer different types of disease.
Funded by the Neurosciences Research Foundation we are looking at the best ways to diagnose, and follow-up the disease, including evaluation of new magnetic resonance imaging (MRI) techniques. Because CADASIL is a rare disease, and progresses slowly, before we can evaluate any new treatments we need to have a method of accurately telling, as quickly as possible, whether any drug works. We have decided to do this using MRI. We hope this will allow us to test whether drugs work over time periods of a year or two and we are currently developing the best MRI techniques.
We may ask you whether you would be prepared to take part in these, and other studies. If you are interested, we will explain the specific details of any individual study and it is always entirely up to you as to whether you take part. Before we plan any study, it is always approved by the local hospital ethics committee
If you wish to support the work at St George's donations can be made to the Neuroscience's Research Foundation and sent to Professor Markus at the address at the end of the leaflet

Fig. 13.7 (continued)

How can I find out more information about CADASIL?

Because CADASIL is a rare disease, and because much of the information on it is very new, it is quite difficult to find out information about CADASIL. As far as I know there are no books for the general public about CADASIL. There is an internet site in the United States, which has been set up by a CADASIL sufferer. The address for this is http://home.earth-link.net/~cadasil/lin.htm. This may be a good way to get in touch with other sufferers from CADASIL. This site also gives some links to other web sites with information on CADASIL. A further site which gives details about medical aspects of CADASIL is: http://www.geneclinics.org. Further copies of this leaflet and information about CADASIL at St George's can be downloaded from the St George's Hospital Medical School address: http://www.sghms.ac.uk/depts/cn/cad.html. If you have any specific questions about CADASIL you are always welcome to write to me at St. George's at the following address:

Professor Hugh Markus
Clinical Neuroscience
St. George's Hospital Medical School
Cranmer Terrace
London
SW17 0RE
United Kingdom

Fig. 13.7 A patient information leaflet for CADASIL which we use as part of the genetic counselling process. Copies of this leaflet can be obtained from the following World Wide Web address: *http://www.sghms.ac.uk/depts/cn/cad.html*

diagnosis the implications can be discussed in detail and appropriate advice on treatment and follow-up provided. The possibility of testing other family members can be discussed, although it is important to explain that whether other family members are tested is entirely their decision and that they would have to undergo a similar counselling procedure. Either routine follow-up should be provided, or the patient should be given a contact number and address if they feel they would like to discuss things further, or are finding the diagnosis difficult to come to terms with. Due to the rarity of monogenic causes of stroke many patients may attend a specialist clinic from a long distance. In such cases it is helpful to send copies of information sheets about the appropriate diseases to the family doctor so that he can provide informed advice. Many of these conditions are so rare that the average family doctor is unlikely to see more than one case during his lifetime.

In practice the procedure for counselling individuals with well-established symptomatic disease is quite different from that counselling asymptomatic family members. In the former category it is often clinically important to establish a diagnosis quickly. The genetic diagnosis being tested for is often already suspected. Alternatively in other

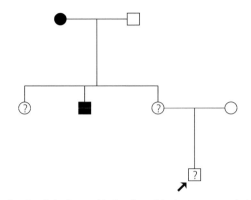

Fig. 13.8 Genetic testing by default. In this family, with the autosomal dominant form of stroke CADASIL, the asymptomatic arrowed member has requested genetic testing. His maternal grandmother and maternal uncle are both affected. If he is found to carry the same notch 3 mutation, his mother who is currently asymptomatic, must also carry the mutation.

cases, its probability is low and the test is being sent off as many screening tests such as in a patient being screened for MELAS. In such cases a fairly rapid process can be appropriate. In contrast in asymptomatic members of a family with a known autosomal dominant genetic disease, more careful counselling with a period of a few weeks for contemplation is required.

Without appropriate counselling problems can arise. One of the few problems encountered in our clinic is that of a patient who presented with complex migraine to another clinic and in whom an MRI scan was performed. This showed appearances typical of CADASIL. The patient found the possible diagnosis difficult to come to terms with and wished he had not had the MRI scan in the first place. This emphasizes that tests which do not involve DNA mutation analysis, such as MRI, can in fact be a 'genetic' test. A different problem can arise in families with autosomal dominant inheritance in whom, for example, one of the grandparents, has symptomatic and diagnosed disease. If the grandson or granddaughter request genetic testing, and this turns out to be positive, it implies that transmission has occurred through the probands daughter (i.e. the grandchild's parents). Essentially the grandchild's parent is having genetic testing without consent. A typical example is shown in Fig. 13.8. This is a difficult situation but is usually best resolved by discussion amongst different family members.

We do not routinely perform genetic testing for any individuals under 18 years of age unless they are already symptomatic. Sometimes parents with diagnosed disease request genetic testing for their children but we explain that this should wait until the individual is an adult and can make an informed decision. Although many cases of stroke occur in individuals who are post-childbearing age, prenatal testing can occasionally be an issue. This requires knowledge of the underlying mutation, and establishing the mechanism for rapid testing, prior to pregnancy. Therefore, in patients of childbearing age it is advisable to discuss this possibility at the time of diagnosis and certainly prior to conception.

References

Auer, D., Putz, B., Gossl, C., Elbel, G., Gasser, T., and Dichgans, M. (2001). Differential lesion patterns in CADASIL and sporadic subcortical arteriosclerotic encephalopathy: MR imaging study with statistical parametric group comparison. *Radiology*, **218**, 443–51.

Berciano, J. (1988). Sneddon syndrome: another mendelian etiology of stroke. *Annals of Neurology*, **24**, 586–7.

Brandt, T., Orberk, E., Weber, R., Werner, I., Busse, O., Muller, B.T., Wigger, F., Grau, A., Grond-Ginsbach, C., and Hausser, I. (2001). Pathogenesis of cervical artery dissections: association with connective tissue abnormalities. *Neurology*, **57**, 24–30.

Ciafaloni, E., Ricci, E., Shanske, S., *et al.* (1992). MELAS: clinical features, biochemistry, and molecular genetics. *Annals of Neurology*, **31**, 391–8.

Desmond, D.W., Moroney, J.T., Lynch, T., Chan, S., Chin, S.S., and Mohr, J.P. (1999). The Natural History of CADASIL a pooled analysis of previously published cases. *Stroke*, **30**, 1230–3.

Dichgans, M., Filippi, M., Bruning, R., Iannucci, G., Berchtenbreiter, C., Minicucci, L., Uttner, D.P., Crispin, A., Ludwig, H., Gasser, T., and Yousry, T.A. (1999). Quantitative MRI in CADASIL, correlation with disability and cognitive performance. *Neurology*, **52**, 1361–7.

Dong, Y., Hassan, A., Zhang, Z., Huber, D., Dalageorgou, C., and Markus, H.S. (2003). The yield of screening for CADASIL mutations in lacunar stroke and leukoaraiosis. *Stroke*, **34**, 203–6.

Ebke, M., Dichgans, M., Bergmann, M., Voelter, H.U., Rieger, P., Gasser, T., and Schwendemann, G. (1997). CADASIL: skin biopsy allows diagnosis in early stages. *Acta Neurologica Scandinavia*, **95**, 351–7.

Fukutake, T. and Hirayama, K. (1995). Familial young-adult-onset arteriosclerotic leukoencephalopathy with alopecia and lumbago without arterial hypertension. (Review) *European Neurology*, **35**, 69–79.

Greenberg, S.M., Vonsattel, J.P., and Stekes, J.W. (1993). The clinical spectrum of cerebral amyloid angiopathy: presentations without lobar hemorrhage. *Neurology*, **43**, 2073–9.

Haan, J., Lanser, J.B., Zijderveld, I., van der Does, I.G., and Roos, R.A. (1990). Dementia in hereditary cerebral hemorrhage with amyloidosis—Dutch type. *Archives of Neurology*, **47**, 965–7.

Hassan, A., Sham, P.C., and Markus, H.S. (2002). Planning genetic studies in human stroke: sample size estimates based on family history data. *Neurology*, **58**, 1483–8.

Iglesias, S., Chapon, F., and Baron, J.-C. (2000). Familial occipital calcifications, hemorrhagic strokes, leukoencephalopathy, dementia, and external carotid dysplasia. *Neurology*, **55**, 1661–7.

Joutel, A., Vahedi, K., Corpechot, C, *et al.* (1997). Strong clustering and stereotyped nature of Notch3 mutations in CADASIL patients. *Lancet*, **350**, 1511–5.

Labauge, P., Laberge, S., Brunereau, L., Lévy, C., Tournier-Lasserve, E. and the Société française de Neurochirurgie. (1998). Hereditary cerebral cavernous angiomas: clinical and genetic features in 57 French families. *Lancet*, **352**, 1892–7.

Mackie, I., Colaco, C., and Machin, S. (1987). Familial lupus anticoagulant. *British Journal of Haematology*, **67**, 359–63.

Markus, H.S., Martin, R.J., Simpson, M.A., Dong, Y.B., Ali, N., Crosby, A.H., and Powell, J.F. (2002), Diagnostic strategies in CADASIL. *Neurology*, **59**, 1134–8.

Mead, S., James-Galton, M., Revesz T., *et al.* (2000). Familial British dementia with amyloid angiopathy. Early clinical, neuropsychological and imaging findings. *Brain*, **123**, 975–91.

O'Sullivan, M., Jarosz, J.M., Martin, R.J., Deasy, N., Powell, J.F., and Markus, H.S. (2001). MRI hyperintensities of the temporal lobe and external capsule in patients with CADASIL. *Neurology*, **56**, 628–34.

Pavlakis, S., Prohovnik, I., Pionelli, S., and De Vivo, D.C. (1989). Neurologic complications of sickle cell disease. *Advances in Pediatrics*, **36**, 247–76.

Plant, G.T., Revesz, T., Barnard, R.O., Harding, A.E., and Gautier-Smith, P.C. (1990). Familial cerebral amyloid angiopathy with non-neuritic amyloid plaque formation. *Brain*, **113**, 721–47.

Schon, F., Martin, R.J., Prevett, M., Clough, C., Enevoldson, T.P., and Markus, H.S. (2003). Acute encephalopathy; an underdiagnosed presentation of CADASIL. *Journal of Neurology Neurosurgery and Psychiatry*, **74**, 249–52.

Taillia, H., Chabriat, H., Kurtz, A., Verin, M., Levy, C., Vahedi, K., Tournier-Lasserve, E., and Bousser, M.G. (1998). Cognitive alterations in non-demented CADASIL patients. *Cerebrovascular Diseases*, **8**, 97–101.

Vidal, R., Frangione, B., Rostagno, A., Mead, S., Revesz, T., Plant, G., and Ghiso, J. (1999). A stop-codon mutation in the BRI gene associated with familial British Dementia. *Nature*, **399**, 776–81.

Chapter 14

Useful web sites for stroke genetics

Hugh S. Markus

The World Wide Web offers access to a large number of sites relevant to both research and clinical aspects of stroke genetics. A number useful for research studies are covered in Chapter 2. The ones listed below are primarily of use to the clinician looking after patients with monogenic stroke disorders, and to the patients themselves.

(A) General clinical, patient, and professional information sites

1. GeneTests.GeneClinics website
http://www.geneclinics.org/

This is an excellent website which contains a lot of useful information for health professionals working with genetic disorders, including a number of causes of monogenic stroke. It is free. It has a number of sections.

1. *Gene reviews.* There are detailed reviews of the clinical features, and molecular basis, of many monogenic disorders including: CADASIL, MELAS, Marfan syndrome, Ehlers–Danlos Syndrome Type IV, Neurofibromatosis 1, Pseudoxanthoma Elasticum, Fabry disease, Hereditary haemorrhagic telangectasia, and Familial hemiplegic migraine. This section includes very useful links to the relevant patient support groups.

2. *The Clinic Directory.* This is a voluntary listing of US and international genetics clinics providing genetic evaluation and genetic counselling.

3. *The Laboratory Directory.* This is a voluntary listing of international laboratories offering molecular genetic testing, specialized cytogenetic testing, and biochemical testing for inherited disorders.

There is also an introduction to genetic testing and counselling, including teaching tools such as a downloadable slide show on aspects of genetic counselling.

2. Online Mendelian Inheritance in Man (OMIM)
http://www.ncbi.nlm.nih.gov/

Online Mendelian Inheritance in Man (OMIM) is a catalogue of human genes and genetic disorders, with links to literature references, sequence records, maps, and related databases. It is authored and edited by Dr Victor McKusick and his colleagues at Johns

Hopkins and elsewhere, and developed for the World Wide Web by the National Centre for Biotechnology Information (NCBI). It has links to many other genetic databases both for clinical information and for gene localization. It provides an excellent first step when looking for clinical and molecular details of a particular disorder although the clinical reviews are not always as comprehensive or up to date as the gene reviews above.

3. Genetic Alliance
http://www.geneticalliance.org/index.html
This site has lists of patient support groups, mostly confined to the USA, for a number of genetics disorders including monogenic causes of stroke.

4. Dolan DNA learning centre
http://www.dnalc.org/
This site has a number of multimedia teaching and professional resources.

1. In 'multimedia site to genetic disorders' (http://www.yourgenesyourhealth.org/ygyh/mason/index) there are multimedia presentations for patients on Marfan syndrome, Neurofibromatosis and Sickle cell disease, which include information and interviews with sufferers.

2. In 'DNA from the Beginning' there an introduction to genetics suitable for the lay person. Organized around key concepts, the science behind each concept is explained by animation, an image gallery, and video interviews.

5. List of genetics databases
http://www.cdc.gov/genomics/info/database.htm
Links to a large number of genetic databases covering both research and clinical aspects.

6. Office of Rare Diseases
http://rarediseases.info.nih.gov/index.html
The Web site of the Office of Rare Diseases (ORD). Here you can find information on more than 6000 rare diseases, including current research, publications from scientific and medical journals, completed research, ongoing studies, and patient support groups.

7. Genetics statistical software
http://linkage.rockefeller.edu/soft/
A very extensive list of genetic statistical analysis software.

8. Human Gene Mutation Database
http://www.hgmd.org/
This is an attempt to collate known (published) gene lesions responsible for human inherited disease run from the Institute of Medical Genetics in Cardiff, UK.

9. Orphanet
http://www.orpha.net/

ORPHANET is a French database (but also in English) dedicated to information on rare diseases and orphan drugs. Its access is free of charge. It has entries for most of monogenic causes of stroke such as CADASIL, Fabry disease and cavernous angiomas, and under each includes genetic clinics and laboratories in France and patient support groups.

(B) Disease specific websites

Many patient groups can be accessed via gene reviews at the GeneTests·GeneClinics website, via the Genetic Alliance site, and via OMIM, all listed above. There are many rare disorders which occasionally cause stroke as part of a systemic disease. Patient groups for these diseases, such as Marfan syndrome, and Neurofibromatosis can be accessed via these addresses. The resources below are for conditions where stroke is the major, or one of the major, complications.

(i) Cerebral amyloid angiopathy (CAA)

1. CAA Research Laboratory website, Massachusetts General Hospital
http://neuro-oas.mgh.harvard.edu/caa/
This website is intended as a resource for both patients and families suffering from CAA, and investigators and clinicians who work in this field. It has been organized by Dr Steven Greenberg at the Massachusetts General Hospital in Boston.

(ii) CADASIL

1. Patient Information leaflet
http://www.sghms.ac.uk/depts/cn/cad.html
This website provides a downloadable patient information sheet for CADASIL.

2. Patient CADASIL website
http://home.earthlink.net/~cadasil/index.htm
This website was established by the wife of a CADASIL sufferer. It gives some useful information and an opportunity to contact other CADASIL patients and their relatives. The husband is severely disabled and some patients find this site rather frightening.

3. The Association of CADASIL Francais
http://association.cadasil.free.fr/index.php
The Association of CADASIL Francais provides information for health professionals and patients. It is mostly in French although some bits are translated into English.

(iii) Sickle cell disease

1. The Sickle Cell Society
http://www.sicklecellsociety.org/
The sickle cell society, is a UK patients charity providing information, counselling and caring for those with sickle cell disorders and their families.

2. **Sickle Cell professional and patient information**
http://www.emory.edu/PEDS/SICKLE/
This site provides sickle cell patient and professional education, news, and research updates.

3. **Multimedia site to genetic disorders: Sickle cell disease**
http://www.yourgenesyourhealth.org/ygyh/mason/index
A multimedia presentations for patients with sickle cell disease, which includes information and interviews with sufferers.

(iv) Fabry disease

1. **Fabry Support and Information Group**
www.Fabry.org
An information site for Fabry patients.

(v) Moya–Moya

1. **http://www.ninds.nih.gov/health_and_medical/moyamoya.htm**
This site provides a good overview of the causes and treatment of Moya–Moya.

2. **http://cpmcnet.columbia.edu/dept/nsg/PNS/moyamoya.html**
This site discusses surgical treatment options, although the role of surgery is very controversial.

3. **http://www003.upp.so-net.ne.jp/moya-moya/**
This site from Japan has a lot of information and pictures, although the English has lost a little in the translation.

Index